Multiple Sclerosis

W0050441

Multiple Sclerosis

A Critical Conspectus

Edited by E. J. Field

Multiple Sclerosis Research Unit
The Royal Victoria Infirmary
Newcastle upon Tyne

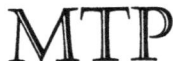

Published by
MTP Press Limited
St Leonard's House
Lancaster
England

Copyright © 1977 MTP Press Limited
Softcover reprint of the hardcover 1st edition 1977

First published 1977

No part of this book may be reproduced
in any form without permission from the
publisher except for the quotation of
brief passages for the purpose of review

ISBN 978-94-010-9536-5   ISBN 978-94-010-9534-1 (eBook)
DOI 10.1007/978-94-010-9534-1

Contents

List of Contributors

Milton Alter
Department of Neurology,
School of Medicine,
Temple University,
Philadelphia,
Pennsylvania 19140, *USA*

P. R. Carnegie
The Russell Grimwade School of Biochemistry,
University of Melbourne,
Parkville,
Victoria 3052,
Australia

Richard I. Carp
Department of Microbiology and Animal Experimentation,
Institute for Basic Research in Mental Retardation,
Staten Island,
New York 10314, *USA*

E. J. Field
Department of Experimental Neuropathology,
Multiple Sclerosis (MS) Research Unit,
The Royal Victoria Infirmary,
Newcastle upon Tyne, NE1 4LP

Torben Fog
Kommunerhospitalitet København,
DK-1399 *Copenhagen, Denmark*

J. F. Kurtzke
Department of Neural Epidemiology,
Veterans Administration Hospital,
Washington D.C. 20422, *USA*

P. C. Licursi
Department of Microbiology and Animal Experimentation,
Institute for Basic Research in Mental Retardation,
Staten Island,
New York 10314, USA

A. Löwenthal
Department of Neurochemistry,
Borne-Bunge Institute,
B-2600 Berchem-Antwerp, Belgium

G. S. Merz
Department of Microbiology and Animal Experimentation,
Institute for Basic Research in Mental Retardation,
Staten Island,
New York 10314, USA

P. A. Merz
Department of Microbiology and Animal Experimentation,
Institute for Basic Research in Mental Retardation,
Staten Island,
New York 10314, USA

N. R. Sims
Department of Biochemistry,
University of Melbourne,
Parkville,
Victoria 3052, Australia

A. D. Smith
Courtauld Institute of Biochemistry,
Middlesex Hospital Medical School,
London, W1P 3PR

R. H. S. Thompson
Courtauld Institute of Biochemistry,
Middlesex Hospital Medical School,
London, W1P 3PR

Preface

Although a strikingly modern account of multiple (disseminated) sclerosis was given by Charcot more than one hundred years ago, we are still not sure of the precise nature of the disease, still less of any precise mode of management. Even diagnosis is at best 'probable'. This collection of essays examines the particular difficulties which beset the problem and have militated against the solution—problems of data collection and evaluation; clinical and biochemical vagaries and unanswered questions; laboratory test prediction of the disease, etc. Experts in their fields have set out the difficulties and way forward as *they* see them, and there must necessarily be overlap or contradictions which underline our lack of knowledge. Clearly no attempt can be made to cover more than a very few aspects of the problem (a further volume is planned to review other areas not covered here, in particular the relationship between multiple sclerosis and experimental allergic encephalomyelitis)—but it is hoped that the 'softness' of much of the data we have to work upon will become apparent.

It is intended that this volume should clearly differ from the large number of monographs and reports of symposia dedicated to multiple sclerosis in bringing out the *shortcomings* of our approaches, and in some respects our naïvities rather than our individual brilliancies. It may help to answer the general physician's question why neurologists have been so long in coming to grips with multiple sclerosis and above all it is hoped that it may direct younger workers coming into the field of neurology towards what is now a central problem medically, socially, economically and intellectually.

'Kreutzigen sollte man jeglichen Schwärmer im dreissigsten Jahre,
Kennt er nur einmal die Welt, wird der Betrogene der Schelm.'

Goethe: Venedige Epigramme

'Si quelquefois les savants ont moins de préjugés que les autres hommes ils tiennent, en revanche, encore plus fortement à ceux qu'ils ont.'

Jean-Jacques Rousseau, 1765

'Zu alten Zeiten sind der Entwicklung der Medizin hauptsächlich zwei Hindernisse entgegengetreten, die Autoritäten und die Systeme.'

R. Virchow, 1856

'The most difficult things to explain are those which are not true.'

A. S. Wiener, 1956

'Those who fetch from hypothesis the foundation on which they build their speculations may form indeed an ingenious romance, but a romance it will still be.'

Roger Cotes. Preface to 2nd edition of Newton's 'Principia Mathematica', 1713

'Der Geist der Medizin ist leicht zu fassen;
Ihr durchstudiert die gross' und kleine Welt,
Und es am Ende gehen zu lassen,
Wie's Gott gefällt.'

Goethe: Faust 1

Foreword

Although multiple sclerosis has been known for more than 100 years, we still have no real knowledge of the fundamental nature of the illness and still less of any rational method of handling it. The hope expressed by Charcot at the time of his classic description, that the physician would one day learn the secret of the spontaneous remission and harness it to therapeutic purposes, has so far remained quite unfulfilled.

The great hopes and expectancies raised by the discoveries of Rivers and his associates in the mid-30s of what soon came to be called 'experimental allergic encephalitis (EAE)' have not solved the riddle of MS. Although EAE has proved to be a powerful stimulus for investigations of immunologic phenomena considered analogous to those developing in the course of MS, a heuristic experimental model which rapidly yields results applicable to the human situation has yet to be found.

Even the diagnosis is never certain until thorough post-mortem examination of the brain and spinal cord has been completed, so that the real extent of the disease, the data derived from epidemiological and genetic studies, as well as the results of immunological and biochemical investigations necessarily carry a built-in 'uncertainty principle'. This situation is not unique to MS; medical research in many fields requires that we recognize clearly the obstacles which stand in the way of gathering firm data on which to build, whilst at the same time keeping an open mind upon new and speculative ideas, provided always that they are open to refutation and therefore of scientific validity.

The selection of essays presented here makes no pretence to cover the vast field of MS studies. Necessarily restricted to topics of particular interest, it will be of value not only as an explanation of the special hazards in this research, but also in bringing them once more before many of those who are themselves engaged in the effort and need from time to time to be reminded of some of the assumptions upon which they work. Of course many readers will find their particular interest not discussed or inadequately treated. I hope they will be indulgent and accept this as inherent in the nature of this book, which may engender considerable discussion and reassessment of premises accepted as the valid basis in many areas of current MS-research.

H. J. BAUER,
Professor and Director, Department of Neurology,
University of Göttingen, Germany
Chairman, Medical Advisory Board of the
International Federation of Multiple Sclerosis Societies

Special difficulties of the multiple sclerosis problem

E. J. Field

More than one hundred years have gone by since Charcot gave a strikingly modern, clinical and pathological account of multiple sclerosis (MS). Indeed, as Fog points out (Chapter 2), a very great deal of subsequent writing amounts to little more than expansion of Charcot's descriptions as detail has been filled in, and recognition of the truly protean manifestations of the disease. 'Ideas about the cause of multiple sclerosis have long been the weathercock of medicine swinging from one fashionable and unproven theory to another, pointing most recently towards a virus infection which seems to be related to measles' (Lancet[1]); still more recently the small transmissible agent first described by Carp et al.[2] has also been adopted as a contender by the same journal (Lancet[3])—though both Carp and Henle et al.[4] are very far from making such claims. Burnett[5], remarking that 'more than one editor interested in the changing pattern of medical science has commented on the influence of fashion in the interpretation of disease', singles out MS as 'an example which, at the moment, is moving from autoimmunity to slow virus infection without any really legitimate reason for the change'. Perhaps it is true today that 'slow virus' gives the verbal satisfaction which 'autoimmunity' did a decade ago. The twin ideas of 'autoimmunity' (rather broadly interpreted) and 'slow' infection remain the pivotal ideas (with various combinations) around which modern thinking about aetiopathogenesis has evolved. Genetic aspects of MS have been relatively neglected[6], though it would be remarkable if, practically alone amongst diseases known to medicine, 'diathesis' (a term which used to conceal our ignorance of human genetic mechanisms) played no role in the evolution of the disorder.

It is of interest transcending the immediate problem of MS, to examine the causes, general and special, that have so long delayed real advance in our understanding of the disease, and to single out some for more detailed study since they continue to operate.

Untestable hypotheses (*aus der Luft gegriffen*) abound in the literature of MS, many being based on uncritical acceptance of 'soft' facts and data. Every possible category of disease process has had its advocate, and the modern rush to expound phenomena in terms of molecular biology, with its accompanying aura of 'science', has generated its own speculations. Whilst the making of hypotheses is often an essential preliminary to insight, only those which offer refutable predictions will guard against degeneration into an encumbering mythopoiesis[7]. Above all, such exercises must be grounded on 'hard' facts and for a variety of special reasons these are particularly difficult to establish in the field of MS investigation. The situation is compounded by the tendency, by no means limited to MS (or even medicine as a whole), to confuse observation (even when accurately made) with interpretation and hypothesis. Amongst the reminders which should be prominently displayed in the research worker's laboratory is one to the effect that 'of all scientific instruments available, reasoning is perhaps the least reliable': and facing him as he enters his laboratory might be Claude Bernard's aphorism, 'Put off your imagination, as you put off your overcoat, when you enter the laboratory. But put it on again, as you put on your overcoat, when you leave.'

Some of the more important difficulties will be briefly introduced, their explanation being considered in detail in individual chapters.

Important difficulties in MS

Diagnosis

First and foremost stands the *difficulty in recognition*—in other words, *diagnosis*. The truly protean picture of the disease, especially in the early stages, has been commented upon by Fog (Chapter 2). To this must be added the problems posed by *formes frustes*—cases which after initial symptoms or signs never apparently progress (Charcot) so that the classic 'dissemination in time and space', which makes six or seven cases out of ten so simple to diagnose, is absent. Indeed McAlpine[8] pointed out that approximately one patient in 20 is free from fresh symptoms for 15 or more years following the first symptoms, and this initial latent phase tends to be especially long after an onset with retrobulbar neuritis. Experienced neurologists have estimated a 20% revision rate of their primary diagnosis[9, 10], and something over 4 years generally goes by between initial symptoms and definitive diagnosis. Diagnosis, indeed, is only assured at autopsy (and may then well depend upon thoroughness of examination), so that many cases are classed as 'probable' or 'possible'. The essentially benign character of MS in many patients ('If a remission may last 30 years, why not a lifetime?'[11]) with minimal presenting symptoms makes it probable that what comes to the neurologist is the 'tip of an iceberg' of cases.

The problem is made worse by uncertainty as to the nature of retrobulbar neuritis (RBN) unaccompanied by other signs, since the proportion who later develop symptoms and signs of MS has been variously reported between 11·5% and 85%[12, 13]. Optic neuritis, especially in older patients, may, of course, arise from a number of causes (diabetes, vascular disease, pernicious anaemia, and others) and, in the absence of a distinguishing laboratory test for MS (see *British Medical Journal*[14]), presents problems of prognosis. To RBN may be added neuromyelitis optica (Devic's disease) and obscure encephalitis in childhood where diagnosis is often made only reluctantly because of the rarity of the condition (see brief review by Field[15]).

Laboratory tests (spinal fluid, especially oligoclonal IgG bands [see Chapter 6], flicker fusion tests, etc.) give no absolute diagnosis and the recent linoleic acid depression (LAD) test[16] may yet provide rare exceptions (see section below).

Epidemiological ascertainment

Allied to diagnostic difficulties are those of *epidemiological ascertainment* which make the precise magnitude and distribution of the problem imprecise. This problem has been dealt with both at the fundamental and detailed level in a masterly fashion by Doctors John Kurtzke and Milton Alter. Differences in interpretation and 'acceptability' of evidence come to light and the reader may well have the feeling that, as with archaeological discoveries, some new finding may appreciably alter outlook.

It is well recognized, for example, that the number of cases uncovered depends very much upon the enthusiasm and obsession of the investigator. There are also differences in opinion as to the most efficient (or even correct) manner of handling the statistics once they are obtained (see discussion by Hyllested[17], Kurtzke[18], Leibowitz[19] and others). Kurtzke[20] has recently evaluated critically accepted surveys of world distribution and classified studies according to the standards of ascertainment observed. His excellent papers should be considered for details. Such an established observation as the variation in frequency of MS with latitude requires modification and reassessment. Kurtzke writes '. . . there is little evidence for a direct correlation . . . (of distribution of MS) with latitude, and such correlations, to be meaningful, need to consider longitude as well. At latitude 40° north, for example, MS is of high frequency in America, medium in Europe, and low in Asia. Accordingly, the worldwide distribution of MS is best regarded as comprising three bands or zones of high, medium and low risk or frequency. . . .'

To the *forme fruste* referred to above, cases of MS totally undiscovered during life, but revealed at postmortem examination, add further inaccuracy to the ascertainment of cases. Whilst every neuropathologist has encountered instances of misdiagnosis, their extent is indicated by the oft-quoted series of Georgi[21], who found only 69·7% of MS cases correctly diagnosed at autopsy (out of a series of 15 644 postmortem examinations). In 18·2% it was an adventitious finding. Two of his 66 cases were, indeed, accident deaths unsuspected of the disease during life. Vost *et al.*[22] found 5 of 440 brains examined for the presence of infarcts following heart disease to have MS (only one having had any neurological disturbance recorded). Ghatak *et al.*[23] have also recorded unsuspected MS at autopsy. Clearly there must be many more cases than diagnosed, and much will depend upon the enthusiasm with which the brain is studied (likely to be low!) in subjects who die from non-neurological disease. These circumstances underline the element of uncertainty which necessarily attaches to even the best epidemiological studies, especially those involving comparisons of prevalence upon which aetiological theories are constructed, for example the occurrence or nature of some exogenous infective agent.

Earliest lesion of MS

Opportunities for the direct study of the earliest lesions in clinically recent MS cases are few, though this difficulty is in some measure alleviated by the frequent occurrence of clearly 'young' lesions even in established cases. Charcot[24] had no doubts when he wrote: 'Incontestablement, la multiplication des noyaux et l'hyperplasie concomitante des fibres réticulées de la névroglie sont le fait initial, fondamental, l'antécédent nécessaire; l'atrophie dégénérative des éléments nerveux est secondaire, consécutive; elle a déjà commencé à se produire lorsque la névroglie fait place au tissu fibrillaire, bien qu'elle marche alors d'un pas plus rapide.' Others, too, have been impressed with the precocious and seemingly disproportionately large activation of macroglia[25-28]. It is of special interest that Lumsden[29], in his beautiful review of the neuropathology of MS based upon direct personal experience, also combats the 'tradition' teaching that gliosis—commonly qualified as reparative gliosis—follows demyelination and maintains that 'gliosis probably begins simultaneously with the demyelination' (p. 278). (Incidentally, his illustration (Figure 64) shows minimal perivascular infiltration, though it is elaborated at some length.) A central 'hard' fact relating to MS lesions is their undoubted development around small blood vessels[30-33]. None of the clear and detailed descriptions of lesions[29, 34, 35] stress perivascular infiltration of small veins with lymphocytes or plasma cells, and indeed Adams and Kubik[36] found no such perivascular exudate in the earliest lesion they studied with an estimated age of 2 days, nor did Zimmerman and Netzky[37]. The author has seen early lesions with no more than sudanophilic macrophage accumulation and no small round cell infiltration. The very beautiful but highly selected photographs offered by electronmicroscopists, purporting to show direct lymphocytic attack upon myelin, cannot be evaluated without some indication of the frequency with which such appearances (themselves open to interpretational differences) can be seen (see, for example, Lampert and Kies[38] and Field and Raine[39, 40]) —the latter authors examined 84 representative lesions in the guinea-pig and 130 blocks in the rhesus monkey. Field and Raine[40] point out that 'seldom is some estimate given in a description of the frequency with which a given phenomenon has been encountered, and photographic evidence of one good example may lead to quite misleading estimates of the regularity of a process'. They found cellular attack upon myelin sheaths (though not necessarily an initiatory phenomenon) much more common in the monkey than in the guinea-pig. This may, of course, merely be an expression of the insult to the nervous tissue which could have been damaged by some immunological reaction going on in the vicinity as an 'innocent bystander' in much the same way as platelets may be affected under similar conditions[41]. Certainly the frequency with which direct cellular attack upon myelin sheaths can be seen unequivocally either in the light or electronmicroscope does not suggest that it can be a frequent or important primary event in myelin destruction, and it is chiefly those who are most attracted to the delayed hypersensitivity EAE model of MS who see the primacy of lymphocytic action (see below).

Genetic studies in MS

Despite our long-standing awareness that MS is 5 to 20 times more common in the near relatives of a patient than in the surrounding general population, genetic studies have been much neglected in the Anglo-American literature, though many papers have appeared from continental European authors.

Indeed, it is the monograph by Curtius[42] which has served as the point of departure for modern studies.

Twin studies, which might be expected to shed clear light on any genetic component in MS, are 'beset by ascertainment and diagnostic difficulties and are . . . inconclusive' (Myrianthopoulos[6]). With the 'most rigid diagnostic standards' 15·4% of monozygotic twins have been reported concordant whilst 10·3% of dizygotic twins were also concordant. However, as Mackay and Myrianthopoulos[43] point out, even if MS were completely genetic in origin, monozygotic twins could not be expected to show more than 50% concordance at any particular time, because of the distribution of age of onset. Moreover, in making a twin study it is necessary to follow the non-MS member throughout life and verify the absence of lesions at autopsy—something which has certainly never been done.

However, the growth of HLA-typing methods associated with organ transplantation has stimulated much work on the association of specific diseases with a known tissue type. Fog (Chapter 2) reviews some of this work which promises to make a major contribution to our knowledge of the backcloth against which MS evolves. Here it may only be noted that this work again underlines the importance of the LD (lymphocyte-determined) rather than the SD (serum-determined) factors.

Coupled with the study of tissue type preponderance in MS has been the realization over the past few years that immunological response is genetically controlled[44] by Ir gene(s), which are closely allied to the MLC (mixed lymphocyte culture) and MHS (major histocompatibility system) complexes, and that they are susceptible of experimental analysis. Since it is difficult to evade the conclusion that an immunological reaction contributes in some measure to the clinical picture of MS at some stage of the disease, it appears likely that, as long recognized in the case of so many diseases, MS develops against a background predisposition, which itself may (in part at least) be determined by immunological responsiveness.

Cellular sensitization studies in man

These have been hampered by the absence of a reliable, quantitative and reproducible means of estimation[45]. The well-tried lymphocyte transformation method is too coarse, whilst the macrophage migration inhibition method[46] and its descendant, the leukocyte migration method of Søborg and Bendixen[47] and Søborg[48], is insufficiently sensitive[49] to pick up sensitization readily demonstrable by the macrophage electrophoretic mobility (MEM) test[50, 51]. This method, depending upon a recruitment phenomenon amongst lymphocytes, which did not belong to the original very small percentage of specifically sensitized cells[52] is exquisitely sensitive and discriminatory. It has the disadvantages, however, that it is totally dependent upon a supply of healthy non-sensitized guinea-pigs and makes (especially in the training stages) considerable demands upon the patience of the observer as he acquires skill. (However, it may be possible to substitute tanned red blood or even other cells for normal guinea-pig macrophages as indicator cells, and this will greatly simplify the whole procedure.) On the other hand, the MEM method can evaluate with assurance the uniformly low MLR between unrelated MS subjects as compared with non-MS[53], which is made out only 'on average' by classical lymphocyte co-cultivation[54].

Experimental allergic encephalomyelitis (EAE)

This is commonly regarded as the animal model for MS, and a statement to this effect often introduces papers on the subject (and applications for grants). Certainly the mechanism of EAE (which remains elusive) may well be relevant to the development of MS, though there are considerable species differences in the degree of 'demyelination' produced. Carnegie (Chapter 6) has indicated the complexity of the 'encephalitogenic antigen' in EAE and (putatively) in MS, and the advanced chemical techniques and concepts which have in recent years been recruited to the study of myelin components and enzymes. In guinea-pigs, for example, demyelination has been said not to occur[55], though the author has seen it on rare occasions in the spinal cord (with persistence of axis cylinders)[56], whilst in monkeys it is commonly a destructive process leading to granuloma formation. Much depends upon the tempo of the process, and recently it has indeed been possible to produce experimental lesions in rhesus monkeys, more closely resembling MS plaques than any previously reported, by repeated administration of small doses of human encephalitogenic factor (EF) with Freund's complete adjuvant, over a period of 18 months[15]. More experiments along these lines (preferably in chimpanzees) need to be carried out, since the regular establishment of real MS-type lesions in an experimental model would be a major step forward, though, as Kersting and Pette[57] point out, true MS changes may be species-specific and the most we may hope for from animal experimentation is insight into the mechanisms at work. Certainly the pathological findings of Uchimura and Shiraki[58] and Shiraki and Otani[59] in patients who had survived the acute phase of a neuroparalytic accident during the Pasteur prophylactic treatment for rabies show that the human nervous system is able to react in much the same way as that of experimental animals, though the striking lesions so closely resembling MS plaques were rejected by Lumsden[60] largely on the grounds that they were monophasic and represented the closed episode of EAE rather than the continuing MS pathological process. The same may be said of the massive lesions described by Jellinger and Seitelberger[61] in the brain of a man who had been treated for Parkinsonism with repeated injections of bovine brain.

The clinical course of MS

This introduces special difficulties in the assessment of any therapy which might itself throw light upon the causation of the disease (as for example, liver and B_{12} therapy in pernicious anaemia and subacute combined degeneration of the spinal cord).

Double-blind trials of ACTH in the long term[62-64] have not shown the drug to be of benefit. Despite this, long-term treatment with ACTH (sometimes not in very small doses) is still employed by some physicians. Any 'double-blind' trial is necessarily prolonged, time-consuming and tedious. However, quite recently Millar et al.[65] established an important landmark in the history of MS in reporting that supplementation of the diet with sunflower seed oil, in a properly controlled double-blind trial over the space of 2 years, had a statistically significant effect in reducing the number and severity of attacks of MS (though not the gradual downward trend). In the 100 years the disease has been known, this is the only long-term treatment, properly tested, from which any benefit has been shown (although, of course, claims for untested treatments abound). As such, Millar's[65] findings are in urgent need of testing (and retesting), but they do appear to indicate a way forward, and will be considered in some detail below. If substantiated they may indeed be said to have transformed the therapeutic outlook in MS, and perhaps, as will appear, herald a rational prophylactic therapy (Chapter 9).

Not least amongst the difficulties inherent in MS research are two which stem from human nature. 'Cure' or even 'amelioration' and still more prophylaxis for a disease which has been pronounced for 100 years to be 'incurable', immediately engenders considerable scepticism and a heavy onus of proof is allotted to anyone who proposes new ideas. Only patient clinical research can overcome this scepticism and this takes time.

The second factor is the need to obtain funds for research and the 'partial view' which may be (quite unconsciously) taken in presenting the facts of MS. An outstanding example of this recently has been the very great emphasis laid upon measles as a causative agent in MS. At the time of writing, the Carp–Henle agent has engendered much (not very substantially based) optimism.

The difficulties outlined above, ranging from so fundamental a step as the certain recognition of MS cases through 'softness' of many of the facts, to failure to develop an unequivocal experimental model of the disease either from the angle of an immunological reaction or a 'slow' infection of the nervous system, account for our tardiness in making progress. However, what would appear to be a real step forward has been made in the last five years, and where this leads will be considered in the chapters devoted to unsaturated fatty acids and their significance.

References

1. *Lancet* (1974). Measles and multiple sclerosis, **i**, 247
2. Carp, R. I., Licursi, P. C., Merz, P. A. and Merz, G. S. (1972). Decreased percentage of polymorphonuclear neutrophils in mouse peripheral blood inoculation of material from multiple sclerosis patients. *J. Exp. Med.*, **136**, 618
3. *Lancet* (1976). A milestone in multiple sclerosis, **i**, 459
4. Henle, G., Koldovsky, U., Koldovsky, P., Henle, W., Ackermann, R. and Haase, G. (1975). Multiple sclerosis-associated agent: neutralisation of the agent by human sera. *Infect. Immunol.*, **12**, 1367
5. Burnett, Sir McF. (1972). *Autoimmunity and Autoimmune Disease*, p. 170 (Lancaster: MTP)
6. Myrianthopoulos, N. C. (1970). Genetic aspects of multiple sclerosis. In P. J. Vinken and G. W. Bruyn (eds.) *Handbook of Clinical Neurology*, vol. 9. Chapter 5, p. 86 (Amsterdam: North-Holland)
7. Popper, K. R. (1965). *Conjectures and Refutations; The Growth of Scientific Knowledge*, 2nd edition (London: Routledge and Kegan Paul)
8. McAlpine, D. (1955). In D. McAlpine, N. D. Compston and C. E. Lumsden (eds.) *Multiple Sclerosis*, (Edinburgh and London: E. and S. Livingstone)
9. Tourtelotte, W. A. (1974). International symposium on multiple sclerosis. O. Andersen, L. Bergmann, and T. Broman (eds.). *Acta Neurol. Scand.*, **50**, suppl. 58, 63
10. Fog, T. (1974). International symposium on multiple sclerosis. O. Andersen, L. Bergmann, and T. Broman (eds.). *Acta Neurol. Scand.*, **50**, suppl. 58, 63
11. Brain, W. R. (1936). Prognosis of disseminated sclerosis. *Lancet*, **ii**, 866
12. Kurland, L. T., Beebe, G. W., Kurtzke, J. R., Nagler, B., Auth, T. L., Lessell, S. and Nefzger, M. D. (1966). Studies on the natural history of multiple sclerosis. The progression of optic neuritis to multiple sclerosis. *Acta Neurol. Scand.*, **42**, 157
13. McAlpine, D., Lumsden, C. E. and Acheson, E. D. (1972). *Multiple Sclerosis: A Reappraisal*, 2nd edition. (Edinburgh: Churchill Livingstone)
14. *British Medical Journal* (1975). Leading article, **3**, 265
15. Field, E. J. (1975). Multiple sclerosis: relation to scrapie and slow infection, ageing and measles. *Acta Neurol. Scand.*, **51**, 285
16. Field, E. J., Shenton, B. K. and Joyce, G. (1974). Specific laboratory test for multiple sclerosis. *Brit. Med. J.*, **1**, 412
17. Hyllested, K. (1972). Discussion of the epidemiology of multiple sclerosis. In

E. J. Field, T. M. Bell and P. R. Carnegie (eds.). *Multiple Sclerosis. Progress in Research* (Amsterdam: North-Holland)

18. Kurtzke, J. F. (1972). Discussion of the epidemiology of multiple sclerosis. In E. J. Field, T. M. Bell and P. R. Carnegie (eds.). *Multiple Sclerosis. Progress in Research* (Amsterdam: North-Holland)

19. Leibowitz, U. (1972). Discussion of the epidemiology of multiple sclerosis. In E. J. Field, T. M. Bell and P. R. Carnegie (eds.). *Multiple Sclerosis. Progress in Research* (Amsterdam: North-Holland)

20. Kurtzke, J. F. (1975). A re-assessment of the distribution of multiple sclerosis. Part I, II. *Acta Neurol. Scand.*, **51**, 110, 137

21. Georgi, W. (1961). Multiple Sklerose. Pathologisch–anatomische Befunde multipler Sklerose bei klinisch nicht diagnostizierten Krankheiten. *Schweiz. Med. Wochenschr.*, **91**, 605

22. Vost, A., Wolochow, A., and Howell, D. A. (1964). Incidence of infarcts of the brain in heart disease. *J. Pathol. Bact.*, **88**, 463

23. Ghatak, N. R., Hirano, A., Littmaer, H., and Zimmerman, H. M. (1974). Asymptomatic demyelinated plaque. *Arch. Neurol.*, **30**, 484

24. Charcot, J. M. (1872). Maladies du système nerveux, I: de la sclérose en plaques disséminée. *Anat. Pathol.* (Paris: Delahaye)

25. Müller, E. (1904). *Die multiple Sklerose des Gehirns und Rückenmarks.* (Jena: Fischer)

26. Anton, G. and Wohlwill, F. (1912). Multiple nicht eitrige Encephalomyelitis und Multiple Sklerose. *Z. Ges. Neurol. Psychiatr.*, **12**, 31

27. Jacob, H. (1969). Tissue process in multiple sclerosis and para-infections and post-vaccinal encephalomyelitis. *Int. Arch. Allergy*, **36**, suppl. 22

28. Field, E. J. (1967). The significance of astroglial hypertrophy in scrapie, kuru, multiple sclerosis and old age, together with a note on the possible nature of the scrapie agent. *Dtsch. Z. Nervenheilkd.*, **192**, 265

29. Lumsden, E. C. (1970). The neuropathology of multiple sclerosis. In P. J. Vinken and G. W. Bruyn (eds.) *Handbook of Clinical Neurology*, vol. 9, p. 217 (Amsterdam: North-Holland)

30. Rindfleisch, E. (1863). Histologisches Detail zu der grauen Degeneration von Gehirn und Rückenmark. *Virch. Arch. Pathol. Anat.*, **26**, 474

31. Putnam, T. J. (1937). Evidences of vascular occlusion in multiple sclerosis and 'encephalomyelitis'. *Arch. Neurol. (Chicago)*, **37**, 1298

32. Fog, T. (1964). On the vessel–plaque relationship in the brain in multiple sclerosis. *Acta Neurol. Scand.*, **40**, suppl. 10, 9

33. Fog, T. (1965). The topography of plaques in multiple sclerosis, with special reference to cerebral plaques. *Acta Neurol. Scand.*, **41**, suppl. 15

34. Borst, M. (1903). Die multiple Sklerose des Zentralnervensystems. *Ergeb. Allg. Pathol.*, **9**, 67

35. Dawson, J. W. (1916). The histology of disseminated sclerosis. *Trans. R. Soc. Edin.*, **50**, 517

36. Adams, R. D. and Kubik, C. S. (1952). The morbid anatomy of the demyelinating diseases. *Am. J. Med.*, **12**, 510

37. Zimmerman, H. M. and Netsky, M. G. (1950). The pathology of multiple sclerosis. *Pub. Ass. Res. Nervous and Mental Dis.*, **28**, 271

38. Lampert, P. and Kies, M. W. (1967). Mechanism of demyelination in experimental allergic encephalomyelitis of guinea-pigs. An electron microscopic study. *Exp. Neurol.*, **18**, 210

39. Field, E. J. and Raine, C. S. (1966). Experimental allergic encephalomyelitis: an electron microscopic study. *Am. J. Pathol.*, **49**, 537

40. Field, E. J. and Raine, C. S. (1969). Experimental allergic encephalomyelitis in the rhesus monkey: an electron microscopic study. *J. Neurol. Sci.*, **8**, 397

41. Humphrey, J. H. and Jacques, R. (1955). The release of histamine and 5-hydroxytriptamine (serotonin) from platelets by antigen–antibody reactions (*in vitro*). *J. Physiol.*, **128**, 9

42. Curtius, F. (1933). *Multiple Sklerose und Erbanlage* (Leipzig: Thieme)

43. Mackay, R. P. and Myrianthopoulos, N. C. (1966). Multiple sclerosis in twins and their relations. Final report. *Arch. Neurol. (Chicago)*, **15**, 449

44. Bennaceraff, B. and McDevitt, H. O. (1972). Histocompatibility-linked immune response genes. *Science*, **175**, 273

45. Bloom, B. R. (1971). *In vitro* methods in cell-mediated immunity in man. *N. Engl. J. Med.*, **284**, 1212

46. David, J. R., Al-Askari, S., Lawrence, H. S., and Thomas, L. (1964). Delayed hypersensitivity *in vitro*. *J. Immunol.*, **93**, (2), 264, 274

41. Søborg, M. and Bendixen, G. (1967). Human lymphocyte migration as a parameter of hypersensitivity. *Acta Med. Scand.*, **181**, 247

48. Søborg, M. (1968). *In vitro* migration of peripheral human leucocytes in cellular hypersensitivity. *Acta Med. Scand.*, **184**, 135

49. Hughes, D. and Paty, D. (1971). Lymphocyte sensitivity in cancer. *Br. Med. J.*, **2**, 770

50. Field, E. J. and Caspary, E. A. (1970). Lymphocyte sensitisation: an *in vitro* test for cancer? *Lancet*, **ii**, 1337

51. Caspary, E. A. and Field, E. J. (1971). Specific lymphocyte sensitisation in cancer: is there a common cancer antigen in human malignant neoplasia? *Br. Med. J.*, **2**, 613

52. Carnegie, P. R., Caspary, E. A., Dickinson, J. P., and Field, E. J. (1973). The macrophage electrophoretic mobility (MEM) test for lymphocyte sensitisation: a study of the kinetics. *Clin. Exp. Immunol.*, **14**, 37

53. Field, E. J., Shenton, B. K. and Meyer-Rienecker, H. (1976). Mixed lymphocyte reaction in multiple sclerosis. *Acta Neurol. Scand.*, **54**, 181

54. Källen, B., Low, B. and Nillson, O. (1975). Mixed leukocyte reaction and HLA specificity at multiple sclerosis. *Acta Neurol. Scand.*, **51**, 184

55. Freund, J., Stern, E. R. and Pisani, T. M. (1947). Isoallergic encephalomyelitis and radiculitis in guinea-pigs after one injection of brain and microbacteria in water-in-oil emulsion. *J. Immunol.* **57**, 179

56. Field, E. J. (1966). Transmission experiments with multiple sclerosis: an interim report. *Br. Med. J.*, **2**, 564

57. Kersting, G. and Pette, E. (1957). Zur Pathohistologie und Pathogenese der

experimentellen, 'allergischen' Encephalomyelitis des Affen. *Dtsch. Z. Nerven-heilkd.* **176,** 387

58. Uchimura, I. and Shiraki, H. (1957). A contribution of the classification and patho-genesis of demyelinating encephalopathies with special reference to the central nervous system lesions caused by preventive inoculation against rabies. *J. Neuro-pathol. Exp. Neurol.*, **16,** 139

59. Shiraki, H. and Otani, S. (1959). Clinical and pathological features of rabies post-vaccinal encephalomyelitis in man. (Relationship to multiple sclerosis and to experimental 'allergic' encephalomyelitis in animals). In M. W. Kies and E. C. Alvord (eds.) *Allergic Encephalomyelitis*, p. 58. (Springfield, Ill.: C. C. Thomas)

60. Lumsden, E. C. (1961). Consideration of multiple sclerosis in relation to the auto-immunity process. *Proc. R. Soc. Med.*, **54,** 11

61. Jellinger, K. and Seitelberger, F. (1958). Akute tödliche Entmarkungsencephalitis nach wiederholten Hirntrokkenzelleninjektionen. *Klin. Wochenschr.*, **36,** 437

62. Miller, H., Newell, D. J., and Ridley, A. (1961). Multiple sclerosis: trials of main-tenance treatment with prednisolone and soluble aspirin. *Lancet*, **i,** 127

63. Fog, T. (1965). The long-term treatment of multiple sclerosis with corticoids. *Acta Neurol. Scand.*, **41,** suppl. 13, 1

64. Millar, J. H. D., Vas, C. J., Naronha, M. J., Liversedge, L. A. and Rawson, M. D. (1967). Long-term treatment of multiple sclerosis with corticotrophin. *Lancet*, **ii,** 429

65. Millar, J. H. D., Zilkha, K. J., Langman, M. J. S., Payling-Wright, H., Smith, A. D., Belin, J. and Thompson, R. H. S. (1973). Double-blind trial of linoleate supplementation of the diet in multiple sclerosis. *Br. Med. J.*, **1,** 765

2

Clues from clinical features

Torben Fog

Introduction

The symptomatology and course of MS as described by Charcot[1] is so complete that subsequent literature may be considered largely as differentiation only regarding type, frequency and quantitation. However, opinions about the unique character of the disease soon began to emerge before the beginning of the twentieth century. The terms primary and secondary sclerosis appeared and with increasing knowledge of clinical neurology and neuropathology a wealth of variation was described, nowadays under the heading demyelinating disease. As regards MS proper, that is, the classical picture, any neurologist with special interest in this unpredictable disease hardly escapes the temptation to differentiate his own MS patients into different subgroups—until now a frustrating procedure, depending largely on the author's opinion. The difference in age and type of initial symptoms, covering a span from below 10 years of age (Allison and Millar[2], Poskanzer et al.[3]: 0·3% below the age of 10) to over 60 years of age (see Kurtzke[4], p. 204); the varied clinical signs and symptoms from any part of the central nervous system; the atypical proved MS cases included; the difference in course and prognosis: all this seems to represent multiplicity rather than unity. The term multiple sclerosis, with stress upon multiple, seems very suitable.

The signs and symptoms of MS have been described in detail over the years in many books and journals, and need not be repeated here. The reader may be referred, for example, to the excellent and detailed description by McAlpine[5, 6] and to Kurtzke's chapter 4 on the clinical manifestations of MS in the *Handbook of Clinical Neurology*[4].

Onset of the disease

The classical type of MS is characterized by two phases, the episodical phenomenon, called attack or relapse, as defined by McAlpine; and the interval between such episodes. To the patient, and to most neurologists who are mostly consulted on account of symptoms of disability during such episodes, stress is laid upon this phenomenon, though it is well known that some cases (according to most authors about 10%), are characterized from the very onset by a progressive course without relapses. In some studies the diagnosis has only been accepted when relapses have occurred. However, studies by different methods during the last few years have clearly proved that much is going on in the central nervous system on a subclinical level. Analysis by more or less sophisticated methods have shown that the attack or relapse may only be considered as the tip of the iceberg. It is possible to demonstrate anomalies in the function of parts of the CNS in patients without any complaints or demonstrable neurological signs or symptoms from such areas. This problem will be discussed later. The episodical phenomenon will be mentioned briefly.

The onset of MS generally occurs in two different ways. One is as an attack or bout, as another expression of an attack, acute or subacute. The second is as a slowly progressing condition. McAlpine[5, 6] has analysed the mode of onset in 219 patients in whom it was recent enough to be recalled in detail, 17% among these 219 cases developed their symptoms fully in a matter of minutes, 22% in a matter of hours, in other words no less than nearly 40% revealed an apoplectiform beginning. Now in cases of hemiplegia as the first bout, however seldom this seems to occur, one wonders how many cases of so-called cerebrovascular accidents in young women are initial symptoms of MS, and not due to suspected contraceptive medication!

The clinical manifestations of the first—and later—attacks or relapses (defined by McAlpine as an appearance of a new symptom at any time after the initial attack or the return of a previous symptom) have been described in full detail by McAlpine[5, 6] and Kurtzke[4] (see above).

Difficulties relating to the type of the onset bout, to the time of the onset bout, as well as to the number of bouts per year—the so-called relapse rate—are worth considering, as both duration of disease and activity of disease is generally based upon such parameters in studies of MS.

Of course, most patients must consider the initial bout as the first manifestation of their disease, especially in the case of a remarkable symptomatology, for example an optic neuritis or a paraparesis. It is a common experience that in retrospective analysis, and this is the most common method in any hospital record, or at the first consultation of the neurologist, the answers given by patients to the question about the first symptom may differ from one time to another. Relatives of the patient may often supply information which deviates from the patient's own opinion. In a disease like MS, characterized by a number of plaques in silent areas of the brain, and with demonstrable subclinical activity, any calculation regarding duration of the disease must be taken with reservation. The tendency in some studies to consider the onset of the disease back to several years before the clearcut clinical manifestations must be taken seriously.

Let us look upon some studies from modern literature and from our own studies. The following tables show the onset of MS as judged by different authors.

Table 2.1

McAlpine[6], p. 135, has given the following incidence of initial symptoms based on figures given in the literature, symptoms occurring alone or in combination roughly as follows:

Motor weakness	40%
Optic neuritis	22%
Paraesthesiae	21%
Double vision	12%
Vertigo/vomiting	5%
Disturbance of micturition	5%
Other types (hemiplegia, trigeminal neuralgia, facial palsy, deafness)	below 5%

Our own material, like most cases from the literature, is also based upon a retrospective analysis, together with some cases, known from the beginning (prospective studies). In all we have determined the onset in 190 computer-designed cases of definite and probable MS cases, 154 with an acute or sub-acute beginning (58 males, 96 females) and 36 cases characterized by a gradual onset (17 males, 19 females).

The symptoms in Table 2.2 were registered as percentages of neurological deficit for each symptom, alone or in combination with other symptoms.

Table 2.2 shows that motor symptoms dominate both in cases with acute onset and of slow progress. Next come sensory symptoms, again representative of long tract involvement. Disturbances in balance are especially

Table 2.2

	Acute onset	Slow onset
	%	%
Optic neuritis	15·58*	2·78
Disturbance of vision	5·84	11·11
Double vision	9·74	0
Trigeminal symptoms	1·95	2·78
Facial paresis	1·30	0
Hearing disturbances	0·65	2·78
Oblongata symptoms	1·30	0
Vestibulocerebellar symptoms	2·60	0
Vertigo (unspecified)	6·49	5·56
Disturbance of balance	7·79	22·22
Motor tracts	26·62	61·11
Sensory tracts	37·01	27·77
Sensory disturbance of trunk	3·90	0
Bladder symptoms	3·25	2·78
Headache	1·30	0
Nausea, vomiting	1·95	0
Mental symptoms	1·30	0
Other cerebral symptoms	3·90	0
Lumbago	0·65	2·78
General sense of malaise	1·30	5·56

* The percentage of neurological deficit for each sign or symptom

seen in cases with a slow progress. This term is used by the patients themselves. Of course, different types of neurological deficit lie behind this complaint. Other symptoms are less frequent except for visual symptoms. In all, 35% of both groups have visual complaints. Some of them may be due to optic neuritis, but the term optic neuritis has only been used in cases with verified optic neuritis.

Both our own and McAlpine's[5, 6] analyses are, as mentioned, based upon retrospective and prospective studies. However, Kurtzke's[4] material is unique. He has studied 572 male patients with definite or possible MS over a period of 20 years. He divided this material into two groups A and B, group A representing those who had a separate bout prior to the bout at which their diagnosis of MS was made, and group B, those in whom the diagnostic bout was the onset bout. Neurological examinations were available for the onset bout in 50 of the 293 men in group A, and in 219 of the 234 in group B.

In Kurtzke's table 17[4], p. 184, the percentage frequencies for types of neurological deficit found at examination in the onset bout was as follows (see Table 2.3).

Table 2.3

Type	Group A	Group B
Pyramidal	45	88
Cerebellar	44	77
Brainstem	47	73
Sensory	42	55
Optic signs	24	23
Bowel/bladder	8	19
Cerebral-total	9	20
Cerebral-mentation	2	2
Other	8	15

Kurtzke discusses these figures. Group B seems to be more severely affected than group A. Again we are seeing the dominance of motor signs, even if brainstem attacks are equal or almost equal to the long tract attacks. What seems remarkable is the high number of cerebellar signs in both groups. Neither in McAlpine's nor in our material is so high a representation of cerebellar symptoms to be found. All Kurtzke's patients were male but, as far as I know, no difference exists in symptomatology between men and women. However, the high percentage of long tract and brainstem symptomatology in Kurtzke's patients, compared to our and McAlpine's series demonstrate the difficulties in drawing conclusions from retrospective compared to a pure prospective quantitative analysis. In our studies in the course of MS[7], the same distribution was found but we had only 73 cases in this study.

The so-called relapse rate, postulated as a parameter for severity of the disease, and indicating the number of relapses per year, is varyingly reported as between 0·2 and 1·15[8], a rather wide range which seems unfitted for statistical analysis. To this may be added the circumstance, that this relapse rate tends to vary with time. A tendency to a decline in relapse rate as time goes by is often mentioned.

Lhermitte et al.[9] have not been able to confirm this postulate in their studies of over 800 cases of MS from the Salpêtrière and it must be accepted that no correlation is demonstrable between number of relapses and severity of disease[7]. On the contrary, in several cases showing only slight or no progress, the number of relapses may be rather high.

'Silent' MS

The lack of correlation between clinically manifest symptomatology and neuropathology is apparent from studies of either so-called 'silent cases' of MS, and from modern electrophysiological studies in MS. Even if some cases of 'silent MS' as described by Mackay and Hirano[10] may be due to only a small number of plaques in the CNS, we all know unexpected cases of MS. Studies of this type are in progress in this country. Particularly remarkable is the study by Georgi[11]. Among 15 644 autopsies at the Basle University Hospital 66 cases of MS were found. Among these 12 cases from the clinical records were unexpected. However, most of these were not studied by a neurologist, but the records deviated in a remarkable way from MS. Cases showing a dominance of cerebral symptomatology, especially progressive dementia, are well-known too. McAlpine[6] mentions such cases (p. 183). One of our own patients was treated in our department under a diagnosis of cryptogenic epilepsy and dilantin intoxication, verified by blood analysis. He died suddenly and was found to have typical MS in the brain. In another case, the clinical picture was dominated by a progressive dementia. The pathological diagnosis of MS was a great surprise to us.

Much activity may take place in the CNS without apparent clinical manifestation in the sense of a relapsing-remitting symptomatology. Modern electrophysiological studies as well as the well-known heat-provoking technique have unveiled such activity.

The recording of evoked potentials in MS patients has been used in demonstrating lesions in the CNS, both by visual, auditory and somatosensory stimulation from the cervical cord and from the bladder, even in patients without knowledge of visual auditory or bladder symptoms. Halliday et al.[12] found, by recording evoked potentials from the scalp using a special photic stimulation, a delay both from the affected eye in optic neuritis patients, even with full clinical recovery as in MS patients. There were delays from one or both eyes in 90% of the patients, including 21 out of 23 patients with normal optic discs. This method is so sensitive that it may be the single most reliable method of detecting optic nerve damage[13-15]. Another 'optical' method which registers the electrically elicited blink reflex may be useful in unveiling silent lesions localized in the pons[16]. Somatosensory-evoked potentials were recorded by Small and Matthews[17] from surface electrodes over the cervical cord and somatosensory cortex in 14 patients with MS, after electric stimulation of the median nerve. For details the reader may be referred to McDonald[13] in which auditory-evoked potentials are mentioned. William E. Bradley has recorded abnormally evoked potentials from the bladder in MS cases, without any known sphincter disturbance (personal communication). A surprising number of auditory and vestibular aberrations have been found in an extensive study by Noffsinger et al.[18] of 61 cases of MS using advanced technical audiological methods. This study proves more activity in the central paths of both the auditory and vestibular pathways, more than in the acoustic nerve itself. Studies of ocular responses to optokinetic stimulation in MS are in progress in Denmark[19] and in England. With electronystagmography subclinical lesions of the median longitudinal fasciculus can be detected.[13]

An especially convincing method of detecting subclinical lesions in MS is the heating procedure. In 1955 Dr Jens Edmund and the author published a paper: Visual and motor instability in MS[20]. We noticed in a suspected MS male patient that his vision declined during walking. We had no knowledge of Uhthoff's sign. We therefore tried to see if physical work had any influence upon visual acuity in other cases of MS. For practical reasons we gave up using a cycle-ergometer. We therefore tried to see if heating had any influence because we knew from the first-mentioned patient that sweating correlated with a decline in visual acuity. We therefore put MS patients in a heat cabin, with electrical light, as used by physiotherapists, and to our surprise not only did vision decline but other signs and symptoms appeared or reappeared. We were able to reproduce a reappearance of reflex abnormalities, for example a Babinski reflex or a disturbance in the position sense. But motor function especially was influenced by heat. We sometimes saw a formidable increase of the degree of paresis, almost imitating a myasthenic crisis. Shortly after cooling these aggravations disappeared. This heating procedure has been studied by Davis et al.[21] and by Michael and Davis[22]. They used an analogous technique but the body temperature was monitored. The authors confirmed the decline in visual acuity, correlated to body temperature, but what is of special interest here is that they have made serial testings in three patients for periods of up to 7 months. These testings revealed marked fluctuations in thermal sensitivity at times when the patients' overt clinical status was essentially stable. In two patients recently recovered from clinical exacerbations, there was a heightened response to hyperthermia that gradually reversed during days or weeks. They concluded that the manifest signs and symptoms only reflect a portion of the extent and activity of the underlying pathology 'like the tip of an iceberg'. This conclusion coincides with our opinion in our own studies. A plaque or a group of plaques exists at a given time. The extent of a plaque and the symptoms it arouses are determined both by topographical localization in the CNS and also by the size of the vein or venules involved. New symptoms

as well as an exaggeration of old symptoms may be due to a flaring up of the
activity in the old plaque, as well as a purely functional disturbance without
inflammations, but may also be a consequence of the formation of new
plaques around the neighbouring veins. The old argument that the fresh
changes are found in the periphery of the plaques may be due to artificial
phenomena. As shown in the drawing which I sent to Lumsden during a discussion a few years ago and which Lumsden, McAlpine *et al.* published in
their book[6], p. 587, a cutting at the periphery of the coalescing veins will
show the fresh changes in the periphery only. The coalescing of the peri-
phlebitic changes produced the same changes as on the borderline between
fresh tissue and the plaque.

Relapses and Fluctuations

In the daily clinic it often seems impossible to differentiate between a 'real'
relapse, due to pathological activity in the tissue, and a flaring-up of old
symptoms, as in temporary exacerbations. A flaring-up of old symptoms
may last for more than some days or even weeks without any proof of a
pathological activity in the tissue. Fluctuations in the function of the CNS
are highly dependent upon both exogenous and internal circumstances, not
least in a diseased tissue. Our chance to have a stable function is highly
dependent on normal functioning nervous tissue. Some patients tell themselves that they feel that their state is fluctuating periodically, over weeks. A
few patients consider this as a more or less rhythmic change. Everyone
acknowledges the fluctuations of both symptoms and signs during the course
of the disease. Most patients talk of differences in their power and ability
during day and at evening time. Many patients feel much better at night
and may even be able to walk, though they have to use a wheelchair during
the day. The same patient is one day able to lift up his stretched leg to
60 or 80°, and the next day to only 30 or 40°. The rhythmic changes have
been mentioned. They are seldom so striking as in one of our female patients
who behaved in a very ladylike way most of the time (her true character),
but whose behaviour changed dramatically with the approach of menstrua-
tion. She then behaved almost like a prostitute, advancing upon unsuspecting
male patients and male personnel in the waiting-room. These episodes got
more and more psychotic as time went on and one day she drank ether
and died during such an episode.

The fluctuations in the clinical state outlined above make it difficult to
draw definite conclusions from single examinations with long intervals in
any study of MS. This problem will be analysed in more detail later. Here
we will discuss the discrepancy between pathological lesions and clinical

manifestations a little more, in relation to our possible failure even to diagnose MS, and attempt to draw some conclusions regarding both prevalence, incidence and duration of the disease.

The presence of abortive cases of MS is worth mentioning in this connection. The well-known problem of optic neuritis as an abortive case of MS may throw some light upon this topic. Several studies have been published in which the problem of the percentage of cases of optic neuritis which eventuate as MS has often been studied. The figures vary from 8% to over 70%. No doubt the only way to clarify this important problem is to make prospective studies. It seems so important because mostly the diagnosis of optic neuritis is so clearcut, in contrast to several episodes in CNS-disease, especially when appearing at the onset of the disease.

A thought-provoking case was demonstrated by Andersen, myself and Hyllested[23] at the MS symposium in Newcastle upon Tyne in June 1971 (more details at the Scandinavian Congress of Neurology, Oslo, 1973). A female had a span of 45 years free from any neurological complaints between an attack of optic neuritis, combined with hemisensory symptoms, which had appeared and remitted one year before the optic neuritis and her death. She died from a coronary thrombosis. The autopsy showed numerous small plaques throughout the whole brain, with the typical localization. In the diseased optic nerve only about 40% of the optic fibres were preserved. Her vision was said to be normal! And as mentioned she had no complaints from the CNS during 45 years.

The problem of the existence of abortive MS cases can be lightened by mentioning the recent studies by Sandberg-Wollheim et al.[24] who in collaboration with the tissue-typing laboratory in Rigshospitalet, Copenhagen, made HLA and LD typing in 54 monosymptomatic optic neuritis cases, in a prospective study. They have found increased frequencies of the HL-A$_3$7 and LD-7a determinants of approximately the same magnitude as in patients with MS. Arnason and Chelmicka-Szorc[25] were unable to confirm an increase in HLA typing 3–7 in optic neuritis patients who did not develop into MS. However, the Scandinavians also studied the LD-7a type; 48% of these 54 optic neuritis cases showed this type, compared to 60% in MS and 18% in the normal population.

In a later publication Sandberg-Wollheim[26] has focused on the changes in the cerebrospinal fluid in 61 patients with acute monosymptomatic optic neuritis and their clinical course. Among these the above-mentioned 47 cases are included. Her conclusion is that in 51% a mononuclear pleocytosis was noted at the onset of the disease, but only in 41% was oligoclonal IgG demonstrable. Among the 11 cases who later developed MS, 5 showed the typical disease-pattern in the fluid. In 5 more patients with subsequent

MS, an oligoclonal IgG appeared in the follow-up, but there was no correlation between the time of appearance of new symptoms and fluid changes. In 6 patients with normal fluid and 4 patients with pleocytosis at onset, the IgG pattern became oligoclonal during the follow-up although the patients had no further symptoms or signs of MS. The patients were between 15 and 55 years at onset, 21 were males and 40 women. The follow-up period ranged from 7 months to 6 years (mean 2·6 years). These figures may be compared with those of Link and Müller[27] where an increase of IgG was found in 73% of 64 cases; and an oligoclonal IgG in 86·9% of 84 definite MS cases[28], and in 94% of 64 MS patients[27]. Sandberg-Wollheim concludes that a normal cerebrospinal fluid in optic neuritis does not preclude later development of MS. Among the 11 later MS cases, 6 did not have an oligoclonal IgG at onset, but in 5 of these this change appeared later.

Possibly the cases with normal spinal fluid are 'younger' than are those with oligoclonal bands and represent the real first onset of the disease. But at present we have no means of determining this point.

Evaluation of clinical condition and prognosis

We must conclude from these studies that the clinician is in a singularly difficult position when studying the duration of the disease and trying to evaluate the intensity of pathological change in the CNS. He may adopt the point of view that they have to define which cases to choose, as has been done by Schumacher et al.[29], and to define the probability of diagnosis as made by Allison and Millar[2], or by McAlpine[6]. This problem was thoroughly discussed at the Göteborg Symposium, 1972[30]. For epidemiological studies it seems necessary to have such clearcut definitions, but it seems too restrictive to accept cases only showing two or more episodes of worsening (relapses) in any clinical study. The different criteria must be taken as a whole, and we must also accept cases as 'possible MS', as defined by McAlpine[6], p. 202. Generally the experience of the clinician will be decisive, and it is always difficult to define or assess it. However, in attempting to understand what is going on in the CNS and how much is going on, it seems necessary to follow the patients during long-term studies. The most important information we may get from such studies is an idea of the intensity of the pathological process, rather than of real duration and only rarely of precise localization.

The diagnostic problem is in itself perhaps more difficult to solve than many neurologists are aware of during their daily work. Some of these have been discussed above, but others remain. The differentiation between some cases of so-called familial MS and pure hereditary central nervous system disease, especially of recessive heritability type, seems to cause much trouble, not least in the genetic field. The important role of spinal fluid changes in MS is well known, but does not seem to have been studied in hereditary CNS disease. However, I want to emphasize the periphlebitis retinae as a useful diagnostic procedure[31] and the retinal striae, described by Hovt[32] and confirmed by McDonald[13], following a retrobulbar neuritis, perhaps undiagnosed, should become a help to the clinician.

Another new diagnostic procedure by using the EMI-scan seems to show a very promising help in the diagnosis of MS. Gyldensted[33] made studies in 110 cases from our clinic and was able to demonstrate areas of low X-ray attenuation, mostly around the anterior and posterior horns of the lateral ventricles in 41 cases (37%). These areas may represent the well-known large periventricular plaques and were never seen in any other neurological disease. They were sometimes found even in isolated areas of the white matter of the hemispheres. The contours of these low-absorption areas correspond beautifully to the plaques, especially by delineating the areas on the computer's maps (Figures 2.1 and 2.2).

What I would like to emphasize is what I call the progressive stage of the disease. I find it most important to document not only relapses but also what is going on between these episodes. The progressive stage may be defined as a more or less fluctuating state but as a whole with a downhill course, rather independent of clinical circumscript periods of new, or flaring-up of old, symptoms, followed by remission.

In our book[7] about the course of MS in 73 computer-designed cases we have tried to study this stage, based upon a semiquantitative documentation of neurological deficits at repeated examinations, with different intervals, usually about 3 months.

In drawing curves of the course we have been able to approximate these curves with different mathematical functions. This was done on account of the demonstrable relatively frequent levelling of the peaks in the curves. This was a surprise because a more stepwise progress would be expected, if the clinical curves should follow a sequelae of relapses. Of course any curve may be made to approximate to a mathematical function, but in studying the slope of the curves, we were able to extrapolate backwards the year which the patient himself had told us that the course had begun to show a rather downhill progress. In making an extrapolation forwards into the future, the curves have foreseen the degree of medical impairment during these future years.

The different mathematical functions need be mentioned only briefly. For details the reader may refer to our book[7]. We have used the following functions: 2 linear, 2 exponential, 1 logarithmic, 1 parabolic, 1 hyperbolic

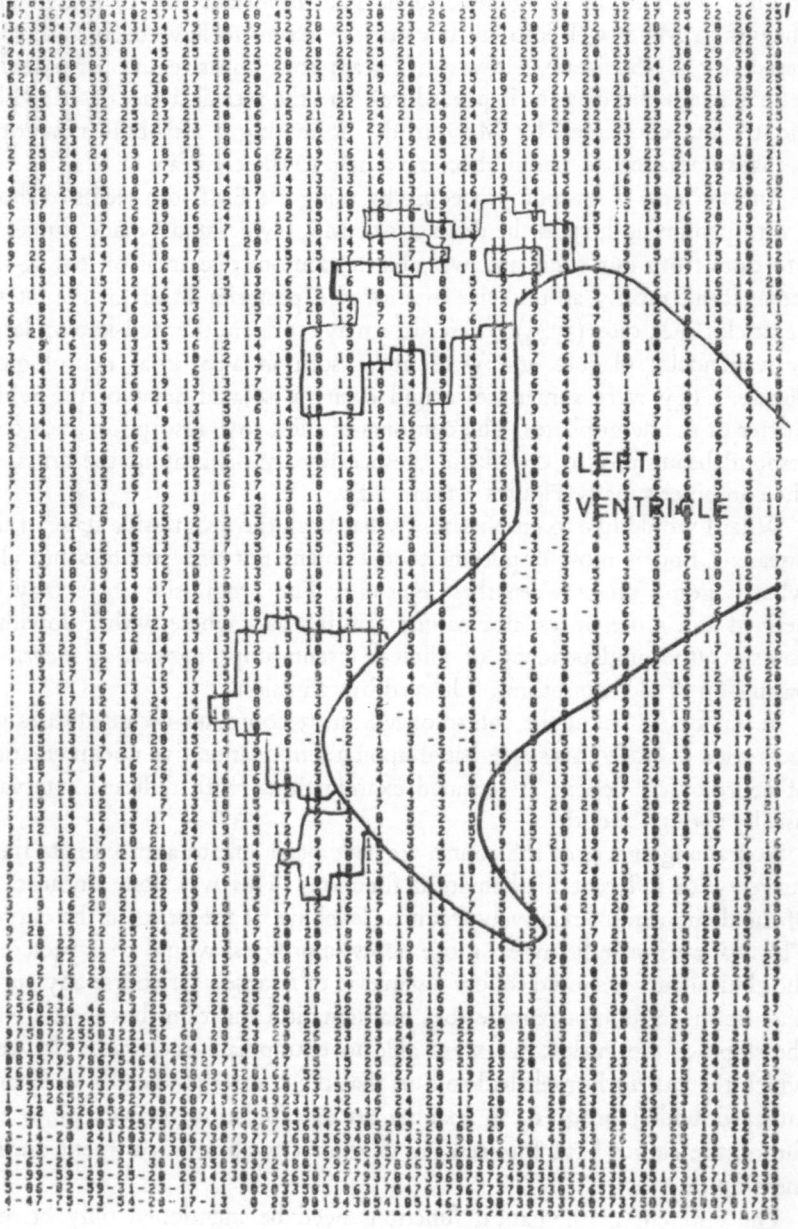

Figure 2.1 EMI-scanning from MS case. Absorption-counts from the computer (see text)

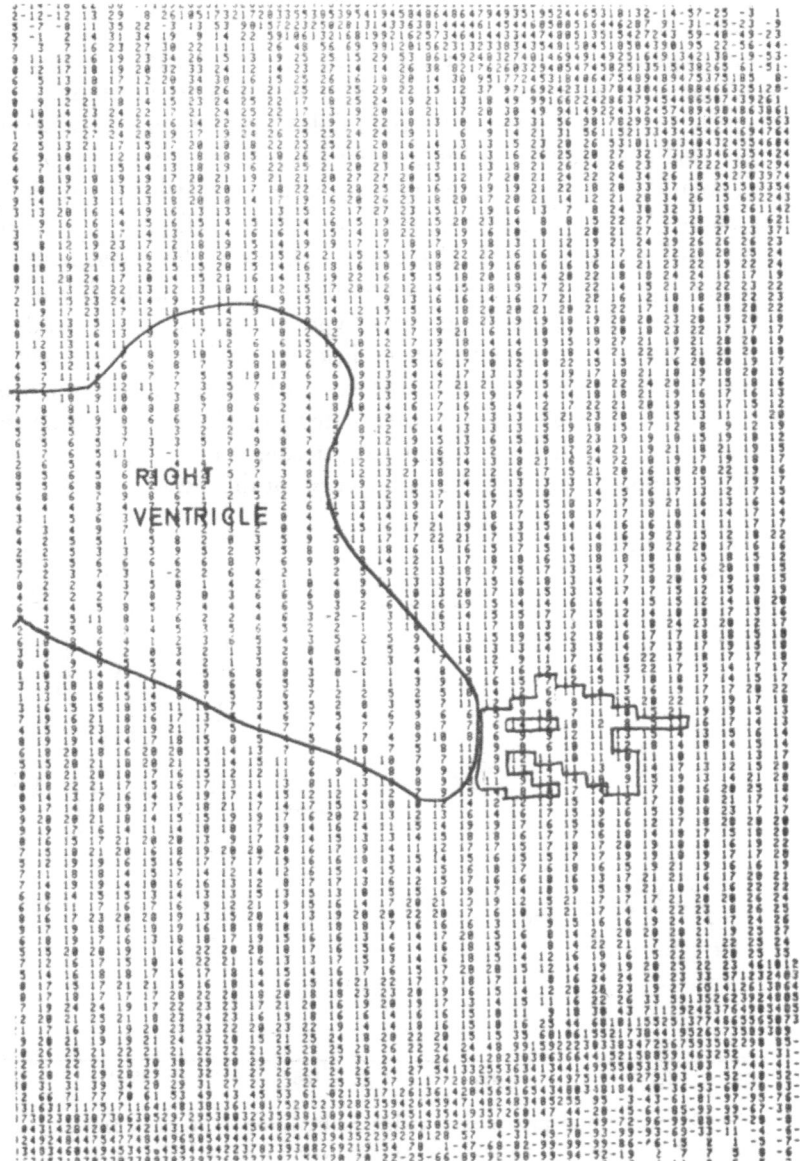

Figure 2.2 EMI-scanning from another MS case (see text)

and 3 polynominal (second, third and fourth degree) curves. We have made correlation determinations and used the curve with the highest correlation coefficient as the 'best'.

In our original work we found that no less than 65 among 73 curves may be determined so precisely that it is possible to conclude something about this type of study. This material has been followed up during the years and has been analysed from a statistical point of view by Linnemann[34]. The course, following the exponential type of curve as used by us originally, seems unsuited to a judgement over the years since it follows too steep a course. Another type of exponential progress curve may, however, be useful. Altogether, 15 out of 18 linear curves followed the original inclination (83·8%), 4 out of 5 of the logarithmic type, and 12 out of 16 parabolic curves continued their course; 23 patients belonged to the exponential curve-type mentioned, but only 6 followed the expected course. The other patients had died or left the study or had deteriorated so badly that a scoring was impossible. This analysis shows the relative steadiness of the progress which may be an important point in the pathogenesis of the disease.

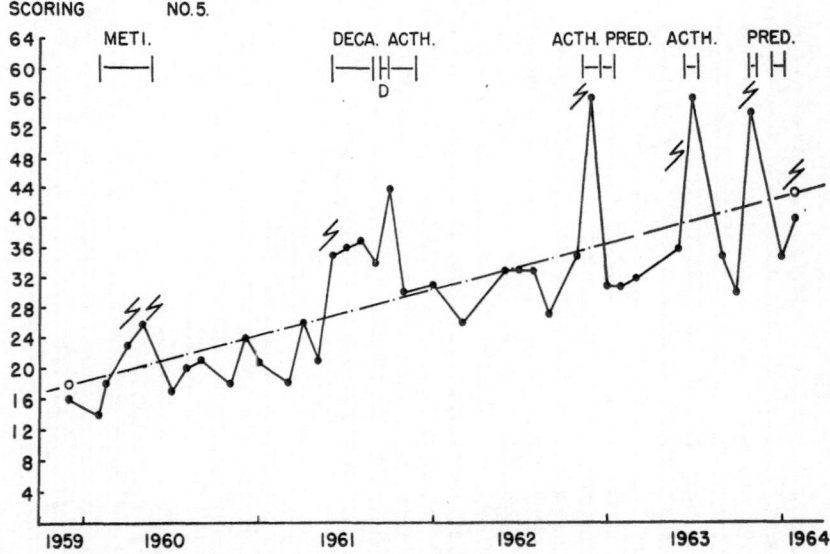

Figure 2.3 Remittant and progressive, rather malign case, registrated from 1959 to 1964. She died 1965 verified by autopsy (adapted from Fog and Linnemann[7])

If the low absorption areas demonstrated by the EMI-scan are identical with the plaques, as they seem to be, the approximation to the low absorption of the fluid in the ventricles may indicate a steady progress in the

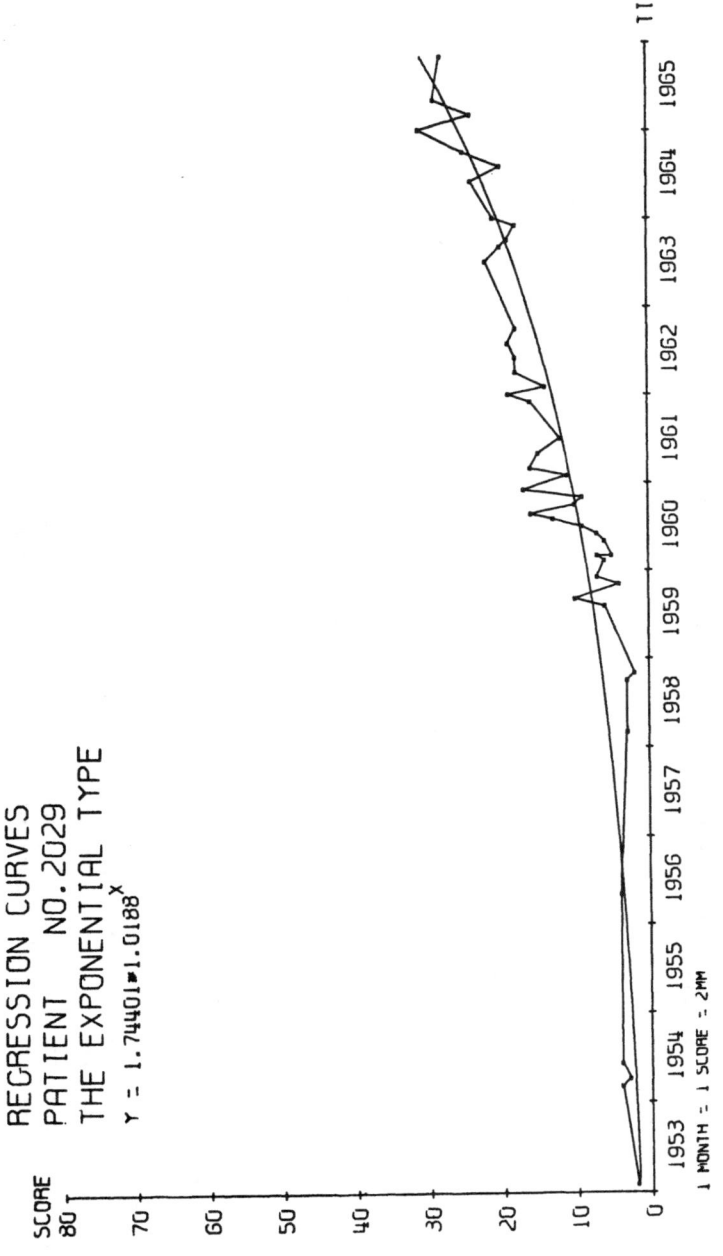

Figure 2.4 Remittant and progressive case, followed from 1953 until 1965. Died 1969 (after a bladder operation), diagnosis verified by autopsy (adapted from Fog and Linneman[7])

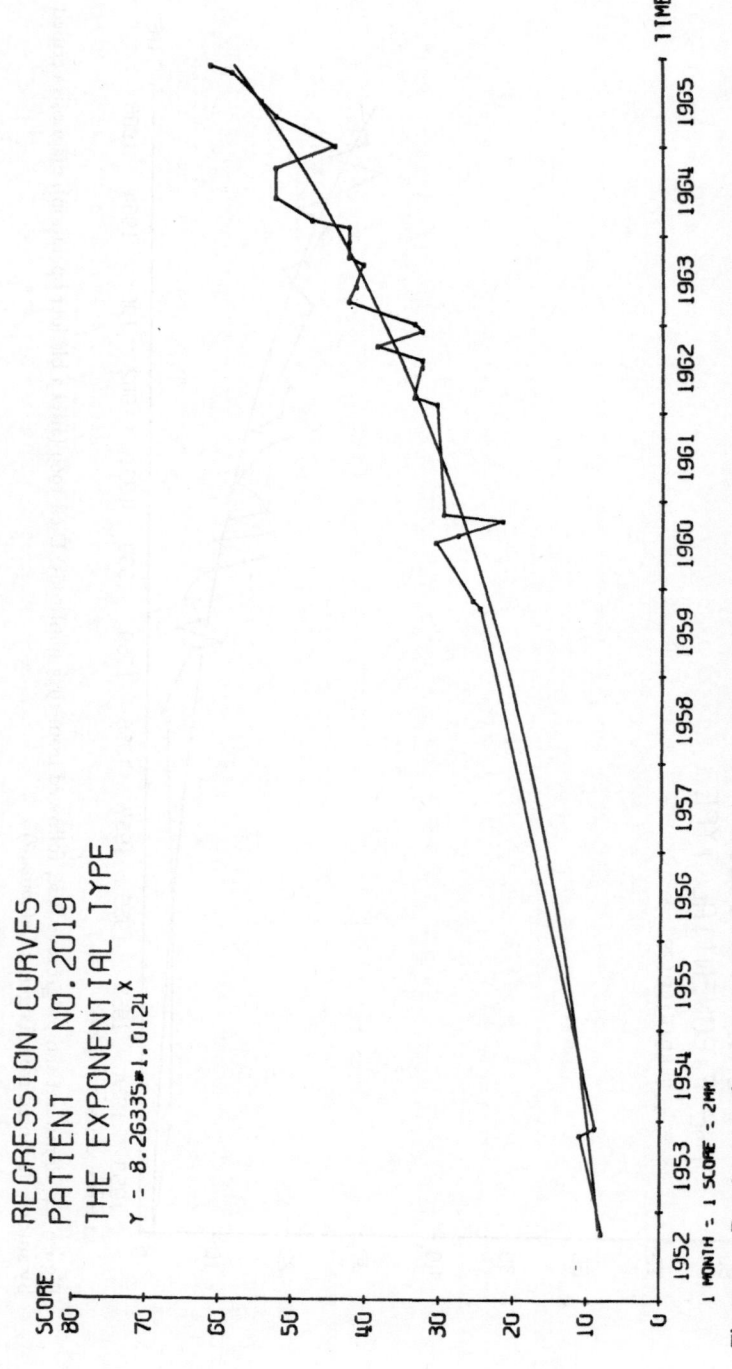

Figure 2.5 Remittant and progressive case, seen three times during 1952–53 and followed from 1959 until 1968 (only 1965 on the curve). The progress continued without demonstrable episodes (adapted from Fog and Linneman[7])

disintegration of the tissues within the plaques. From a neuropathological point of view the cystic type of these old plaques indicates a process which again may determine the even downhill course of the disease. Studies in the morphology of several cerebral plaques, especially the great plaques, seem to disclose a degeneration of both myelin sheaths and many axis cylinders. The glia-proliferation is localized to the periphery of these areas, like any other scar. The old hypothesis by Putnam (for literature see Fog[35]) of a venular obstruction causing the plaque may be reconsidered. Theoretically the outflow may be blocked by immunecomplexes, locally produced.

The histocompatibility system and multiple sclerosis

During June 1976 an international meeting took place in Paris concerning the so-called HLA system and its role in human disease generally. A special session was devoted to neurology and this was dominated by MS, which enables us to give a short view of our knowledge today about this new approach to MS research.

The reader is referred to the report from this meeting concerning the theoretical background of the HLA system and its aspects[36]. A short view may be read in the editorial article in the *Archives of Neurology*[37]. The histocompatibility system is localized to all cell surfaces and is composed of antigens that from a chemical point of view are glycoproteins. A number of experimental studies have shown that these genes control immune responses or they may possibly serve as receptors for viruses.

The histocompatibility system is controlled by genes localized on chromosome number 6. Originally these genes were divided into one group named the LA-locus, another named the FOUR-locus, each representing a number of different genes, determined by serum reactions (therefore named SD antigens) and a third locus, the LD locus, determined by a mixed lymphocyte reaction, that is, genes possibly controlling cellular immunity. These loci have now got a new practical nomenclature as follows: The A, B, C and D-locus, for LA, FOUR and D for LD-locus. The C-locus seems to have only small importance in MS. However, an I-a-like antigen named B-cell alloantigen 'Ag7a' is coding for antibodies to B-lymphocytes (see below, page 30). The D-locus is determined by a so-called one-way mixed lymphocyte reaction and its demonstration is limited by the claim to have homozygous stimulator cells in the MLC procedure, and these homozygous cells are not so easy to obtain.

The following conclusions came from the Paris meeting[36]:

(1) So far studies of HLA antigens in familial MS cases have shown that MS is not a genetic disease in the classical sense. This is in accordance with

the general genetical aspect of MS. However, these studies are still incomplete. Almost no studies in the D-locus exist in families, and the need
of a reliable proof of the diagnosis of MS in the families examined has not
been established versus hereditary CNS diseases, especially the types with
recessive heritability.

(2) A clear association exists between MS and the D-locus, earlier named
the HLA7a, now the DW2. This has been confirmed by several investigators
from different laboratories, studying populations from the Caucasian races
and has even been found among some black MS patients in the USA. The
DW2 allele is found in about 60 to 70% of MS cases among Caucasians
compared to less than 20% in non-MS people.

An association may exist between the course and prognosis of MS and
the presence or absence of the DW2 allele in the patient. The most severe
and fast-progressing cases are found in the DW2 group. These studies must
be enlarged and scrutinized to see if a new classification of MS may be
based on such studies.

(3) An increase in serum antibodies to different viruses, especially measles
virus, shows in some studies an association to, in other studies no association
to, the HLA system in MS. More relevant are studies of the spinal fluid
measles antibody titre and the association to the HLA antigen, especially
the DW2 allele. The number of these studies is too small to permit definite
conclusions.

(4) New promising studies are going on in 4 different laboratories with
the Ag7a antigen coding for antibodies to B-lymphocytes. A high percentage of MS patients have demonstrated the presence of such antibodies.
Further studies are necessary before the presence of such antibodies can be
established in MS, as compared to controls and family members, and in
other neurological diseases. Wernet et al.[38] found this antigen present in 92
out of 100 cases of MS.

(5) The following hypothesis concerning the coding of an MS-associated
gene is given as follows: HLA-SDA3—HLA-SDB7—HLA-LDW2—
HLA-Ag7a, in the order of increasing binding to MS, all more frequent
than could be expected by chance in the Caucasian population.

The interpretation of the studies of the HLA system in MS is difficult
and open to many speculations. An analogy to the demonstration of the
HLA-A8a (DW2) type in a special category of myasthenia gravis is evident.
Possibly this sytem determines the susceptibility towards certain exogenous
influences (virus?). Nevertheless, this association seems to be a well-established
fact.

References

1. Charcot, J. M. (1886). Leçons sur les maladies du système nerveux. Œuvres complètes de J. M. Charcot, Tome 1, pp. 258–263 (Paris: Bournevill)
2. Allison, R. S. and Millar, J. H. D. (1954). Prevalence of disseminated sclerosis in Northern Ireland. *Ulster Med. J. Suppl.* **2, 23,** 5
3. Poskanzer, D. C., Schapira, K. and Miller, H. (1963). Epidemiology of multiple sclerosis in the counties of Northumberland and Durham. *J. Neurol. Neurosurg. Psychiatry* **26,** 368
4. Kurtzke, J. F. (1970). Clinical manifestation of multiple sclerosis. P. J. Binken and G. W. Bruyn (eds.). *Handbook of Clinical Neurology,* Vol. IX (Amsterdam: North-Holland)
5. McAlpine, D., Compston, N. D. and Lumsden, C. E. (1955). *Multiple Sclerosis* (Edinburgh: Livingstone)
6. McAlpine, D., Lumsden, C. E. and Acheson, E. D. (1972). *Multiple Sclerosis. A Reappraisal,* 2nd edition (Edinburgh: Churchill Livingstone)
7. Fog, T. and Linnemann, F. (1970). The course of multiple sclerosis, in 73 computer-designed curves. *Acta Neurol. Scand.,* **46,** suppl. 47
8. Thygesen, P. (1953). *The course of disseminated sclerosis. A close-up of 105 attacks.* (Copenhagen: Rosenkilde and Bagger, Disputats)
9. Lhermitte, F., Marteau, R., Gazengel, J., Dorda, G. and Deloche, G. (1973). The frequency of relapse in multiple sclerosis. *Z. Neurol.,* **205,** 47
10. Mackay, R. P. and Hirano, A. (1967). Forms of benign multiple sclerosis. Report of two 'silent cases' discovered at autopsy. *Arch. Neurol.,* **17,** 588
11. Georgi, W. (1961). *Multiple Sklerose.* Pathologisch–anatomische Befunde multipler Sklerose bei klinisch nicht diagnostizierten Krankheiten. *Schweiz. Med. Wochenschr.,* **91,** 605
12. Halliday, A. M., McDonald, W. I. and Muskin, J. (1972). Delayed visual evoked response in optic neuritis. *Lancet,* **i,** 982
13. McDonald, W. I. (1975). *What is Multiple Sclerosis? Clinical Criteria for Diagnosis.* Medical Research Council. Multiple Sclerosis Research (London: Her Majesty's Stationery Office) (Amsterdam and New York: Elsevier Scientific Publish. Comp.)
14. Milner, B. A., Regan, D. and Heron, J. R. (1974). Differential diagnosis of MS by visual evoked potential recording. *Brain,* **97,** 755
15. Asselman, P., Chadwick, D. W. and Marsden, C. D. (1975). Visual evoked responses in the diagnosis and management of patients suspected of MS. *Brain,* **98,** (2), 261
16. Kimura, J. (1975). Electrically elicited blink reflex in diagnosis of MS. Review of 260 patients over a seven-year period. *Brain,* **98,** (3), 413
17. Small, D. G. and Matthews, W. B. (1974). Subcortical somatosensory evoked potentials in man. International symposium on central evoked potentials in man. (Brussels) (cited from McDonald, 1974)
18. Noffsinger, D., Olsen, W. O., Carhart, R., Hart, C. W. and Sahgal, V. (1972).

Auditory and vestibular aberrations in multiple sclerosis. *Acta Oto-Laryngol.*, **303**, Suppl.

19. Dam, M., Johnsen, N., Thomsen, J. and Zilstorff, K. (1975). Vestibular aberrations in multiple sclerosis. *Acta Neurol. Scand.* **52**, 407

20. Edmund, J. and Fog, T. (1955). Visual and motor instability in multiple sclerosis, *Arch. Neurol. Psychiat. (Chicago)*, **73**, 316

21. Davis, F., Michael, J. and Neer, D. (1973). Serial hyperthermia testing in multiple sclerosis: a method of monitoring subclinical fluctuations. *Acta Neurol. Scand.*, **49**, 1, 63

22. Michael, J. and Davis, F. (1973). Effects of induced hyperthermia in multiple sclerosis: differences in visual acuity during heating and recovery phases. *Acta Neurol. Scand.*, **49**, 2, 141

23. Andersen, S. R., Fog, T. and Hyllested, K. (1972). Changes in the optic nerve 44 years after retrobulbar neuritis in a benign case of multiple sclerosis. In E. J. Field, T. M. Bell and P. R. Carnegie (eds.). *Multiple Sclerosis. Progress in Research*, Clinical studies, Vol. 3, pp. 166–168 (Amsterdam: North Holland)

24. Sandberg-Wollheim, M., Platz, P., Ryder, L., Nielsen, L. and Thomsen, M. (1975). HLA histocompatibility antigens in optic neuritis. *Acta Neurol. Scand.*, **52**, 161

25. Arnason, B. G. W. and Chelmicka-Szorc, E. (1975). Immunogenetic aspects of demyelinating disease. *Proc. Perspectives in MS*, 10–11 (Bethesda: National Institute of Health)

26. Sandberg-Wollheim, M. (1975). Optic neuritis: studies on the cerebrospinal fluid in relation to clinical course in 61 patients. *Acta Neurol. Scand.*, **52**, 167

27. Link and Müller (1971). Cited by *Sandberg-Wollheim* (1975)

28. Laterre *et al.* (1970). Cited by *Sandberg-Wollheim* (1975)

29. Schumacher, G. A., Beebe, A., Kibler, R. F., Kurland, L. T., Kurtzke, J. F., McDowell, F., Nagler, B., Sibley, W. A., Tourtelotte, W. W. and Willmann, T. L. (1965). Problems on experimental trials of therapy in multiple sclerosis: report by the panel on the evaluation of experimental trials of therapy in multiple sclerosis. *Am. N.Y. Acad. Sci.*, **122**, 552

30. The International Symposium on Multiple Sclerosis, Göteborg, September 1972. O. Andersen, L. Bergmann and T. Broman (eds.). *Acta Neurol. Scand.*, **50**, suppl. 58

31. Møller, P. M. and Hammerberg, P. E. (1963). Retinal periphlebitis in multiple sclerosis. *Acta Neurol. Scand.*, **39**, suppl. 4, 263

32. Frisen, L. and Hoyt, W. F. (1974). Insidious atrophy of retinal nerve fibres in multiple sclerosis. Fundoscopic identification in patients with and without visual complaints. *Arch. Ophthalmol.*, **92**, 91

33. Gyldensted, C. (1976): Computer tomography of the brain in multiple sclerosis. *Acta Neurol. Scand.*, **53**, 386

34. Linnemann, F. (1975). En statistisk forløbsanalyse af sclerosepatienter. *IM SOI* (In Danish)

35. Fog, T. (1948). Rygmarvens patologiske anatomi ved dissemineret sclerose og dissemineret encephalomyelitis. Disputats (Copenhagen: Ejnar Munksgaard)

36. Proceedings of the First International Symposium on HLA and disease. Paris, June 21–24, 1976 (In press)
37. Farlin, P. E. and McFarland, H. F. (1976). Histocompatibility studies and multiple sclerosis *Arch. Neurol. (Chicago)*, **33,** 395
38. P. Wernet (1976): Human ia type alloantigens. *Transplant Rev.* **30,** 271

3

Clues to the cause based upon the epidemiology of multiple sclerosis

Milton Alter

The primary goal of epidemiological research in multiple sclerosis (MS) is to determine the environmental and host factors which are related to the cause of this disease. These factors are sought by analysing MS frequency in different populations and in different parts of the world. Over the last half-century, a large literature has accumulated documenting differences in frequency of MS among peoples and places[1-3] and, if reasons for these differences were known, then the list of possible environmental and host factors related to the cause of MS could at least be narrowed. Therefore, the observed differences in MS frequency can provide important clues to aetiology if their meaning were unravelled.

One consistent finding to emerge from epidemiological research in MS is that this disease has an unequal geographical distribution. Since the mid-1950s, it has been known that MS was more common in temperate than in tropical areas of the world[4, 5]. More recent studies of MS distribution introduced methodological refinements but the general characteristics of the geographical distribution have not been appreciably altered. Today, it is generally accepted that MS increases in frequency with geographical latitude both in the northern[6] and southern hemisphere[7]. Reviews[1, 2, 8] of the geographical distribution of MS have been published and Figure 3.1 summarizes some of this information.

According to one interpretation[9], the geographical distribution of MS resembles a parabolic *gradient* (Figure 3.2) which increases sharply with latitude. An alternative interpretation[10] of these same data is that *zones* of

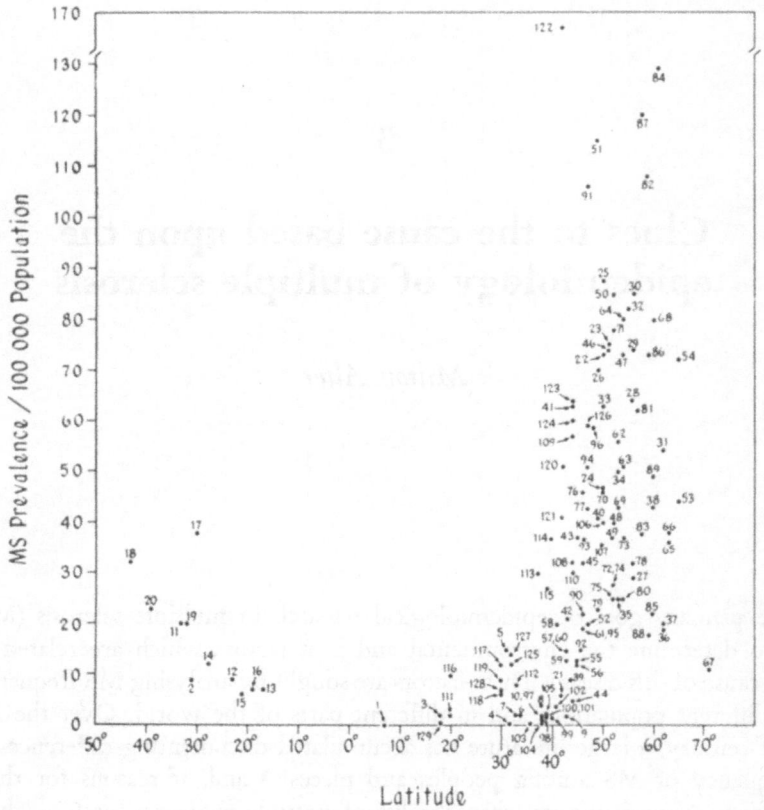

Figure 3.1 Worldwide distribution of multiple sclerosis by latitude (see [9])

varying frequency exist in different parts of the world. The latitude of the zones may overlap considerably (Figure 3.3). According to the gradient interpretation, MS should have the highest frequency at the extremes of latitude. However, available data from communities in northern areas, for example, northern Norway[11] and Canada[12, 13], suggest that MS may actually be lower in frequency at extreme latitudes than in regions farther south[14–16]. In Europe, MS appears to be highest in frequency in the central part[6] and frequency decreases toward the north as well as south (Figure 3.4). An east–west gradient may also exist in Europe[17]. When the prevalence of MS is plotted against geographical latitude in different parts of the world, remarkably similar gradients result (Figure 3.5).

Statistically significant variations in frequency have also been observed over limited geographical areas, giving rise to the suggestion that 'foci' or

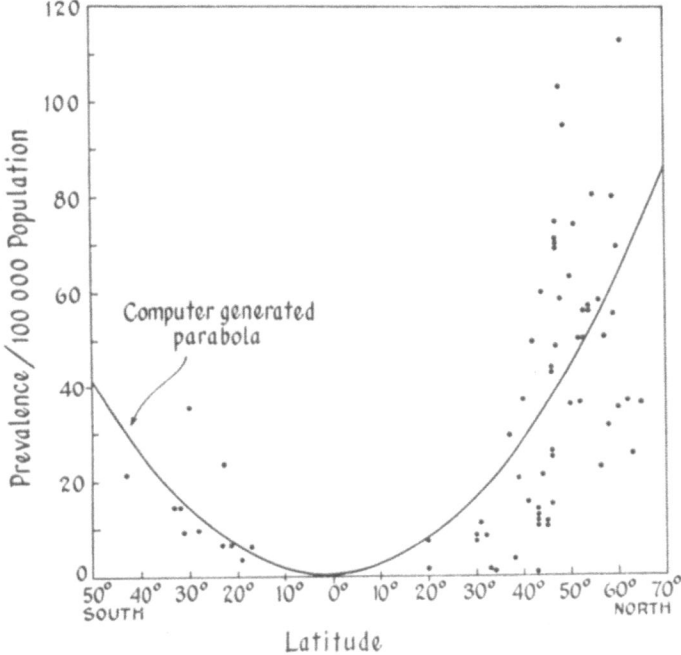

Figure 3.2 Distribution of multiple sclerosis: selected data (see [9])

pockets of unusually high frequency may exist next to areas of much lower frequency[11] (Figure 3.6). A focus in Finland has been described recently by Wikström[18]. His monograph reviews other foci of MS in northern Europe as well. The highest rates of MS in Finland occur in the western and south-western parts of the country, confirming earlier work by Panelius[19]. The Finnish focus was most marked when frequency rates of MS were calculated by place of birth, rather than place of later residence of the patients, suggesting that the period *early in life* may be most important in determining the risk of MS. Wikström found a positive association in Finland between MS frequency and tuberculosis deaths, whereas in Mexico, Japan and the United States[20], high MS rates were associated with *low* tuberculosis mortality. Wikström also reported an association between high MS frequency and high rates of nutritional muscular dystrophy in cattle, a disease attributed to low vitamin E levels. His finding fits in with notions that MS risk is increased in areas where vitamin E levels in the diet are depressed, as for example where the diet contains a large proportion of saturated animal fat[21, 22].

The highest rate of MS in the world may exist in the Shetland and Orkney

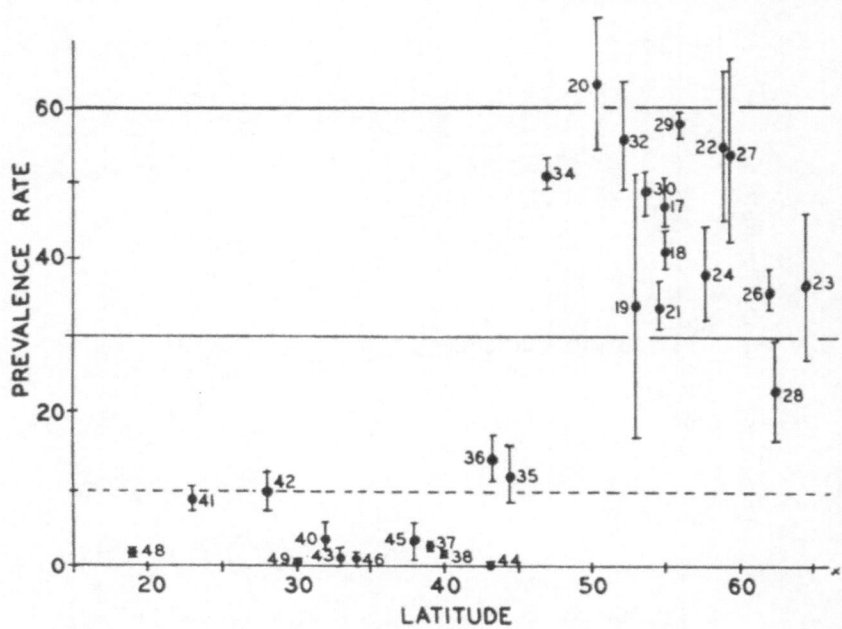

Figure 3.3 Band theory of distribution of multiple sclerosis (see [10])

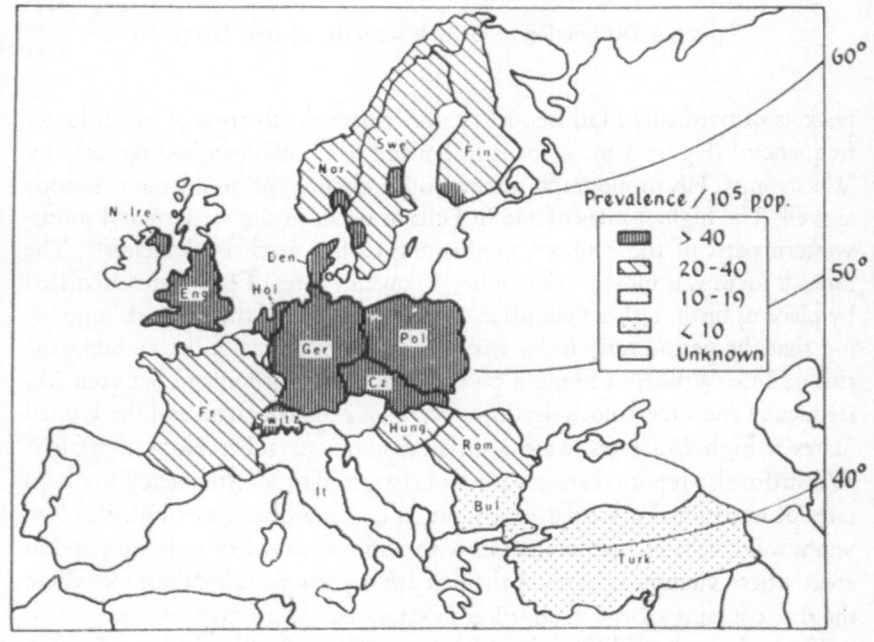

Figure 3.4 Prevalence of multiple sclerosis in Europe (see [17])

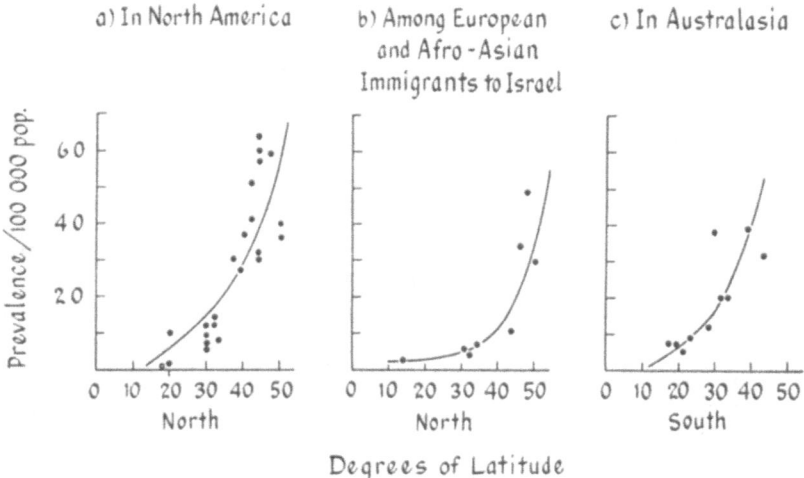

a) In North America   b) Among European   c) In Australasia
                          and Afro-Asian
                          Immigrants to Israel

Degrees of Latitude

Figure 3.5 Prevalence of multiple sclerosis by geographical latitude (*a*) North America, (*b*) among European and Afro-Asian immigrants to Israel and (*c*) in Australasia

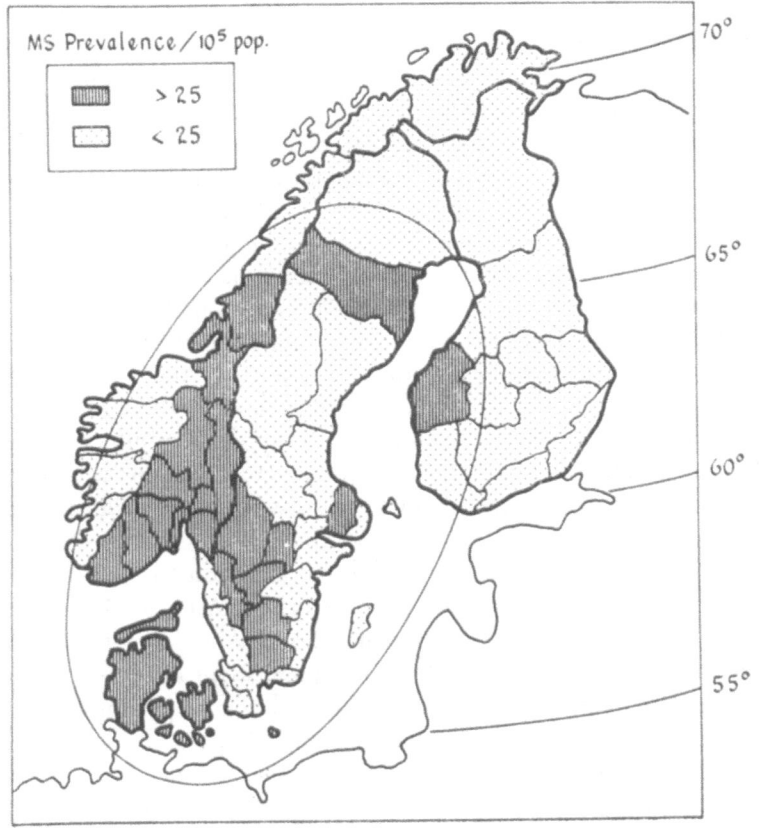

Figure 3.6 Fennoscandian focus of multiple sclerosis (see [11])

Islands, off the coast of Scotland[23]. A study in that area, now ongoing, is seeking to explain the cause of this high rate. Preliminary results indicate that it cannot be attributed simply to an emigration of well people nor to a return of individuals with MS to their families on the Islands.

The notion that zones of varying frequency exist with overlapping geographical latitudes is weakened by recognition of the imprecision of available methods of estimating frequency. Even if differences between areas are 'statistically significant', no amount of statistical manipulation can make up for incomplete case finding, variations in diagnostic criteria and differences in population structure (e.g. sex, age, and race) between different regions. All of these factors can certainly affect the observed frequency and have not often been taken into account. The data shown in Figure 3.1, for example, are based on crude prevalence rates of MS without correction for age and sex differences among the places compared. One attempt to refine the estimate of MS frequency for better comparisons showed that age differences among populations could not account for the observed differences in the distribution of MS[24]. None the less, small differences in reported values of MS frequency among regions should not be taken as necessarily meaningful.

If the 'true' distribution of MS were known, several advantages would accrue: one could predict the frequency of MS in areas not yet studied without conducting a tedious and expensive case-finding effort; it would permit recognition of 'deviant' communities with either abnormally high or abnormally low rates of the disease; and finally, it might suggest a similarly distributed factor which was of aetiological importance.

Alter et al.[9] have examined curves other than the parabola as possibly descriptive of the 'true' distribution of MS and found that a fourth-order curve (Figure 3.7) described the available data well. The fourth-order curve showed low rates near the equator and frequency rose with latitude to a maximum near the 50–60° parallels. Beyond these parallels, MS declined in frequency and at the extreme latitudes to the north and south of the equator, MS was again rare. A fourth-order curve could represent interaction between two aetiological variables, each of which was distributed with latitude as a second-order variable (i.e. $x_a^2 \times x_b^2 = x^4$).

Studies of MS frequency have now been carried out in most of the world but there are still large regions (such as eastern Asia and Central Africa) and even whole continents (for instance, South America) where no formal studies of MS frequency in well-defined populations have, as yet, been reported. These 'dark' regions will, no doubt, also be mapped in the future to determine whether they follow the general distribution pattern for MS found for most other areas or whether they are 'deviant'.

Besides the regional variations which complicate the relationship between

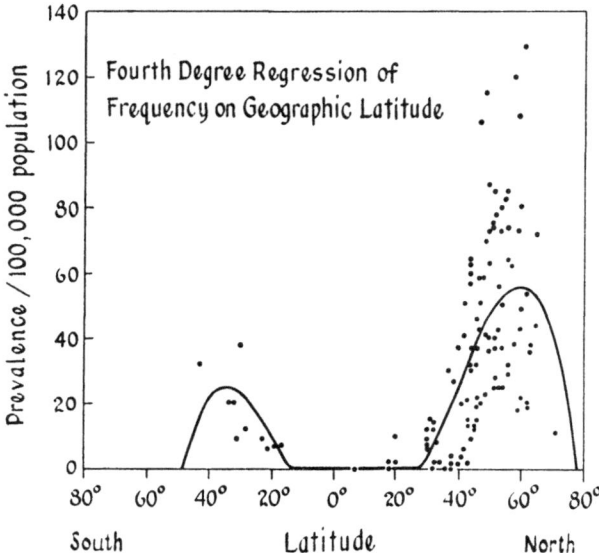

Figure 3.7 Worldwide distribution of multiple sclerosis: fourth degree regression of frequency on geographical latitude (see [9])

MS frequency and latitude, there is evidence that all of Asia may have a low rate of the disease. The best-studied example in Asia is Japan which has a lower rate of MS than would be expected from latitudinal considerations alone. Recent studies[25] using thorough case-finding methods and standardized diagnostic criteria have confirmed earlier reports that MS is rare throughout all of Japan (Figure 3.8). But, even in Japan, a north–south gradient in MS frequency exists[26]. In other regions of eastern Asia[27–30] and among Orientals living in continental United States[31], relatively few cases of MS have been observed. A total of eight Japanese-Americans with MS was found after an intensive search by Detels et al.[32] in two counties in the state of Washington and in Los Angeles, California. This was far lower than expected on the basis of the rate of MS in Caucasians living in these same areas. If the low rate of MS in Orientals were confirmed, then reasons for the Oriental 'resistance' could be sought and another clue to the aetiology of MS might be at hand.

Clinical features of MS in different populations

In view of the marked differences in frequency of MS in various parts of the world, there has been interest in learning whether the disease also

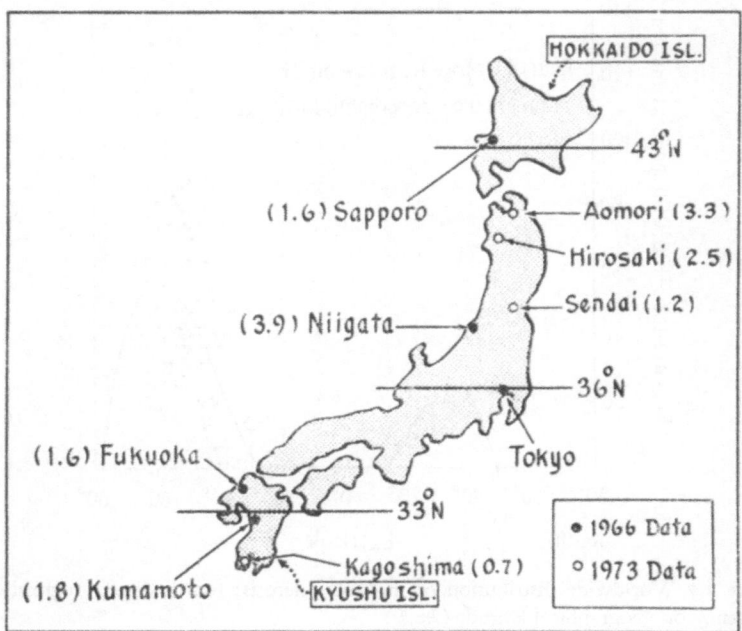

Figure 3.8 Prevalence of multiple sclerosis in Japan (see [26])

differed in its clinical characteristics. However, there is surprising uniformity in the clinical features of MS even in populations which differ markedly in frequency of MS (Table 3.1).

A case series drawn from a particular hospital in Bombay, India[33], included 74 cases diagnosed over a 15-year period; of these, 2 were autopsy proven and 15 (21%) were diagnosed as Devic's disease or possible Devic's disease. Thus, Devic's disease constituted a relatively high proportion of cases with demyelinating disease in this Indian series compared to cases in western and middle-eastern series. Also, in Japan, the proportion of Devic's disease among all demyelinating diseases was believed to be high[34], but recent reports have shown an apparent decline[35].

Changing diagnostic criteria were thought most likely to account for this decline[35]. However, high rates of acute transverse myelopathy during the course of MS and optic nerve involvement at onset in Orientals has been confirmed recently and bilateral optic neuropathy was also more common in Orientals than in Caucasians.

Optic neuritis, as an initial manifestation of MS, also seems to be more common among Orientals in Hawaii[36] and in Japan[37] than in western

Table 3.1 Initial symptoms of multiple sclerosis in diverse populations

Symptom	Japan[1]	Per cent US Army Series[146]		Müller[146]	Israeli immigrants[1] Europe	Afro–Asia
		A*	B†			
Motor	24	40	68	47	41	39
Sensory	15	34	52	22	13	8
Combined motor–sensory	—	—	—	—	16	8
Visual	42	21	30	20	14	8
Diplopia	11	—	—	—	3	3
Cerebellar–vestibular	—	—	—	—	7	8
Sphincter	—	8	23	20	2	3
Mixed	—	—	—	—	12	17

* Onset before induction into Army   † Onset after induction into Army

countries and in Israel[38], perhaps reflecting another difference in clinical manifestation of the disease in different populations. Knowledge of the range in clinical variation of MS among different populations is important because it could explain apparent differences in MS frequency. For instance, if optic neuritis or Devic's disease were excluded and such cases happened to constitute a higher proportion of demyelinating disease in a given area, a spurious low rate of demyelinating disease in that area could result. Available evidence suggests, however, that where MS is common, optic neuritis is common; where MS is rare, optic neuritis is rare[18]. In Finland[18] and other areas[39] the frequency of optic neuritis and MS was significantly correlated. The area with the highest MS rate in Finland (Vassa) was the same as the area with the highest rate of optic neuritis, further supporting the contention of Kahana et al.[38] that optic neuritis cases should be considered in all attempts to estimate the frequency of MS. Inclusion of all optic neuritis cases in an area would probably increase the apparent absolute frequency of MS but would probably not alter the pattern of its geographical distribution. Kahana et al.[38] have shown that about one-third of patients with an initial episode of optic neuritis will develop signs of dissemination within 10 years.

In many respects, the Indian series of MS which Singhal and Wadia[33] reported and the Japanese series reported by Kuroiwa et al.[25] were similar to series reported in other parts of the world, for instance, the average age at onset was close to 30 years, there was a slight female excess of cases, the proportion of severely disabled cases in the series and the spinal fluid findings (total protein, cell count and colloidal gold curve) were all similar to western series (facilities for measurement of γ-globulin in CSF were not available). The basic similarities in clinical manifestation of MS worldwide imply a similarity in aetiology as well.

Factors accounting for the distribution of MS

Investigators have displayed remarkable ingenuity in suggesting possibilities to account for the unequal distribution of MS. Some of these notions will be discussed, but first the validity of the data upon which current concepts of the distribution of MS are based must be examined critically.

It was originally thought that the variation in MS frequency with latitude was an artifact of the quality and availability of neurological care. This suspicion seemed to be supported when gross recording errors were uncovered in mortality statistics on MS, i.e. many cases of cerebral sclerosis (meaning cerebral *arterio*sclerosis) were listed with MS under the same coding rubric[40]. Northern areas, where MS is common, had more trained neurologists, on average, than southern regions where MS was allegedly rare. It was argued that the north–south differences in MS frequency merely reflected differences in number of neurologists. When different neurologists reviewed case material included in the epidemiological studies, there were disagreements among them about diagnosis[41].

To counter such criticism, various refinements in methodology were introduced. At first, classification of cases in different areas was standardized by requiring a review of clinical protocols by experts[42]. Later, the same research team of neurological experts, using identical criteria of diagnosis and the same case-finding techniques, searched for and examined cases in different regions[43]. More recently, comparisons have been made of MS frequency in a given area among populations of diverse origin[7, 44–46]. In the latter group of studies, any differences in frequency of MS among the populations could hardly be attributed to an artifact of diagnosis or to variation in thoroughness of case-finding, as the same group of doctors had examined the patients, from all populations, in the same medical facilities. A notable example of the analysis of MS frequency among diverse populations in a given area is Israel. In Israel, the same medical facilities are available to all segments of the population. When an intensive case-finding study was conducted among the diverse populations of Israel and frequency of MS was plotted, a striking relationship between frequency and the geographical latitude of the region of origin of immigrants to Israel was found (Figure 3.9). The Israeli study did much to win acceptance of the idea that the peculiar distribution of MS was not artifactual.

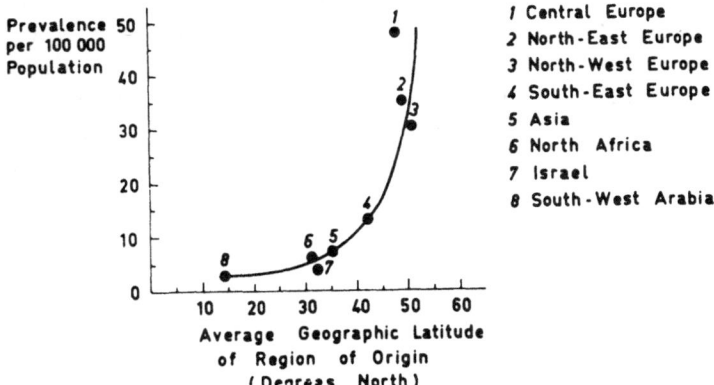

Figure 3.9 Prevalence of multiple sclerosis in Israel among immigrants and native-born by region of origin (see [44])

Environmental factors in Aetiology

Because MS has an unequal geographical distribution, attention has been directed to factors which vary with latitude in seeking additional clues to the cause of MS. A little thought yields a long list of factors which vary with latitude and could be candidates for causing MS. Unravelling which factors are really important and which are only incidentally or fortuitously associated with MS is a difficult task. Therefore, a coherent theory of the cause of MS woven from available epidemiological 'threads' remains a challenge.

Climate

Because MS is common in temperate areas and rare in the tropics, climate comes quickly to mind as one variable which might be important in MS. However, climate is a complex variable and it is not easy to decide which component of climate, if any, might be relevant. Sunlight is one factor which is obviously related to climate and varies with latitude. The average amount of sunlight per year in a given region has a high negative correlation with MS frequency, i.e. the less sunlight per year in the area, the more MS. One such correlation in Australia is illustrated in Figure 3.10. Acheson et al.[47] found that sunlight correlated better than temperature with MS frequency in the United States. Sunshine could exert its effect in a variety of ways: directly, by influencing the viability of an organism causing MS, or indirectly, by affecting the pattern of living in a given area in such a way as to make MS more or less common.

If an inverse relationship between MS frequency and sunlight really exists, then MS should be highest in frequency at the extremes of latitude. However, as mentioned, there is evidence that MS may actually decrease in frequency toward the far north[9]. Therefore, any relationship between sunlight and MS would have to be complex. One would have to conclude that

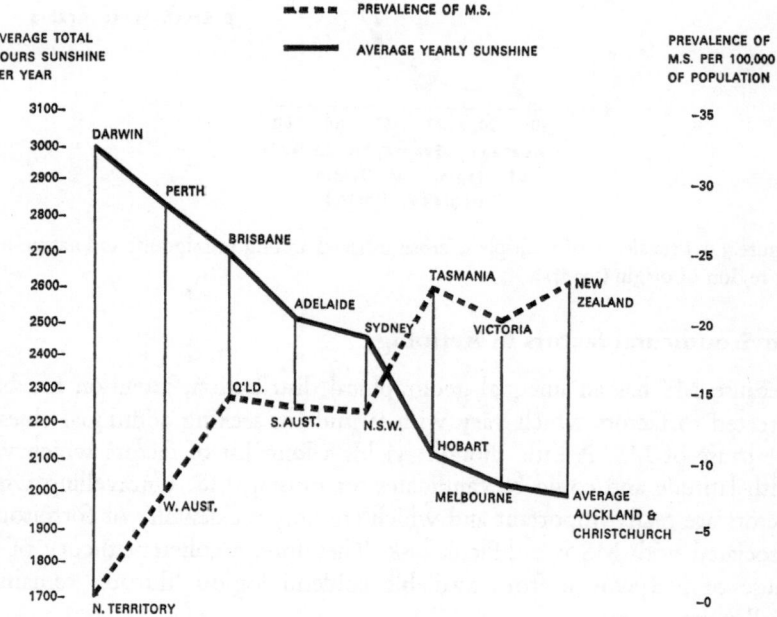

Figure 3.10 Prevalence of multiple sclerosis in Australasia and average hours of sunshine (see [1])

large amounts of sunlight, as occurs nearer the equator, and small amounts, as occurs toward the extreme latitudes, are both associated with low rates of MS. Only a particular amount of sunlight would be associated with high rates of MS. These 'optimally detrimental' amounts of sunlight may be present in temperate zones of latitude.

There are many weaknesses in assuming that even a complex relationship between sunlight and MS exists. If sunlight were important in preventing MS, seasonal variations in MS frequency should be found. There have been several studies of onset and of exacerbation of MS in relation to season[35, 48, 49] but no consistent seasonal pattern has emerged. Sunlight cannot, at present, be eliminated as an important variable in accounting for the distribution of MS, but it does not appear to be a fruitful one upon which to base further investigations designed to find the cause of MS.

Diet

Diet certainly varies from region to region. What people eat influences some disease patterns. It is hardly surprising therefore that diet has often been examined as a possible cause of MS. Alter *et al.*[50] have analysed the geographical distribution of various dietary components: total calories, total grams of protein, the per cent calories of animal origin and the grams of fats and oils consumed *per capita*, are all correlated with latitude (Figure 3.11 *a, b, c, d*). Also, each of these dietary variables has a distribution not unlike MS (Figure 3.2). The highest coefficients of correlation were observed with fats and oil consumption (Table 3.2). Alter *et al.*[50] and Agranoff and

Table 3.2 Correlation between multiple sclerosis prevalence and daily per capita intake

Nutrient	Correlation coefficient for 22 countries*	Correlation coefficient for 13 countries†	Significance
Fats and oils	0·68	0·70	$p < ·01$
Per cent calories animal origin	0·62	0·71	$p < ·01$
Total calories	0·38	0·48	N.S.
Total protein	0·12	0·24	N.S.

* With known MS prevalence and *per capita* intake
† With more reliable MS prevalence and *per capita* intake

Goldberg[21] have discussed the mechanisms whereby diet could influence MS. One of these possible mechanisms includes the effect of fat upon blood flow. A high intake of fat increases vascular sludging. This sludging could produce relative hypoxia distal to plugged arterioles and result in perivascular demyelination[51-54]. The perivascular distribution of plaques in MS is cited as support for such a mechanism[55, 56].

A second mechanism is biochemical. Diet may influence the chemical composition of myelin membranes[57-61]. A high-saturated fat intake, which is characteristic of temperate regions where MS is common, could result in less stable myelin membranes and a greater risk of demyelination. However, chemical studies of central myelin in MS patients have not shown consistent abnormalities[62-65], and some chemical changes which have been found in myelin of MS victims could be secondary to demyelination (see also Chapters 8 and 9).

A third mechanism relates diet to immune responsiveness. Diets rich in animal protein may result in more competent immune responsiveness of the

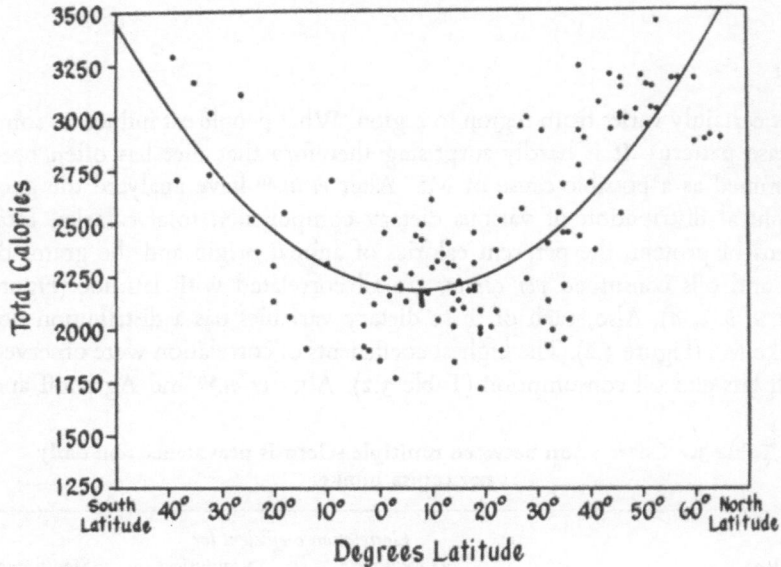

Figure 3.11*a* Daily *per capita* intake of total calories and geographical latitude (120 countries) (see [50])

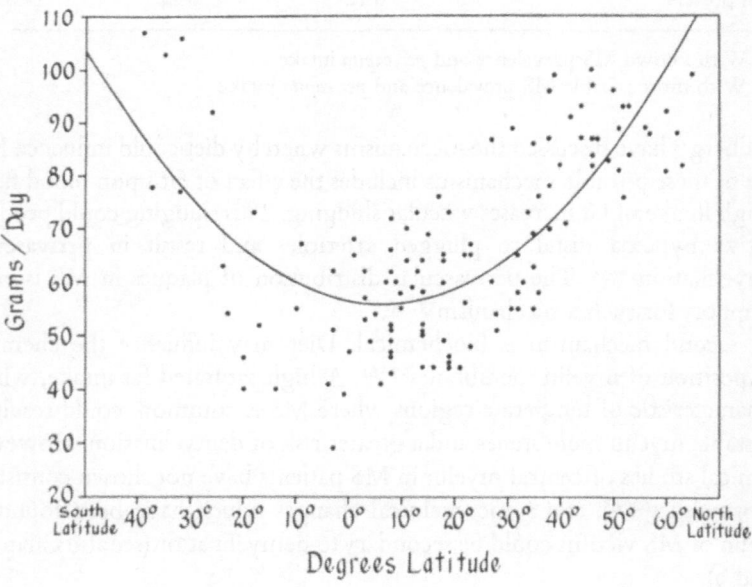

Figure 3.11*b* Daily *per capita* intake of protein and geographical latitude (120 countries) (see [50])

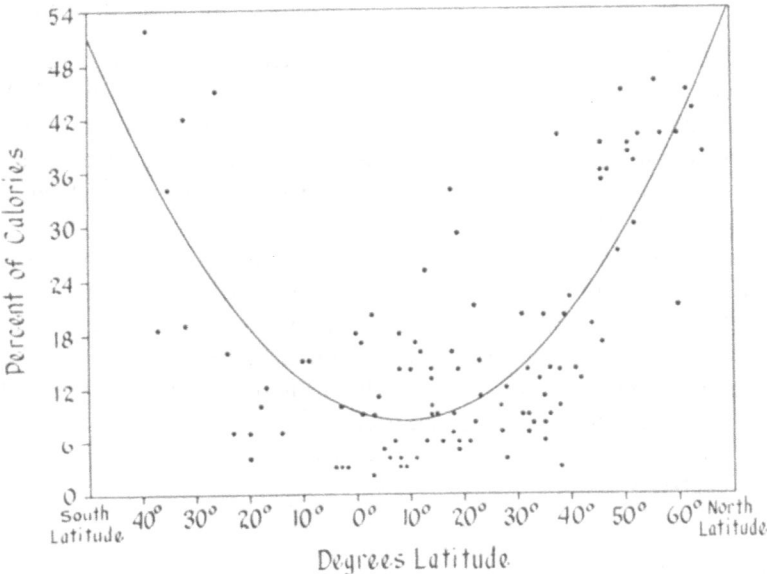

Figure 3.11c Daily *per capita* intake of calories of animal origin and geographical latitude (120 countries) (see [50])

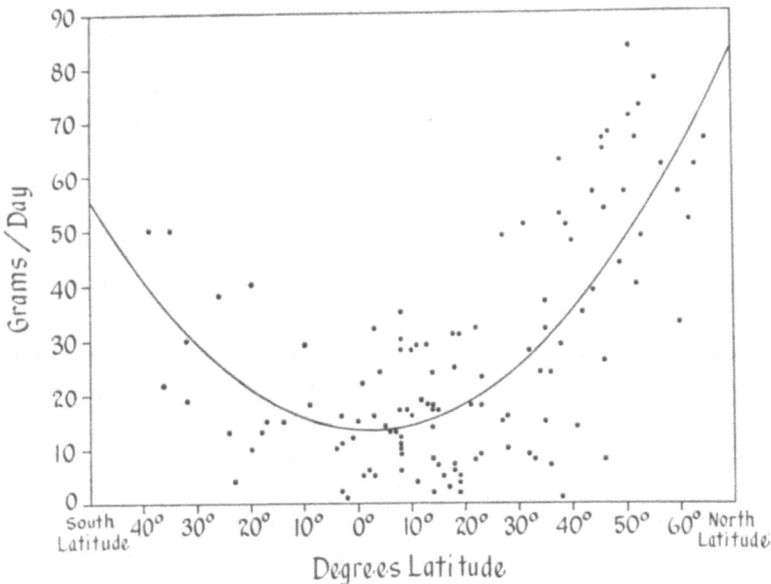

Figure 3.11d Daily *per capita* intake of fats and oils and geographical latitude (120 countries) (see [50])

host[66, 67]. If MS were caused by an immune reaction of the patient against his own myelin, as some investigators suspect[68, 69], then individuals in temperate regions who consume diets containing high proportions of animal protein might be better at forming antibodies and would tend to have a higher rate of MS. In areas where diet is marginal, MS would tend to be low in frequency. Studies of disease patterns have shown an effect upon immune responsiveness and disease susceptibility among marginally nourished individuals[70]. Dutz[71] has suggested that poor diet early in life may profoundly affect the development of host immunity, especially cell-mediated immunity which is believed to be important in MS. A diet-related host immunity could thus operate very early in life to influence the risk of MS. Of all the mechanisms relating diet to MS, the one involving an interaction with immune responsiveness appears to be most worthy of additional study (see Chapters 8 and 9).

Toxins and deficiencies

The geographical distribution of MS has been correlated with geological features of the earth in attempts to implicate a metallic toxin as a cause of the disease[72]. Such efforts were stimulated by observations in animals that metallic content of the soil was a factor in swayback[73], another demyelinating disorder*. Swayback was caused by the possible interaction between copper and lead. Lead itself has been considered[74] and this hypothesis seemed to be supported by regional studies of lead content in the water source of some victims of MS. Even the amalgam of teeth has not escaped attention as a possible cause of MS and must be regarded as having some epidemiological support in that patients, in one study at least, reported a higher frequency of dental work than controls[75]. A more complex theory involving a metallic toxin interacting with vitamin D absorption and the geographical distribution of different food grains deficient in this vitamin has been offered by Goldberg[76].

An industrial pollutant has also been considered responsible for causing MS. Epidemiological data show high correlations between frequency of MS and degree of industrialization of a society[77]. Coefficients of correlation with MS prevalence above 0·7 were found for factors such as steel consumption, automobiles per unit population and electrification. The falloff of MS frequency toward the extremes of latitude and the east–west differences in rate of MS in Europe would fit the notion that some aspects in an industrialized

---

* Editor's note: Few would agree that swayback should be classed as a 'demyelinating disorder'. It may be described as a dysmyelogenesis due to copper (and perhaps other trace elements) in the diet of the ewe. (See p. 209).

society predispose the population to higher rates of MS because the relatively industrialized temperate zones of Europe have the highest rates of MS.

However, Japan would have to be considered an exception as it has a low rate of MS despite the fact that it is highly industrialized. Conceivably, in Japan, some other 'protective' variable such as the high fish diet or genetic 'resistance' could account for the lack of MS in that country.

The hypotheses implicating a toxin or a deficiency as a cause of MS are noteworthy for their ingenuity rather than the weight of supporting evidence. They could gain support or be refuted easily were an animal model of MS available to permit experimental testing. It is difficult to prove or disprove these notions among sufferers of the disease as they are obviously being evaluated 'after the fact'. None the less, it would be helpful in evaluating the idea that a toxin plays a role in MS were patients shown to have a deficiency or excess of a particular metal in serum or CSF or brain, but convincing evidence along these lines is lacking at present.

Sanitation

Interest in the possibility that MS might be an infection of the central nervous system has grown in recent years[78]. Epidemiological data were reviewed for hints as to what the infectious agent might be. Poskanzer and associates[79] focused attention upon similarities between the geographical distribution of MS and poliomyelitis and suggested that an enteric virus, like polio, might cause MS. A detailed analysis of the frequency of MS and of various illnesses due to enteric pathogens was presented by Alter and Olivares[20]. They concurred with Poskanzer and associates[79] that an enteric pathogen could play a role in causing MS and showed that enteric illness and other measures of water sanitation, like the quality of plumbing facilities, had high correlations with MS frequency. Measures of water sanitation correlated better with MS than did measures of air quality (Table 3.3).

Alter and Olivares[20] argued that the important aspect of the environment in so far as the rate of MS was concerned was the quality of water sanitation. It was postulated that in 'sanitary' environments contact with enteric pathogens was delayed until later childhood or even adulthood. As in poliomyelitis, later infection was postulated to be associated with a high incidence of central nervous system involvement and a higher rate of MS.

The attractiveness of the sanitation hypothesis was enhanced by the demonstration that industrialized areas with poor overall levels of sanitation like Japan and Mexico City had *low* rates of MS. Thus, although these communities were like 'developed regions' as regards level of industrialization, they were like primitive areas in level of sanitation and in frequency of MS.

Table 3.3 Frequency of selected diseases in several countries (adapted from[20])

	Country—rate/10^5 population		
	Mexico*	Japan*	United States†
Enteric diseases			
Parasitic and infectious deaths	79	28	9
Gastritis and other enteric deaths	95	13	4
Dysentery deaths	12	2	0·2
Typhoid and paratyphoid cases	13	0·6	0·2
Respiratory diseases			
Deaths due to:			
Bronchitis	31	6	3
Pneumonia	140	24	34
Tuberculosis	22	23	5
Cases due to:			
Tuberculosis	44	37	26
Influenza	299	1	—
Asthma	17	16	23

* Low MS rate
† High MS rate

The sanitation hypothesis was also compatible with observations that MS was more common within a given area among the socially advantaged than among the poorer classes[80–83] and among those with higher intelligence than the less gifted (Figure 3.12). Those with higher socioeconomic status would be expected to have higher levels of sanitation. The slightly but consistently lower frequency of MS among blacks as compared to whites in several communities of the United States could also be interpreted as compatible with a sanitation-related factor in MS as whites, in general, enjoy a higher socioeconomic status (and better sanitary conditions) than blacks in a given area (Figure 3.13). In South Africa, the relatively low rate of MS among whites despite a 'sanitary' environment was explained by the widespread use of black nursemaids who return to their native (less sanitary) enclaves at nights. These 'nannys' introduce the white South African infants early to the factor (infection?) which protects them from MS[84].

In Israel the native-born offspring of Afro-Asian immigrants were exposed to an environment where the sanitary amenities were more European than Levantine. It is noteworthy therefore, that MS frequency in the Afro-Asians born in Israel resembled that of European immigrants (and native-born offspring of Europeans) rather than Afro-Asian immigrants[44].

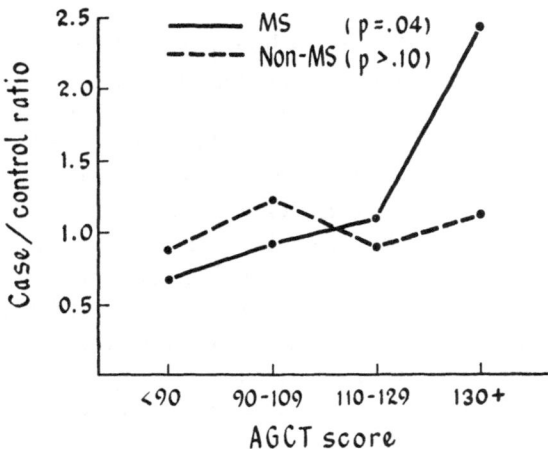

Figure 3.12 Case/control ratios by Army General Classification Test (AGCT) score at induction for US veterans (adapted from [83])

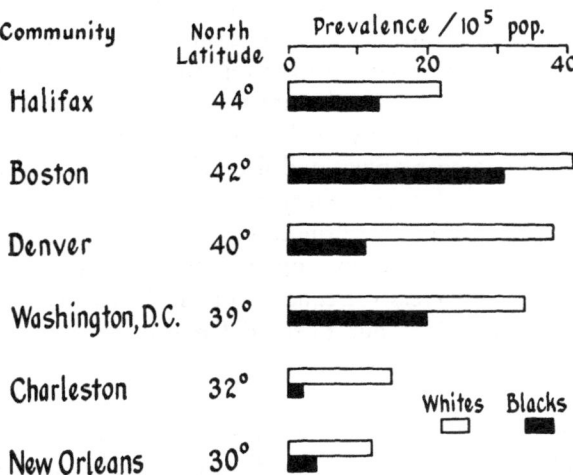

Figure 3.13 Prevalence of multiple sclerosis among blacks and whites by geographical latitude in several North American communities

Lipid peroxide

A novel hypothesis of aetiology has been presented by Mickel[85]. He suggested that the demyelination which produces the syndrome called MS may be attributable to lipid peroxide absorption from the gut. According to the hypothesis, lipid peroxide releases lysosomal peroxidases and enhances autocatalysis of polyunsaturated fatty acids in myelin. Central myelin contains relatively little polyunsaturated fat. Oligodendroglia may have little antioxidant and thus be especially susceptible to the action of lipid peroxides.

Enteric inflammation decreases the natural barrier to lipid peroxide absorption. Enteric viruses constitute a common cause of enteric inflammation and in tropical areas, where MS is rare, enteric infections occur early in life after which immunity to these viral agents exists. In temperate areas, where MS is common, enteric viruses are encountered later and there is an increased chance then of developing MS.

The adverse effect of peroxide absorption is increased where diets rich in animal fat and, therefore, low in natural antioxidants, are eaten. The antioxidants act as free radical acceptors and terminate the chain reaction of lipid oxidation. High animal fat diets are common in regions where MS is common and vice versa.

Where unsaturated fats which are mainly of vegetable origin are eaten, linoleic acid levels in plasma are high, a condition which decreases platelet adhesiveness. Some investigators[86] have reported low plasma linoleic acid levels in MS and increased platelet adhesiveness might result from their absorption of peroxidized fatty acids, especially peroxidized arachidonic acid. The platelet aggregates plug capillaries and venules and account for the perivascular distribution of demyelinated plaques.

Platelet peroxidase could be enhanced by oestrogens, as this hormone has already been shown to enhance myeloperoxidase and uterine peroxidase and thus accounts for the increased frequency of MS in women. The rarity of MS in childhood could be due to the different enzymatic state of oligocytes synthesizing myelin as compared to oligocytes merely maintaining myelin.

Even the increased fragility of red cells[86a,b] and their apparent increased diameter in MS[86c,d] could be accounted for by peroxidation of erythrocyte membranes. Also, peroxidized fatty acids could denature protein by attacking sulph-hydryl groups and give rise to autoimmune reactions. Thus, exacerbations in MS could occur from either or both peroxide absorption or autoimmune reactions.

The above hypothesis is presented in some detail to illustrate how epidemiological data concerning MS were integrated and accounted for. Leaving aside whether or not this particular hypothesis proves to be correct, it will be necessary for any hypothesis to account in similar fashion for the epidemiological 'facts' of MS.

Changing frequency of MS

An epidemiological test of any hypothesis implicating some aspect of developed environments would involve the observation of MS frequency over time. An increasing incidence of MS over time, as industrialization and modernization of a society proceed, would constitute support for the hypothesis. Available information on MS incidence over time, shows remarkable stability in the rate of this disease (Table 3.4). In many of the areas, a stable frequency of MS exists though industrialization has occurred. For example, Israel has changed within a few decades from a rather primitive, agrarian country to one which is quite developed. Yet, the incidence of MS in Israel has been stable for at least the past 15 years.

Bird and Satoyoshi[87] report an apparent increase in MS incidence in greater Johannesburg, South Africa, and in Tokyo, Japan, during the period 1964 to 1970 and suggest that the increase might be due to introduction of an 'infective element' into the community from a high MS risk area. The patients were derived from a private consulting practice in Johannesburg

Table 3.4 Average annual incidence of multiple sclerosis over time[1]

Community	Time period	Rate/10^5 population
Rochester, Minnesota	1905–1914	5·1
	1915–1924	3·6
	1925–1934	5·8
	1935–1944	2·4
	1945–1954	3·2
	1955–1964	3·2
Israelis born in Europe	1950–1954	1·5
	1955–1959	1·3
	1960–1964	1·1
Israelis born in Afro-Asia	1950–1954	0·8
	1955–1959	0·7
	1960–1964	0·8
Israelis born in Israel	1950–1954	1·4
	1955–1959	1·8
	1960–1964	1·3

and from a single hospital in Tokyo and not from a community-wide survey. Therefore, there is no way to exclude the possibility that the apparent increase in MS in each community is not merely a reflection of increased case referral to these neurologists who each admit to a special interest in MS.

A population-wide survey of MS in Japan which included a collection of cases in Tokyo showed a constant rather than an increasing incidence of MS[25] and thus did not agree with the results of Bird and Satoyoshi.[87] Follow-up studies of similar scope in Johannesburg are warranted before the authors' conclusions of an increasing incidence can be accepted.

In Johannesburg, during the last 3 years of the observation period, a slight falling-off of the annual number of new cases of MS was noted but the authors appeared unaware of the fact that such a falling-off is artifactual and due to the cases which have become manifest but have not yet been diagnosed. This artifact in population surveys has been discussed by Leibowitz and Alter[1] and necessitates a 'backdating' of prevalence, say of about 3–5 years in any population study designed to assess frequency, because the average delay from onset to diagnosis in MS is that long.

In an effort to salvage the hypothesis implicating some aspect of development of the environment, it could be argued that insufficient time has elapsed for the effect of modernization upon MS incidence to be discernible. If an industrial pollutant affected risk of MS, and the effect were exerted early in life, it might not be reflected in an increase in incidence of MS until 15 to 30 years had elapsed because the average age at onset of MS is about 30 years. Individuals who manifest MS now might have been affected by an industrial pollutant introduced 15 to 30 years ago. The stable MS incidence rate in Rochester, Minnesota, over some 6 decades[15], does not necessarily refute the industrialization hypothesis because Rochester, Minnesota, has remained essentially a non-industrialized, rather rural type of community. Virtually no heavy industry has been established in Rochester and, in many respects, it is not unlike the rural town it was a half a century ago, though it has grown considerably in size. Continuing and intensive medical surveillance for MS in Rochester and Israel is in progress and future epidemiological reports from these communities may help settle the issue of whether industrialization or other modern developments in a community are associated with an increase in MS frequency.

Immigration and MS

More than 20 years ago[44], it was recognized that immigrant populations offered an opportunity to determine whether an environmental change might affect the risk of developing MS. By studying populations which moved from one area to another, it might be possible to detect a change in the frequency of MS as compared to those which remained in the original environment. Only migration between areas differing in MS frequency would be suitable for detecting an impact of an environmental change on risk of MS. Movement from one MS frequency area to another with the same MS frequency would not be expected to alter risk of MS. Figure 3.14 diagrams possible vectors of migration. Only movement along the diagonal vectors would be expected to alter the risk of MS, whilst the horizontal migration vectors provide control data for the migration 'experiment'.

Original Residence   Later Residence

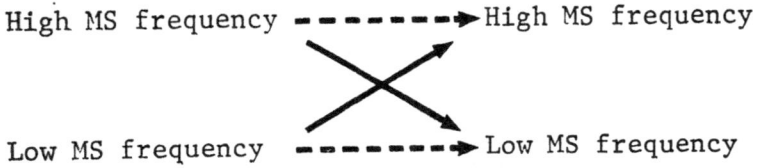

Figure 3.14 Migration vectors

In order for a migrant population to provide suitable data, the population has to fulfil a number of requirements. One of these is that the migrating population must be large enough so that a sufficient number of MS cases for analysis would be expected. Such migrant populations must number at least 100 000 individuals or more. A second requirement is that the immigrants must have access to good medical facilities so that MS cases which occur among them can be recognized and correctly diagnosed. Missing only a few cases of MS could give an erroneous impression about risk of MS in a particular immigrant group. A third requirement is that demographic data on the population be adequate. One must know the age and sex distribution of the migrants as well as their year of immigration. Finally, an appropriate control population is needed, composed of individuals who migrated from the same area at the same time as the patients.

As might be expected, it is not easy to find migrant populations which satisfy all of the above requirements, However, a few suitable populations have been studied (Table 3.5). Most of the migrations listed in Table 3.5 occurred from higher to lower MS frequency areas. In these studies, the migrants who moved from the high-frequency zone to an area of lower frequency had a higher frequency of MS than the native inhabitants of the

**Table 3.5 Frequency of multiple sclerosis among
migrant populations by region of origin
and native-born inhabitants**

| Area | Rate/10^5 population | |
	Migrants	Native-born
Australia[7]		22
High-risk zones	25	
Other zones	12	
Israel[45]		24
European	30	
Afro-Asian	11	
South Africa[147]		6
United Kingdom	51	
Central and northern Europe	48	
South Europe	15	
Elsewhere	9	
United States		
California: Japanese[16]	7	
Other	30	
Washington: Japanese[16]	0	
Other	90	
Hawaii: Caucasian[36]	24	10
Oriental	7	9

new place of residence. Thus, migrants 'carried with them' the risk of their original place of residence.

Populations which migrated from low to higher MS frequency zones (ascending vector) are even less available for study. Kurtzke and Bui-Quoc-Huong[88] have sought cases of MS in France among those who immigrated from southeast Asia. Few cases of MS were found, suggesting that populations migrating along an ascending vector also carried with them the low MS rate of their place of origin.

The results of the latter study were recently confirmed by Dean and associates[89]. They studied MS frequency among immigrants to greater London, England. Those who came to England from parts of the world where MS was uncommon did not have an increased risk of developing MS. Moreover, many from low MS areas who did have MS were offspring of British forebears and might be presumed to have had a lifestyle (and/or genetic constitution) somewhat different from those born in low-risk areas of native forebears.

While the data of Dean *et al.* are consistent with what has been reported heretofore regarding risk of MS among immigrants, there are certain defects in the design of their study. For example, they included patients who already had MS prior to immigration. The average age at immigration was 38 years, whereas average onset of MS was 31 years. Moreover, the reference population was obtained from residents of London in 1966, the midpoint of their study interval, rather than immigrants who left the same areas at the same time as the patients. Only the latter populations can adequately control for differences in length of exposure to the London environment. None the less, the observation of Dean *et al.* is a valuable contribution to our understanding of what may happen to risk of MS among those migrating along an ascending vector. Similar efforts to study MS risk should be encouraged and refined.

Among the migrants to Washington State and California[16], the highest frequency of MS was observed in those who moved from northern United States to Washington State (north–north). Those who moved from the north to Los Angeles (north–south) had lower rates than those who moved from the north to Washington State, suggesting that some protective factor against MS was present in the southern community. Migration from southern United States to Washington State was also associated with a relatively low rate of MS which supports the idea that a protective factor exists in the south. The lowest rates of MS were found in those who migrated from the south to Los Angeles County (south–south).

By studying the rate of MS among migrants who moved at different ages it has been possible to determine the age prior to which migration may affect risk and thus deduce the age at which MS is acquired. The reasoning behind this statement is as follows: if those who migrate before a certain age show a rate of MS like that characteristic of the new environment whilst those who migrate at an older age show the rate of the old environment it would suggest that MS was acquired *before* the age when risk changed. If MS were acquired, for example, in infancy, then no effect upon risk of MS among migrants would be discernible. Merely being born in a given environment would be sufficient to determine risk of MS. On the other hand, if 15 years of age were 'critical' for determining MS risk, then migrants who moved before 15 years' old would show the rate of MS of the new environment whereas those who migrated later would show a rate of MS like that of the original place of residence.

Israel offered many advantages for an analysis of the effect of migration upon risk of MS because of the heterogeneous origin of most of its population. MS in Israel has an intermediate frequency compared to northern Europe and Afro-Asia. Study of MS in migrants to Israel in relation to age at migration has shown that those who immigrated after 15 years of age from high frequency zones had a high rate of MS whereas those who came *before* 15 years had a *lower* rate. Conversely, those who immigrated to Israel after the age of 15 from Afro-Asia and were, in effect, migrating along an ascending vector, had lower rates of MS than are characteristic of Israel whilst younger migrants from Afro-Asia to Israel had higher rates (after appropriate corrections). Thus exposure to the Israeli environment *at an early age* was associated with a decreased rate of MS among young migrants from Europe and an increased rate among young migrants from Afro-Asia (Table 3.6). Careful scrutiny of the data on which the conclusions concerning

Table 3.6 Incidence of multiple sclerosis among
immigrants to Israel by age at immigration
and region of birth[1]

| Age at immigration (years) | Rate/10^5 population Region of Birth | | | |
| | Europe | | Afro-Asia | |
	Crude	Adjusted	Crude	Adjusted
<15	0·7	2·8	0·5	2·0
>15	2·0	—	0·4	—

migration are based revealed very few cases of MS among those who migrated early in life. Thus, small numbers seriously undermine confidence in the conclusions about when MS may be acquired.

Recently, the Israeli study has been repeated on a larger population sample[90]. Sufficient time has elapsed since the earlier study to have allowed more cases of MS among the immigrants to Israel to accumulate.

The data were analysed for patients with 'clinically definite' MS who had immigrated to Israel between 1950 and 1969. Only those whose MS began after immigration were included. The population-at-risk was a sample of all immigrants who had come from the same region at the same time as the patients. The risk of developing MS in Israel, of course, was not identical for those who immigrated during the earlier part of the observation period and those who came later. To compensate for differences in length of exposure to risk among immigrants who came at different times, the population-at-risk was summed for each year of residence to 1969 to yield 'person-years' of exposure. Dividing patients by the person-years of exposure yielded a rate of MS per 100 000 person-years of risk.

No one value could accurately reflect risk of MS because those who migrated while young, between 1950 and 1969, were still young when the observations were terminated; for example, a person who was 10 years old when he came to Israel in 1950 would be only 30 years old in 1969 and he could still develop MS. Therefore, age-specific incidence of MS among immigrants was calculated for different age-at-immigration cohorts. The results are illustrated in Figure 3.15 for those who immigrated before 5 years, between 5 and 14 years, and after 15 years.

It has already been shown that MS among European immigrants to Israel was higher than among Afro-Asian immigrants (Figure 3.16a), whilst MS was virtually identical in frequency among the native-born Israeli offspring of those two different ethnic groups (Figure 3.16b). Both groups had equal access to health care facilities.

When MS frequency was compared among the immigrants in different age-at-immigration cohorts, those who came from Afro-Asia between 5 and 14 years or after 15 years of age still had lower rates of MS than European who immigrated at comparable ages. However, Afro-Asians who immigrated before 5 years of age showed MS rates as high if not higher than European. Thus, only immigration *prior to age 5 years* affected risk of developing MS. By leaving the Afro-Asian environment very early and moving to Israel, the risk of MS was increased and became comparable to that of European. Migration along an ascending vector (from a low- to a high-risk area) *increased* the risk of MS among those who migrated early in life, before 5 years of age. These data may be interpreted to mean that MS is 'acquired' very early in life, perhaps by 5 years of age, even though clinical signs of the disease may not be evident until several decades later (see Chapter 9).

The period during which MS could be acquired according to the above analysis cannot be infancy for then one would expect the mere fact of birth in an area to determine risk of MS and no effect of 'immigration' upon risk would be discernible. MS must, therefore, be acquired after infancy but before 5 years of age. If these migration data are valid, then an event in a narrow timespan of early childhood, perhaps between age 1 and 5 years, may determine the risk of MS.

Review of the migration data requires that conclusions be cautious because the number of cases upon which even the more recent Israeli analysis is based is still small and more time must elapse before additional cases of MS in immigrants become available.

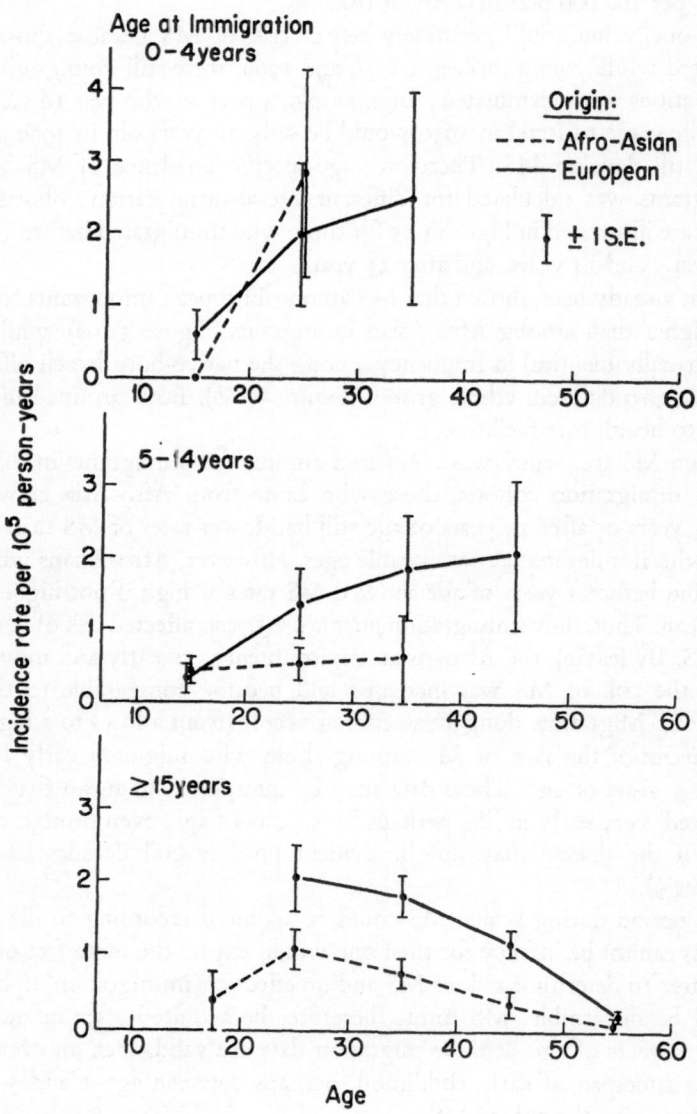

Figure 3.15 Multiple sclerosis incidence rates by age at immigration and origin (1950–1969) (see [90])

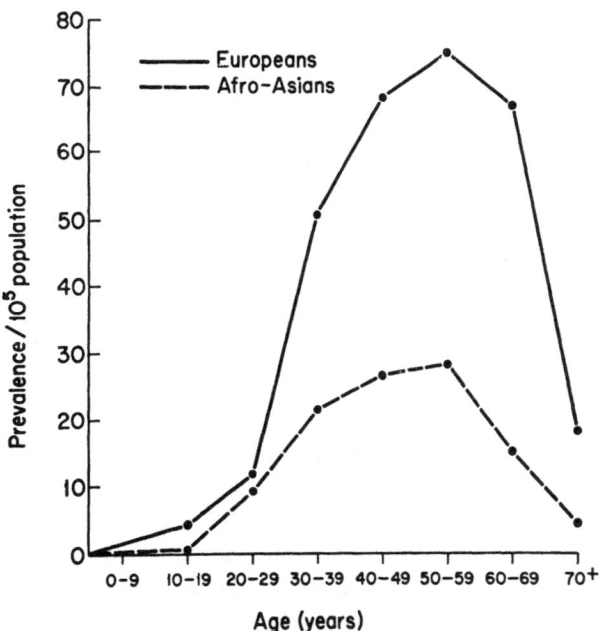

Figure 3.16*a* Age-specific prevalence rates of multiple sclerosis in Israel among immigrants (January 1, 1965) (see [45])

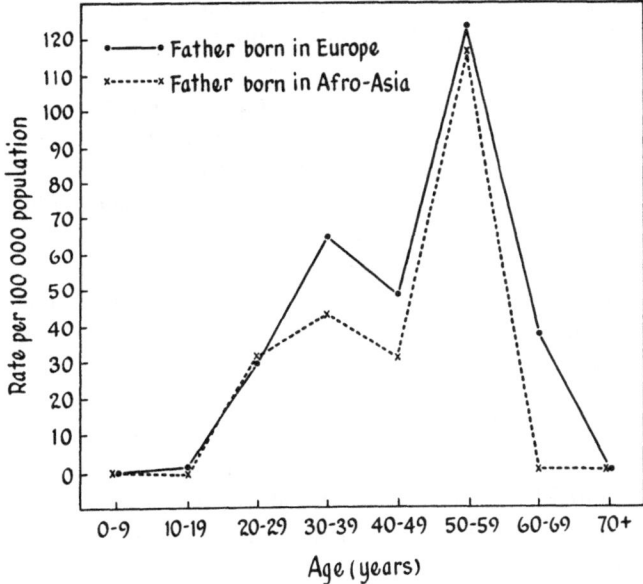

Figure 3.16*b* Age-specific prevalence rates of multiple sclerosis among native-born Israelis, by region of birth of father (January 1, 1965) (see [45])

Childhood illness and age-dependent host immunity

From epidemiological studies of migrants, as well as work on proximity of places of residence of MS cases during childhood compared to later life[18, 83, 91], the early childhood period appears to be when the causative factor in MS is operating. Therefore, the childhood period is the interval during which efforts to identify the cause of MS are being concentrated. In recent years, a childhood infection has been postulated as a likely cause of MS[92, 93]. Efforts to find direct evidence of such an infection are proceeding. Some tantalizing glimmers of successful identification of infectious agent in MS brain have actually appeared in the literature, but investigators who have been working on MS for any length of time recall previous enthusiastic reports of identification of 'infective agents' in MS, such as spirochetes[94] and rickettsia[95]. Later, these enthusiastic reports proved to be unfounded.

Recent reports of viral identifications in MS brain include electron-microscopic visualization of virus-like inclusion bodies[96], isolation of a viral agent by co-cultivation techniques[97], and, most recently, evidence[98] that mouse polymorphonuclear (PAM) cells indicate presence of an infective agent when injected with MS material. Of particular interest to the epidemiologist was the report by Koldovsky et al.[99] and Henle et al.[100] that high titres of an infective agent described first by Carp[98] was present *early in life* in an East African population among whom MS is rare[101]. The implication of these results is that *early* acquisition might render an individual less susceptible to MS.

An illustration of an age-dependent host response to infection is provided by hepatitis B which, if acquired early in life, tends to produce persistent infection whereas later infections are more readily cleared by the host's immune system[102]. The Epstein–Barr (EB) virus also produces different host responses depending on the age of acquisition[103]. Measles (rubeola) virus provides yet another example in that acquisition of this virus under the age of 2 years is apparently associated with an increased risk of subacute sclerosing panencephalitis (SSPE)[104] whereas later infection is associated with an increase in encephalitic complications (Figure 3.17)[105]. There are also experimental data for measles showing differences in host response depending on age of infection[106]. Epidemiological data suggest that regions where measles is acquired very early in life are low in MS frequency whilst regions where measles is acquired later have higher rates of MS[107, 108]. Far northerly communities with high MS rates are relatively isolated and measles tends to occur in widely separated epidemics. The average age of measles acquisition in such communities may be quite high[109]. In contrast, communities nearer the equator, where MS is low in frequency, tend to show a high level of

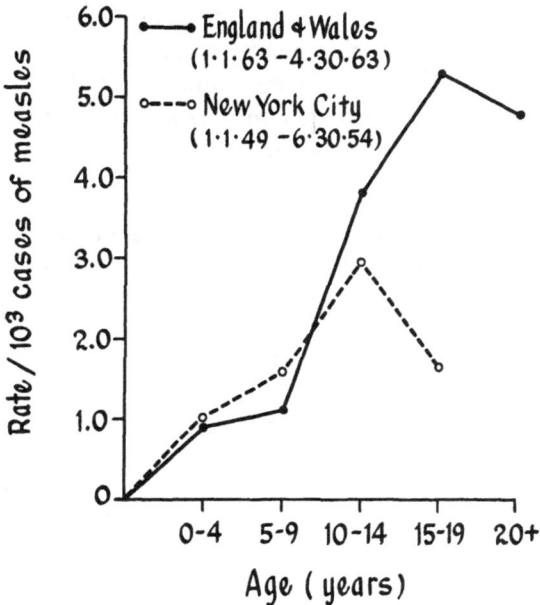

Figure 3.17 Frequency of measles encephalitis by age in two populations (see [105])

'herd immunity' to measles by 3 years of age. Morley[107] has reported that virtually the entire population of Nigeria, a region where MS would be expected to be low, had measles antibodies at the age of 3 years, whereas in England and Wales, where MS is common, more than half the population had no detectable measles antibodies even by 5 years of age (Figure 3.18).

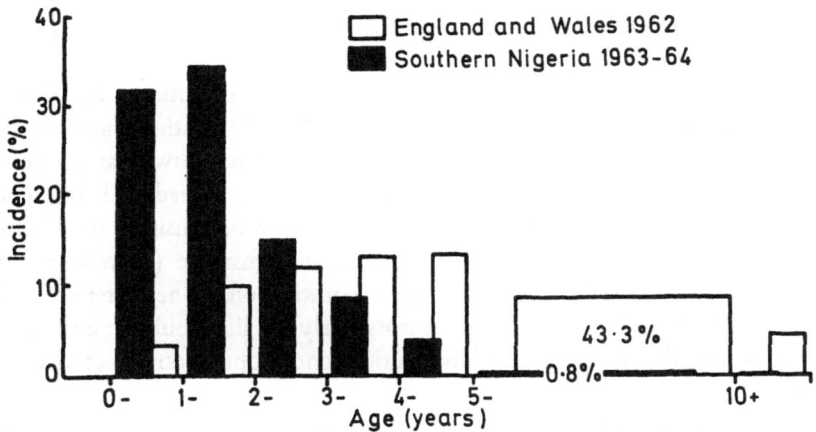

Figure 3.18 Incidence of measles by age in England and Wales and Nigeria (see [107])

Also, in Guatemala, where MS is rare[110], a large proportion of the population had immunity to measles by the age of 3 years[109].

Interesting contrasts between the epidemiology of SSPE, a known complication of measles, and MS, where measles *may* play a role, are shown in Table 3.7. On the basis of these contrasts, it was postulated that MS might

Table 3.7 Contrasts between SSPE and multiple sclerosis

Factor	SSPE[148]	Multiple sclerosis[1]
Sex	M > F	F > M
Socioeconomic status	Poor > rich	Rich > poor
Residence	Rural > urban	Urban > rural
Ethnic distribution	Black > white Arab > Afro-Asian > Euro-American	White > black Euro-American > Afro-Asian > Arab
Measles	Acquired earlier (before age two years)	Acquired later (? near adolescence)

represent an age-dependent host-immune response to later childhood infection with measles, just as SSPE is a response to very early infection. If the migration data implicating the age of 5 years as the 'critical age' by which MS is acquired are not interpreted too literally, the migration data could readily be reconciled with the hypothesis that a childhood infection elicits an age-dependent host-immune response which gives rise to the clinical symptoms of MS.

In light of the above epidemiological research, more attention is being paid to the immune system in MS as important in the pathogenesis of the disease. A great deal of evidence has accumulated to show that immune responses in patients with MS, particularly the cell-mediated immune responses, are altered[69]. The immune profile may be sensitive to dietary factors[71], and influenced by socioeconomic circumstance (crowding, for example), family size, and inherited constitution. The interplay of these environmental and genetic factors early in life could conceivably account for the geographical distribution and population selectivity of MS.

An infection (probably viral) to which a host is exposed at a particular age (probably early in life) is a tenable theory of the cause of MS. Cohen and Bannister[111] were among the first to demonstrate synthesis of immuno-globulins IgG and IgA by cells from the cerebrospinal fluid (CSF) of an MS patient. These early observations have been confirmed[112]. These immuno-globulins are oligoclonal[113] and could be produced in response to a viral antigen. It need not be a single infectious agent such as measles virus but any infection which encounters a susceptible host at a particular time, perhaps when the host's cell-mediated immunity may be depressed[71]. Viral infections can depress cell-mediated immunity for long periods. If another viral infection comes hard upon an earlier one, the host's immune defences could perhaps be more readily breached, and easier entry of the agent into the central nervous system (CNS) may be possible. A persistent, latent infection of the CNS could then be established. A stable state in which the hypothetical virus lies dormant in the CNS could be upset years later by non-specific triggers. The host's immune system might then attack and destroy the chronically infected cells. If these cells are oligocytes, their destruction would result in a plaque of demyelination. Repeated exacerbations and remissions of demyelination could occur in this hypothesized pathogenetic system. Such a system is also compatible with much that is known today about the epidemiology of MS.

Genetic factors in MS

Genetic factors play a role in virtually every disease process, and MS is no exception. It remains to be determined, however, how the genetic factors in MS are expressed and what genetically controlled mechanisms are operative. Most instances of MS are sporadic and often even intensive inquiries fail to disclose anyone else in the family with a similar disorder. However, familial aggregations of MS do occur and the frequency of multiple instances of MS within families is perhaps 20 times greater than would be expected from the frequency of the disease in the general population[114, 115]. Moreover, heritability estimates in MS are as high as 0·86[115]. In some families, the disease appears to follow a recessive inheritance pattern whilst in others, a dominant mode of inheritance[108] seems to fit the familial pattern. Care must be taken in interpreting the significance of reports of familial aggregation because often the families were reported *because* of the aggregation or they may have been otherwise selected and, therefore, genetic data may be biased. Moreover, in instances of familial aggregation of MS a healthy scepticism as to the correctness of the diagnosis is warranted because, not infrequently, 'familial MS' turns out, on close scrutiny, to be progressive spinocerebellar degeneration or Leber's optic atrophy, both of which mimic some features of MS. Finally, familial aggregation could represent a 'common exposure' to an environmental factor rather than a genetic effect because family members certainly have many more shared environmental experiences than the population at large[116].

One should also consider the possibility that the clinicopathological entity now called MS may not be a single disease. There may be several types of MS just as there are now thought to be several types of amyotrophic lateral sclerosis[117]. In one type of MS, hereditary factors may be particularly important.

Despite alternative interpretations of familial aggregation in MS, most investigators still believe that a genetic factor (or factors) is important. The adherents of this view have derived support in recent years from studies of histocompatibility genes and MS[118, 119].

Genes controlling histocompatibility are located close together on a particular chromosome. These genes control the mechanism which allows recognition of tissue which is 'self' from tissue which is 'non-self'. The mechanism is believed to be immunological. Thus, tissues with the same histocompatibility markers will not be rejected if transplanted from one individual to another (as between identical twins). Other tissues, with different histocompatibility characteristics, will evoke a host-versus-graft immune reaction and the 'foreign' tissue will be rejected unless immunosuppression is achieved through drugs or radiation. There are at least four major histocompatibility loci and these are closely linked[120, 121]. Three are determinable using serological techniques (A, B, C) and the fourth is detected using lymphocyte reactions (D). These genetic loci are inherited as dominant traits. A set of loci is inherited from each parent and the two haplotypic sets which an individual inherits constitute his histocompatibility genotype. The large number of alleles present at each histocompatibility locus[121] makes it very unlikely that any two individuals (except identical twins) will have exactly the same histocompatibility genotype, a situation which obviously has advantages if an individual must differentiate self from non-self tissue. The frequency distribution of these alleles varies from population to population[118]. At least one of these alleles appears to have a distribution similar to the distribution of MS (Figure 3.19).

In patients with MS, it has been shown that there is an excess of certain histocompatibility determinants, and a deficiency of others[122-124]. There is general, though not universal, agreement that the histocompatibility determinants which are increased in MS are A3, at the HLA-A locus and B7, at the HLA-B locus. As shown in Table 3.8, the excess of A3, B7 is not large. Therefore, the association between specific HLA determinants and MS is weaker than between HLA determinants and ankylosing spondylitis (B27 in 95%) or gluten-sensitive enteropathy (A8 in 75%).

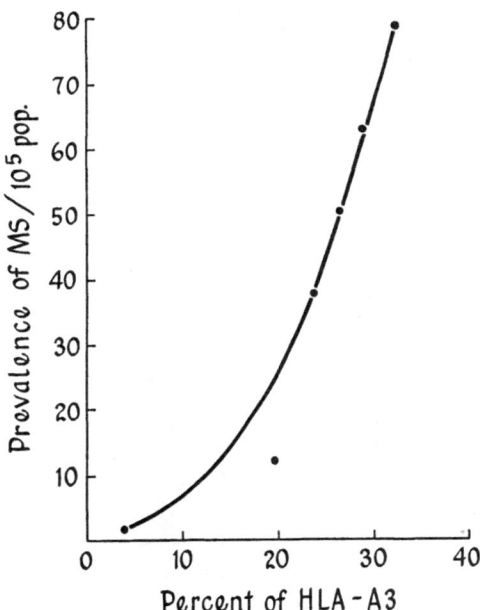

Figure 3.19 Frequency of multiple sclerosis and HLA-A3 in several populations

Table 3.8 Frequency of HLA-A3 and B7 among patients with multiple sclerosis and controls

| | Number | | Per cent with antigen | | | |
| | | | A3 | | B7 | |
Population	Patient	Control	Patient	Control	Patient	Control
Denmark[118]	209	1967	36	27	40	27
Germany[123]	393	255	40	27	36	31
Israel[125]						
Ethnic origin:						
Europe	152	292	14	18	10	9
Afro-Asia	46	167	20	24	4	17
United States						
California[122]	94	871	36	24	36	24
Minnesota veterans[124]	59	401	30	23	31	24

One large population study of HLA and MS in Israel failed to show an excess of A3 or B7[125]. The frequency of the latter two HLA specificities was actually lower in MS patients than in controls (Figure 3.20). Also, in Japan, the HLA specificities associated with MS appear to be different from those in the United States and in northern European populations[118].

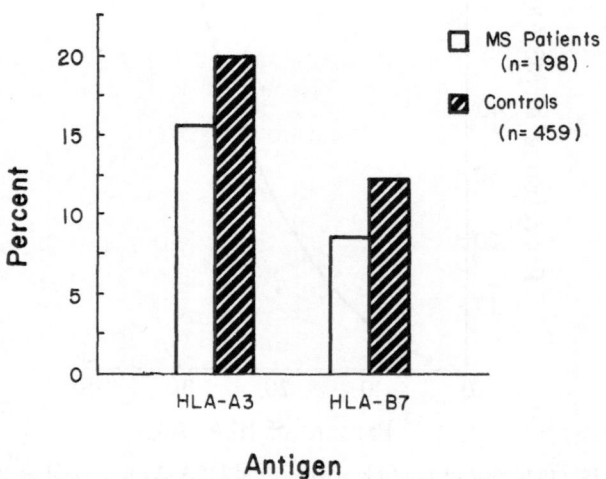

Figure 3.20 HLA-A3 and B7 among multiple sclerosis patients and controls in Israel

The failure to find universal excess of the same serum determinable histo-compatibility determinants in all MS patients and the differences in HLA specificities among MS populations in different parts of the world raised the possibility that another gene, closely linked to the HLA genes, but not identical with them, was associated with MS. This line of thinking appeared to be supported by the findings of Jersild et al.[126] that the D locus is more closely associated with MS than the three serum-determinable loci. They found that about 60% of MS patients had the specificity DW2 (formerly called LD-7a) compared to only 18% of controls. Even some of the MS patients without B7 were DW2 positive (32% compared to only 8% in controls). Thus, A3 and B7 could be thought of as 'markers' for the DW2 locus and the latter was, in turn, associated more closely with MS. Very recently, B-cell antigens have come under close scrutiny and the B-cell antigen Ag-7a has been observed in MS patients with even higher frequency than the DW antigen[127].

One additional line of genetic investigation appeared to strengthen the relationship between the histocompatibility loci and risk of MS. These additional studies were carried out in families where more than one individual had MS. In many instances, the affected individuals in these families 'shared' particular sets of HLA specificities which non-affected members of these families did not inherit[108].

The study of histocompatibility factors and MS is under active investigation at the present time and, as might be expected in so new a field, there is controversy as to the meaning of the results. Drachman and associates[128], for example, concluded that 'neither the inheritance of a particular parental HLA chromosome nor the occurrence of any specific HLA antigen could be shown to be necessary or sufficient for the development of MS in family members'. On the other hand, Alter et al.[108], Jersild et al.[126], and Bird[129] found that individuals with MS showed a particular HLA haplotype far more often than non-affected members in the same family. The selection of families by Drachman et al.[128] has been criticized[119].

The association between given parental haplotypes and MS appears to be a promising lead at present to the genetic factor(s) involved in MS. In the largest of these family studies[108], the association between a given parental haplotype and MS approached but did not reach statistical significance. Therefore, additional work needs to be done before the meaning of the association is resolved and its validity is established.

One reason that the work involving the HLA antigens and MS seems so exciting is that the histocompatibility locus in animals contains genes which control immune responsiveness[130]. The region between the serum-determinable loci in mice contains Ir (immune response) genes which specify responsiveness to certain synthetic polypeptides. Thus, an association between the HLA complex and MS seems compatible with the theory that MS involves an immune response of the host, a view which is widely held[131]. It is important in studying different populations to establish whether the DW2 antigen and, perhaps even more to the point, the Ag-7a B-cell antigen, is a 'universal' marker of MS or whether these traits, like the HLA specificities, are merely associated with yet another gene, which is involved in determining the risk of MS. This hypothetical gene has been labelled 'MSS' for MS susceptibility[108].

According to current thinking, MS occurs in individuals genetically predisposed by virtue of having inherited certain histocompatibility specificities but these specificities alone are, probably, not sufficient to cause the disease. It is not unusual for an inherited disorder to require an environmental trigger to become clinically manifest. An example is diabetes mellitus which, in the absence of a carbohydrate load, can go undetected clinically. Sharp separation in thinking about the environmental factor and the genetic substrate of MS is not warranted.

In view of the idea now in vogue that a viral agent might represent the environmental factor important in the aetiology of MS, it is worth observing that elevated antimeasles antibodies have been observed in the serum of MS patients in many parts of the world[132-136]. Whilst these titres are nowhere near as high as has been observed in SSPE[137-141], the elevation could represent some special experience with the measles virus among affected individuals.

Alternatively, the titre elevation could mean that the individuals are simply 'better' at producing antibodies. Lehrich and Arnason[142] have shown that MS patients who have higher titres to herpes simplex (but not to para-influenza) may possess A3 or B7 determinants more often than those with lower titres. Jersild et al.[143] found increased titres to measles in MS patients with A3 and B7 determinants and Arnason et al.[144] observed the same phenomenon in MS patients with A3. These investigators postulated that the increased measles titres might therefore be incidental and no aetiological role for measles virus in MS need be inferred. Bertrams et al.[143], on the other hand, found no correlation between measles antibody titres and presence of the A3 or B7 determinants and Whitaker et al.[124] found that MS patients with the B7 antigen actually had a *lower* level of measles antibody than did those who were B7 negative. Obviously, the relationship between these histocompatibility markers and measles antibody titres still needs clarification and the role of the measles virus in MS is still uncertain.

Conclusion

The search for clues to the cause of MS through the study of its epidemiology has been characterized as the 'shoe-leather' approach. This search has yielded considerable broadening of our knowledge about the disease and has helped direct research in the laboratory as well. It is clear from studies of geographical distribution that MS increases in frequency with distance from the equator, at least in western countries, up to perhaps the 50th (North America) or 60th (Europe) parallel and then probably decreases in frequency. The same relationship between MS frequency and latitude exists in Australia and New Zealand. All of Japan, the far-eastern Asian continent and the Indian subcontinent have a low frequency of MS, suggesting an Oriental 'resistance' to the disease. The apparent lower rate in Orientals may be due to genetic or environmental factors. It is not due to significant differences in clinical manifestations, although Orientals have a higher rate of optic neuritis as an initial manifestation of MS and both Orientals and Indians may have a higher rate of transverse myelopathy compared to western patients. The low rate among Orientals even in western United States favours a genetic basis for their resistance. Analysis of the fine structure of MS distribution has revealed foci of higher frequency of MS which exist next to areas of lower frequency, suggesting that the causative agent may be concentrated in some areas while 'deficient' in adjacent areas. All of South America and much of Africa are still 'dark' territories in so far as MS frequency is concerned.

Efforts to account for the distribution and population selectivity of MS have spawned an ingenious array of hypotheses, some of which implicate the role of climate (sunlight), diet (animal fats or protein), toxins (metals or industrial pollutants), and even intestinal absorption of abnormal amounts of naturally occurring noxious substances (lipid peroxides). Recently an infectious agent has attracted the most attention as a possible cause of MS. It is thought to be a virus, perhaps one with special properties such as the ability to produce latent, persistent infection of the central nervous system.

The apparent stability of the frequency of MS over many decades and in many areas of the world makes it unlikely that the introduction of modern amenities alone is sufficient to affect the rate of MS, although it is conceded that not enough time may have elapsed for the effects of modern development to be discernible in terms of increased MS frequency. Ongoing medical surveillance for MS in several communities may help resolve this issue.

Study of MS in populations which have migrated from one region to another suggests that migrants 'carry with them' the risk of MS of their original place of residence unless they migrate as youngsters, before adolescence (about the age of 15 years). A new study suggests that the critical age may be in early childhood, perhaps even before the age of 5 years. These results can mean that a childhood viral infection plays a role in causing MS. It has recently been suggested that the infection need not be specific for MS but could be due to any of a variety of infectious agents which happen to gain access into the central nervous system at a particular time, early in life. According to this hypothesis, MS is looked upon as an age-dependent host *response* to infection rather than due to the effect of any specific infecting agent.

The shift in emphasis to some characteristic of the host rather than upon an environmental agent as the 'cause' of MS has intensified efforts to identify constitutional (genetic) factors which could be important in aetiology. The current vogue among investigators is the histocompatibility complex which in animals and probably in man too encompasses chromosomal areas controlling immune responsiveness. The histocompatibility specificities HLA-A3 and B7 are increased in MS patients in certain populations (North America and Europe) but not in others (Israel and Japan). DW2, a lymphocyte-determinable HLA specificity, is associated more strongly with MS than the serum-detectable HLA determinants, and the B cell specificity Ag-7A is the genetic factor most strongly associated with MS which has so far been detected. These histocompatibility determinants may be markers for a closely linked immune response gene (Ir or MSS) which is required to confer genetic susceptibility to MS upon the host. The results generated by several decades of intensive field work coupled with coordinated laboratory efforts may certainly be regarded as fruitful even if still fragmentary. Though these 'threads' cannot yet be woven into a complete theory of aetiology, their pattern, pointing to the 'cause' of MS, is beginning to be discernible.

References

1. Leibowitz, U. and Alter, M. (1973). *Multiple Sclerosis: Clues to its Cause*, p. 148 (Amsterdam: North-Holland)

2. McAlpine, D., Lumsden, C. E. and Acheson, E. D. (1972). *Multiple Sclerosis. A Reappraisal*, 2nd edition, p. 23 (Baltimore: Williams and Wilkins)

3. Vinken, P. J. and Bruyn, G. W. (1975). *Handbook of Clinical Neurology.* (Amsterdam: North-Holland)

4. Limburg, C. C. (1950). The geographic distribution of multiple sclerosis and its estimated prevalence in the United States. *Res. Publ., Assoc. Res. Nerv. Ment. Dis.*, **28**, 15

5. Kurland, L. T. and Westlund, K. B. (1954). Epidemiologic factors in the etiology and prognosis of multiple sclerosis. *Ann. N.Y. Acad. Sci.*, **58**, 682

6. Behrend, R. C. (1969). Multiple sclerosis in Europe. *Eur. Neurol.*, **2**, 129

7. McCall, M. G., Brereton, T. L., Dawson, A., Millingen, K., Sutherland, J. M. and Acheson, E. D. (1968). Frequency of multiple sclerosis in three Australian cities – Perth, Newcastle, and Hobart. *J. Neurol., Neurosurg. Psychiatry*, **31**, 1

8. Kurtzke, J. F. (1975). A reassessment of the distribution of multiple sclerosis. *Acta Neurol. Scand.*, **51**, 110

9. Alter, M., Loewenson, R. and Harshe, M. (1973). The geographic distribution of multiple sclerosis: an examination of mathematical models. *J. Chronic Dis.*, **26**, 755

10. Kurtzke, J. F. (1966). An epidemiologic approach to multiple sclerosis. *Arch. Neurol.*, **14**, 213

11. Kurtzke, J. F. (1974). Further features of the Fennoscandian focus of multiple sclerosis. *Acta Neurol. Scand.*, **50**, 478

12. White, D. N. and Wheelan, L. (1959). Disseminated sclerosis: a survey of patients in the Kingston, Ontario, area. *Neurology*, **9**, 256

13. Alter, M., Allison, R. S., Talbert, O. R., Godden, J. O. and Kurland, L. T. (1960). The geographic distribution of multiple sclerosis. II. Prevalence in Halifax County, Nova Scotia. *N.S. Med. Bull.*, **39**, 203

14. Siedler, H. D., Nicholl, W. and Kurland, L. T. (1958). The prevalence and incidence of multiple sclerosis in Missoula County, Montana. *J. Lancet*, **78**, 358

15. Percy, A. K., Nobrega, F. T., Okazaki, H., Glattre, E. and Kurland, L. T. (1971). Multiple sclerosis in Rochester, Minnoseta. A 60-year appraisal. *Arch. Neurol.*, **25**, 105

16. Detels, R., Visscher, B., Coulson, A., Malmgren, R. and Dudley, J. (1974). Multiple sclerosis in Japanese-Americans. A preliminary report. *Int. J. Epidemiol.*, 3, 341

17. Morariu, M., Alter, M. and Harshe, M. (1974). Multiple sclerosis in Transylvania: A zone of transition in frequency. *Neurology*, 24, 673

18. Wikström, J. (1975). *Studies on the clustering of multiple sclerosis in Finland*, 7 (Thesis) (Helsinki: University of Helsinki)

19. Panelius, M. (1969). Studies on epidemiological, clinical and etiological aspects of multiple sclerosis. *Acta Neurol. Scand.*, 45, suppl. 39, 1

20. Alter, M. and Olivares, L. (1970). Multiple sclerosis in Mexico: an epidemiologic study. *Arch. Neurol.*, 23, 451

21. Agranoff, B. W. and Goldberg, D. (1974). Diet and the geographic distribution of multiple sclerosis. *Lancet*, ii, 1061

22. Thompson, R. H. S. (1966). A biochemical approach to the problem of multiple sclerosis. *Proc. R. Soc. Med.*, 59, 269

23. Poskanzer, D. C., Walker, A. M., Yokondy, J. and Sheridan, J. L. (1976). Studies in the epidemiology of multiple sclerosis in the Orkney and Shetland Islands. *Neurology*, 26 (2), 14

24. Alter, M. and Morariu, M. (1973). Distribution of multiple sclerosis. *Lancet*, i, 1126

25. Kuroiwa, Y., Igata, A., Itahara, K., Koshijima, S., Tsubaki, T., Toyokura, Y. and Shibasaki, H. (1975). Nationwide survey of multiple sclerosis in Japan: clinical analysis of 1084 cases. *Neurology*, 25, 845

26. Kuroiwa, Y. and Shibasaki, H. (1976). Epidemiologic and clinical studies of multiple sclerosis in Japan. *Neurology*, 26 (2), 8

27. Barlow, J. S. (1967). Multiple sclerosis in North Korea and China. Translations of original papers from the Bulgarian and the Chinese. *Neurology*, 17, 802

28. Kurtzke, J. F., Park, C. S. and Oh, S. J. (1968). Multiple sclerosis in Korea. Clinical features and prevalence. *J. Neurol. Sci.*, 6, 463

29. Hung, T.-P. and Lin, T.-Y. (1957). Multiple sclerosis in Taiwan. *J. Formosan Med. Assoc.*, 55, 578

30. Hung, T. (1970). Multiple sclerosis in Taiwan. *Clin. Neurol. (Tokyo)*, 10, 33

31. Kurland, L. T. and Newman, H. W. (1953). Multiple sclerosis: its frequency and distribution, with special reference to San Francisco. *Calif. Med.*, 79, 381

32. Detels, R., Brody, J. A. and Edgar, A. H. (1972). Multiple sclerosis among American, Japanese and Chinese migrants to California and Washington. *J. Chronic Dis.*, 25, 3

33. Singhal, B. S. and Wadia, N. H. (1975). Profile of multiple sclerosis in the Bombay region on the basis of critical clinical appraisal. *J. Neurol. Sci.*, 26, 259

34. Shibasaki, H., Kuroda, Y. and Kuroiwa, Y. (1974). Clinical studies of multiple sclerosis in Japan: classical multiple sclerosis and Devic's disease. *J. Neurol. Sci.*, 23, 215

35. Satoyoshi, E., Saku, A., Sunohara, N. and Kinoshita, M. (1976). Clinical manifestations and the diagnostic problems of multiple sclerosis in Japan. *Neurology*, 26 (2), 23

36. Alter, M., Okihiro, M., Rowley, W. and Morris, T. (1971). Multiple sclerosis among Orientals and Caucasians in Hawaii. *Neurology*, **21**, 122
37. Shibasaki, H., Okihiro, M. and Kuroiwa, Y. (1976). Multiple sclerosis among Caucasians and Orientals in Hawaii. *Neurology*, **26** (2), 13
38. Kahana, E., Alter, M. and Feldman, S. (1976). Optic neuritis in relation to multiple sclerosis. *J. Neurol.*, **213**, 87
39. Kurland, L. T., Beebe, G. W., Kurtzke, J. F., Nagler, B., Auth, T. L., Lessell, S. and Nefzger, M. D. (1966). Studies on the natural history of multiple sclerosis. 2. The progression of optic neuritis to multiple sclerosis. *Acta Neurol. Scand.*, **42**, suppl. 19, 157
40. Kurland, L. T. and Moriyama, I. M. (1951). Certification of multiple sclerosis as a cause of death. *J. Am. Med. Assoc.*, **145**, 725
41. Stazio, A., Kurland, L. T., Bell, L. G., Saunders, M. G. and Rogot, E. (1964). Multiple sclerosis in Winnipeg, Manitoba: Methodological considerations of epidemiologic survey. Ten-year followup of a community-wide study, and population resurvey. *J. Chronic Dis.*, **17**, 415
42. Westlund, K. B. and Kurland, L. T. (1953). Studies on multiple sclerosis in Winnipeg, Manitoba and New Orleans, Louisiana; prevalence. I Comparison between the patient groups in Winnipeg and New Orleans. *Am. J. Hyg.*, **57**, 380
43. Alter, M., Allison, R. S., Talbert, O. R. and Kurland, L. T. (1960). Geographic distribution of multiple sclerosis. *World Neurol.*, **1**, 55
44. Alter, M., Halpern, L., Kurland, L. T., Bornstein, B., Leibowitz, U. and Silberstein, J. (1962). Multiple sclerosis in Israel. Prevalence among immigrants and native-born inhabitants. *Arch. Neurol.*, **7**, 253
45. Leibowitz, U., Kahana, E. and Alter, M. (1973). The changing frequency of multiple sclerosis in Israel. *Arch. Neurol.*, **29**, 107
46. Dean, G. (1967). Annual incidence, prevalence, and mortality of multiple sclerosis in white South-African-born and in white immigrants to South Africa. *Br. Med. J.*, **2**, 724
47. Acheson, E. D., Bachrach, C. A. and Wright, F. M. (1960). Some comments on the relationship of the distribution of multiple sclerosis to latitude, solar radiation, and other variables. *Acta Neurol. Scand.*, **35**, suppl. 147, 132
48. Sibley, W. A. and Foley, J. M. (1965). Seasonal variations in multiple sclerosis and retrobulbar neuritis in northeastern Ohio. *Trans. Am. Neurol. Assoc.*, **90**, 295
49. Wuthrich, R. and Rieder, H. P. (1970). The seasonal incidence of multiple sclerosis in Switzerland. *Eur. Neurol.*, **3**, 257
50. Alter, M., Yamoor, M. and Harshe, M. (1974). Multiple sclerosis and nutrition. *Arch. Neurol.*, **31**, 267
51. Swank, R. L. (1954). Effect of high fat feedings on viscosity of the blood. *Science*, **120**, 427
52. Cullen, C. F. and Swank, R. L. (1954). Intravascular aggregation and adhesiveness of the blood elements associated with alimentary lipemia and injections of large molecular substances: effect on blood-brain barrier. *Circulation*, **9**, 335
53. Courville, C. B. (1959). Multiple sclerosis as an incidental complication of a disorder of lipid metabolism. I. Close resemblance of the lesions resulting from fat

embolism to the plaques of multiple sclerosis. *Bull. Los Angeles Neurol. Soc.*, **24,** 60

53a. Field, E. J. and Caspary, E. A. (1964). Behaviour of blood platelets in multiple sclerosis. *Lancet*, **ii,** 876

53b. Caspary, E. A., Prineas, J., Millar, H. and Field, E. J. (1965). Platelet stickiness in multiple sclerosis. *Lancet*, **ii,** 1108

54. Wright, H. P., Thompson, R. H. S. and Zilkha, K. J. (1965). Platelet adhesiveness in multiple sclerosis. *Lancet*, **ii,** 1109

55. Fog, T. (1951). On the pathogenesis of multiple sclerosis. *Acta Psychiatr. Neurol. Scand.*, suppl. **74,** 22

56. Lumsden, C. E. (1972). An outline of the pathology of multiple sclerosis. In D. McAlpine, C. E. Lumsden and E. D. Acheson (eds.) *Multiple Sclerosis: A Reappraisal*, 2nd edition, p. 134 (Baltimore: Williams and Wilkins)

57. Dobbing, J. (1964). The influence of early nutrition on the development and myelination of the brain. *Proc. R. Soc. Lond. (Biol.)*, **159,** 503

58. Culley, W. J. and Mertz, E. T. (1965). Effect of restricted food intake on growth and composition of preweanling rat brain. *Proc. Soc. Exp. Biol. Med.*, **118,** 233

59. Chase, H. P., Dorsey, J. and McKhann, G. M. (1967). The effect of malnutrition on the synthesis of a myelin lipid. *Pediatrics*, **40,** 551

60. Galli, C., White, H. B., Jr. and Paoletti, R. (1970). Brain lipid modifications induced by essential fatty acid deficiency in growing male and female rats. *J. Neurochem.*, **17,** 347

61. Davison, A. N. (1972). Biosynthesis of the myelin sheath. In Ciba Foundation Symposium: *Lipids, Malnutrition and the Developing Brain*, 71 (Amsterdam: Excerpta Medica)

62. Gerstl, B., Eng, L. F., Tavaststjerna, M. G., Smith, J. K. and Kruse, S. L. (1970). Lipids and proteins in multiple sclerosis white matter. *J. Neurochem.*, **17,** 677

63. Cumings, J. N. and Goodwin, H. (1968). Sphingolipids and phospholipids of myelin in multiple sclerosis. *Lancet*, **ii,** 664

64. Clausen, J. and Hansen, I. B. (1970). Myelin constituents of human central nervous system. *Acta Neurol. Scand.*, **46,** 1

65. Suzuki, K., Kamoshita, S., Eto, Y., Tourtellotte, W. W. and Gonatas, J. O. (1973). Myelin in multiple sclerosis. Composition of myelin from normal-appearing white matter. *Arch. Neurol.*, **28,** 293

66. Frank, J. A., Kumagai, L. F. and Dougherty, T. F. (1953). Studies on the rates of involution and reconstitution of lymphatic tissue. *Endocrinology*, **52,** 656

67. Jose, D. G. (1973). The cancer connection with immunity and nutrition. *Nutr. Today*, **8,** 4

68. Paterson, P. Y. (1973). Multiple sclerosis: an immunological reassessment. *J. Chronic Dis.*, **26,** 119

69. Lisak, R. P. (1975). Multiple sclerosis: immunological aspects. *Ann. Clin. Lab. Sci.*, **5,** 324

70. Hendrickse, R. G. (1967). Interactions of nutrition and infection: experience in Nigeria. In G. E. W. Wolstenholme and M. O'Connor (eds.) *Nutrition and Infection, CIBA Foundation Study Group 31*, p. 98 (Boston: Little, Brown and Co.)

71. Dutz, W. (1975). Immune modulation and disease patterns in population groups. *Med. Hypotheses*, **1**, 197

72. Warren, H. V., Delavault, R. E. and Cross, C. H. (1966). Geological considerations in some disease patterns. *Arch. Environ. Health*, **13**, 412

73. Campbell, A. M. G., Daniel, P., Porter, R. J., Russell, W. R., Smith, H. V. and Innes, T. R. M. (1947). Disease of the nervous system occurring among research workers on swayback in lambs. *Brain*, **70**, 50

74. Campbell, A. M. G., Herdan, G., Tatlow, W. F. T. and Whittle, E. G. (1950). Lead in relation to disseminated sclerosis. *Brain*, **73**, 52

75. Currier, R. D., Martin, E. A. and Woosley, P. C. (1974). Prior events in multiple sclerosis. *Neurology*, **24**, 748

76. Goldberg, P. (1974). Multiple sclerosis: vitamin C and calcium as environmental determinants of prevalence (a viewpoint). Part 1. Sunlight, dietary factors and epidemiology. *Int. J. Environ. Stud.*, **6**, 19

77. Leibowitz, U., Sharon, D. and Alter, M. (1967). Geographical considerations in multiple sclerosis. *Brain*, **90**, 871

78. Johnson, R. T. (1975). Virological data supporting the viral hypothesis in multiple sclerosis. In A. N. Davison, J. H. Humphrey, A. L. Liversedge, W. I. McDonald and J. S. Porterfield (eds.). *Multiple Sclerosis Research*, p. 155 (Amsterdam: Elsevier)

79. Poskanzer, D. C., Schapira, K. and Miller, H. (1963). Multiple sclerosis and poliomyelitis. *Lancet*, **ii**, 917

80. Russell, W. R. (1971). Multiple sclerosis: occupation and soical group at onset. *Lancet*, **ii**, 832

81. Miller, H., Ridley, A. and Schapira, K. (1960). Multiple sclerosis. A note on social incidence. *Br. Med. J.*, **2**, 343

82. Antonovsky, A., Leibowitz, U., Medalie, J. M., Smith, H. A., Halpern, L. and Alter, M. (1967). Epidemiological study of multiple sclerosis in Israel. III. Multiple sclerosis and socio-economic status. *J. Neurol., Neurosurg. Psychiatry*, **30**, 1

83. Beebe, G. W., Kurtzke, J. F., Kurland, L. T., Auth, T. L. and Nagler, B. (1967). Studies on the natural history of multiple sclerosis. 3. Epidemiologic analysis of the Army experience in World War II. *Neurology*, **17**, 1

84. Dean, G. Multiple sclerosis in South Africa (unpublished)

85. Mickel, H. S. (1975). Multiple sclerosis: a new hypothesis. *Perspect. Biol. Med.*, **18**, 363

86. Belin, J., Pettet, N., Smith, A. D., Thompson, R. H. S. and Zilkha, K. J. (1971). Linoleate metabolism in multiple sclerosis. *J. Neurol., Neurosurg. Psychiatry*, **34**, 25

86a. Laszlo, S. (1964). Fragilité osmotique des globules rouges dans la sclerose en plaques. *Acta Neurol. Belg.*, **64**, 529

86b. Caspary, E. A., Sewell, F. and Field, E. J. (1967). Red blood cell fragility in multiple sclerosis. *Br. Med. J.*, **2**, 610

86c. Plum, C. M. and Fog, T. (1959). Studies in multiple sclerosis. *Acta Neurol. Scandanav.*, **128**, suppl., 34

86d. Prineas, J. (1968). Red blood cell size in multiple sclerosis. *Acta Neurol. Scandanav.*, **44**, 81

87. Bird, A. V. and Satoyoshi, E. (1975). Comparative epidemiological studies of multiple sclerosis in South Africa and Japan. *J. Neurol., Neurosurg. Psychiatry*, **38**, 911

88. Kurtzke, J. F. and Bui-Quoc-Huong (1974). Multiple sclerosis in a migrant population. 1. Hospital data. *Eur. Neurol.*, **12**, 1

89. Dean, G., McLoughlin, H., Brady, R., Adelstein, A. M. and Tallett-Williams, J. (1976). Multiple sclerosis among immigrants in Greater London. *Br. Med. J.*, **1**, 861

90. Alter, M., Kahana, E. and Loewenson, R. Migration and risk of multiple sclerosis (unpublished)

91. Kurtzke, J. F. (1966). The distribution of multiple sclerosis and other diseases. *Acta Neurol. Scand.*, **42**, 221

92. Millar, J. H. D. (1971). *Multiple Sclerosis. A Disease Acquired in Childhood* (Springfield, Ill.: C. C. Thomas)

93. Dean, G. (1976). Epidemiology: what is new and what remains to be done. In A. N. Davison, J. H. Humphrey, A. L. Liversedge, W. I. McDonald and J. S. Porterfield (eds.) *Multiple Sclerosis Research*, p. 39 (Amsterdam: Elsevier)

94. Newman, H. W., Purdy, C., Rantz, L. and Hill, F. C., Jr. (1958). The spirochete and multiple sclerosis. *Calif. Med.*, **89**, 387

95. LeGac, P., Giroud, P. and Dumas, N. (1960). On a possible rickettsial and neorickettsial etiology of multiple sclerosis. *C. R. Acad. Sci. (Paris)*, **250**, 1937

96. Prineas, J. (1972). Paramyxovirus-like particles associated with acute demyelination in chronic relapsing multiple sclerosis. *Science*, **178**, 760

97. ter Meulen, V., Koprowski, H., Iwasaki, Y., Käckell, Y. M. and Müller, D. (1972). Fusion of cultured multiple sclerosis brain cells with indicator cells: presence of nucleocapsids and virions and isolation of parainfluenza-type virus. *Lancet*, **ii**, 1

98. Carp, R. I., Licursi, P. C., Merz, P. A. and Merz, G. S. (1972). Decreased percentage of polymorphonuclear neutrophils in mouse peripheral blood after inoculation with material from multiple sclerosis patients. *J. Exp. Med.*, **136**, 618

99. Koldovsky, U., Koldovsky, P., Henle, G., Henle, W., Ackermann, R. and Haase, G. (1975). Multiple sclerosis-associated agent: transmission to animals and some properties of the agent. *Infect. Immun.*, **12**, 1355

100. Henle, G., Koldovsky, U., Koldovsky, P., Henle, W., Ackermann, R. and Haase, G. (1975). Multiple sclerosis-associated agent: neutralization of the agent by human sera. *Infect. Immun.*, **12**, 1367

101. Georgi, F. and Hall, P. (1960). Studies on multiple sclerosis frequency in Switzerland and East Africa. *Acta Neurol. Scand.*, **35**, suppl. 147, 75

102. Szmuness, W. and Prince, A. M. (1971). The epidemiology of serum hepatitis (SH) infections: a controlled study in two closed institutions. *Am. J. Epidemiol.*, **94**, 585

103. Henle, W. and Henle, G. (1972). Epstein–Barr virus: the cause of infectious mononucleosis—a review. In P. M. Biggs, G. de-The and L. N. Payne (eds.) *Oncogenesis and Herpes Viruses*, p. 269 (Lyon: International Agency of Research on Cancer)

104. Detels, R., McNew, J., Brody, J. A. and Edgar, A. H. (1973). Further epidemiological studies of subacute sclerosing panencephalitis. *Lancet*, **ii**, 11
105. Miller, D. L. (1964). Frequency of complications of measles, 1963. Report on a national inquiry by the Public Health Laboratory service in collaboration with the Society of Medical Officers of Health. *Br. Med. J.*, **2**, 75
106. Byington, D. P. and Johnson, K. P. (1972). Experimental subacute sclerosing panencephalitis in the hamster. Correlation of age with chronic inclusion-cell encephalitis. *J. Infect. Dis.*, **126**, 18
107. Morley, D. C. (1974). Measles in the developing world. *Proc. R. Soc. Med.*, **67**, 1112
108. Alter, M., Harshe, M., Anderson, V. E., Emme, L. and Yunis, E. J. (1976). Genetic association of multiple sclerosis and HLA determinants. *Neurology*, **26**, 31
109. Black, F. L. (1962). Measles antibody prevalence in diverse populations. *Am. J. Dis. Child.*, **103**, 242
110. González Ramírez, L. E. (1975). *Esclerosis multiple: una enfermedad exótica en Guatemala?* (Thesis) (Guatemala City: University of San Carlos)
111. Cohen, S. and Bannister, R. (1967). Immunoglobulin synthesis within the central nervous system in disseminated sclerosis. *Lancet*, **i**, 366
112. Sandberg-Wollheim, M. (1974). Immunoglobulin synthesis *in vitro* by cerebrospinal fluid cells in patients with multiple sclerosis. *Scand. J. Immunol.*, **3**, 717
113. Link, H. (1972). Oligoclonal immunoglobulin G in multiple sclerosis brains. *J. Neurol. Sci.*, **16**, 103
114. Mackay, R. P. and Myrianthopoulos, N. C. (1966). Multiple sclerosis in twins and their relatives. Final report. *Arch. Neurol.*, **15**, 449
115. Berry, R. J. (1969). Genetical factors in the aetiology of multiple sclerosis. *Acta Neurol. Scand.*, **45**, 459
116. Schapira, K., Poskanzer, D. C. and Miller, H. (1963). Familial and conjugal multiple sclerosis. *Brain*, **86**, 315
117. Alter, M. and Schaumann, B. (1976). Hereditary amyotrophic lateral sclerosis. A report of two families. *Eur. Neurol.*, **14**, 250
118. Jersild, C., Dupont, B., Fog, T., Platz, P. J. and Svejgaard, A. (1975). Histocompatibility determinants in multiple sclerosis. *Transplant. Rev.*, **22**, 148
119. McFarlin, D. E. and McFarland, H. F. (1976). Histocompatibility studies and multiple sclerosis. *Arch. Neurol.*, **33**, 395
120. Katz, D. H. and Benacerraf, B. (1975). The function and interrelationships of T-cell receptors, Ir genes and other histocompatibility gene products. *Transplant. Rev.*, **22**, 175
121. Carpenter, C. B. (1976). The new HLA nomenclature. *N. Engl. J. Med.*, **294**, 1005
122. Naito, S., Namerow, N., Mickey, M. R. and Terasaki, P. I. (1972). Multiple sclerosis: association with HLA3. *Tissue Antigens*, **2**, 1
123. Bertrams, J., Kuwert, E. and Liedtke, U. (1972). HLA antigens and multiple sclerosis. *Tissue Antigens*, **2**, 405
124. Whitaker, J. N., Herrmann, K. L., Rogentine, G. N., Stein, S. F. and Kollins, L. L. (1976). Immunogenetic analysis and serum viral antibody titers in multiple sclerosis. *Arch. Neurol.*, **33**, 399

125. Brautbar, C., Alter, M. and Kahana, E. (1976). HLA antigens in multiple sclerosis. *Neurology*, **26** (2), 50

126. Jersild, C., Fog, T., Hansen, G. S., Thomsen, M., Svejgaard, A. and Dupont, B. (1973). Histocompatibility determinants in multiple sclerosis with special reference to clinical course. *Lancet*, **ii**, 1221

127. Winchester, R. J., Ebers, G., Fu, S. M., Espinosa, L., Zabriskie, J. and Kunkel, H. G. (1975). B-cell alloantigen Ag7a in multiple sclerosis. *Lancet*, **ii**, 814

128. Drachman, D. A., Davison, W. C. and Mittal, K. K. (1976). Histocompatibility (HLA) factors in familial multiple sclerosis. *Arch. Neurol.*, **33**, 406

129. Bird, T. D. (1975). Apparent familial multiple sclerosis in three generations. Report of a family with histocompatibility antigen typing. *Arch. Neurol.*, **32**, 414

130. McDevitt, H. O., Oldstone, B. A. and Pincus, T. (1974). Histocompatibility-linked genetic control of specific immune responses to viral infection. *Transplant. Rev.*, **19**, 209

131. Paterson, P. Y. (1972). Experimental allergic encephalomyelitis and multiple sclerosis as immunologic diseases: a critique. In F. Wolfgram, G. W. Ellison, J. G. Stevens, J. M. Andrews (eds.) *Multiple Sclerosis: Immunology, Virology and Ultrastructure*, p. 539 (New York: Academic Press)

132. Adams, J. M. and Imagawa, D. T. (1962). Measles virus antibodies in multiple sclerosis. *Proc. Soc. Exp. Biol. Med.*, **111**, 562

133. Adams, J. M., Brooks, M. B., Fisher, E. D., and Tyler, C. S. (1970). Measles antibodies in patients with multiple sclerosis and with other neurological and non-neurological diseases. *Neurology*, **20**, 1039

134. Brody, J. A., Sever, J. L. and Henson, T. E. (1971). Virus antibody titers in multiple sclerosis patients, siblings, and controls. *J. Am. Med. Assoc.*, **216**, 1441

135. Ammitzbøll, T. and Clausen, J. (1972). Measles antibody in serum of multiple sclerosis patients, their children, siblings and parents. *Acta Neurol. Scand.*, **48**, 47

136. Panelius, M., Salmi, A., Halonen, P. E., Kivalo, E., Rinne, U. K. and Penttinen, K. (1973). Virus antibodies in serum specimens from patients with multiple sclerosis from siblings and matched controls. A final report. *Acta Neurol. Scand.*, **49**, 85

137. Brody, J. A. and Detels, R. (1970). Subacute sclerosing panencephalitis: A zoonosis following aberrant measles. *Lancet*, **ii**, 500

138. Jabbour, J. T., Duenas, D. A., Sever, J. L., Krebs, H. M. and Horta-Barbosa, L. (1972). Epidemiology of subacute sclerosing panencephalitis (SSPE): A report of the SSPE registry. *J. Am. Med. Assoc.*, **220**, 959

139. Baguley, D. M. and Glasgow, G. L. (1973). Subacute sclerosing panencephalitis and Salk vaccine. *Lancet*, **ii**, 763

140. Davidson, N. M. (1973). S.S.P.E. in New Zealand. *Lancet*, **ii**, 1332

141. McDonald, R., Kipps, A. and Leary, P. M. (1974). Subacute sclerosing panencephalitis in the Cape Province. *S. Afr. Med. J.*, **48**, 7

142. Lehrich, J. R. and Arnason, B. G. W. (1976). Histocompatibility types and viral antibodies. *Arch. Neurol.*, **33**, 404

143. Jersild, C., Svejgaard, A., Fog, T., and Ammitzbøll, T. (1973). HLA antigens and diseases. I. Multiple sclerosis. *Tissue Antigens*, **3**, 243

144. Arnason, B. G., Fuller, T. C., Jr., Lehrich, J. R. and Wray, S. H. (1974).

Histocompatibility types and measles antibodies in multiple sclerosis and optic neuritis. *J. Neurol. Sci.*, **22**, 419

145. Bertrams, J., Fisenne, E. V., Höher, P. G. and Kuwert, E. (1973). Lack of association between HLA antigens and measles antibody in multiple sclerosis. *Lancet*, **ii**, 441

146. Kurtzke, J. F. (1970). Clinical manifestations of multiple sclerosis. In P. J. Vinken and G. W. Bruyn (eds.) *Handbook of Clinical Neurology*, Vol. 9 (Amsterdam: North-Holland)

147. Kurtzke, J. F., Dean, G. and Botha, D. P. J. (1970). A method for estimating the age at immigration of white immigrants to South Africa, with an example of its importance. *S. Afr. Med. J.*, **44**, 663

148. Soffer, D., Rannon, L., Alter, M., Kahana, E. and Feldman, S. (1976). Subacute sclerosing panencephalitis: An epidemiologic study in Israel. *Am. J. Epidemiol.*, **103**, 67

4

Multiple sclerosis from an epidemiological viewpoint

John F. Kurtzke

Introduction

Felix qui potuit rerum cognoscere causas (Virgil, Georgics ii, 490)

It may seem unlikely to many that one could even hope to learn the causes of things such as diseases by means of that discipline labelled epidemiology. There are a very few clinicians and research workers who accept with gusto any published item so classified, as if it were graven on two stone tablets; there are perhaps some greater number who will automatically discount all such observations with the comment that they are 'only epidemiological'. But the majority of medical scientists have seemed to regard epidemiology as a not-quite-disreputable method by which a handful of investigators manage to avoid meaningful toil while speaking to each other in arcane symbols on matters with little relevance to the real world.

It is my view not only that epidemiology is important in medicine, but that, in so far as clinical medicine is a science, it is applied epidemiology. Although anatomy and chemistry and the like are basic sciences of themselves which have obvious application to human (and other) diseases, epidemiology is *the* basic science of clinical medicine. This modest statement may require some elaboration, however.

Epidemiology

While there are indeed other definitions, a useful one is that *epidemiology is the study of the natural history of disease* (Figure 4.1). This is based upon an

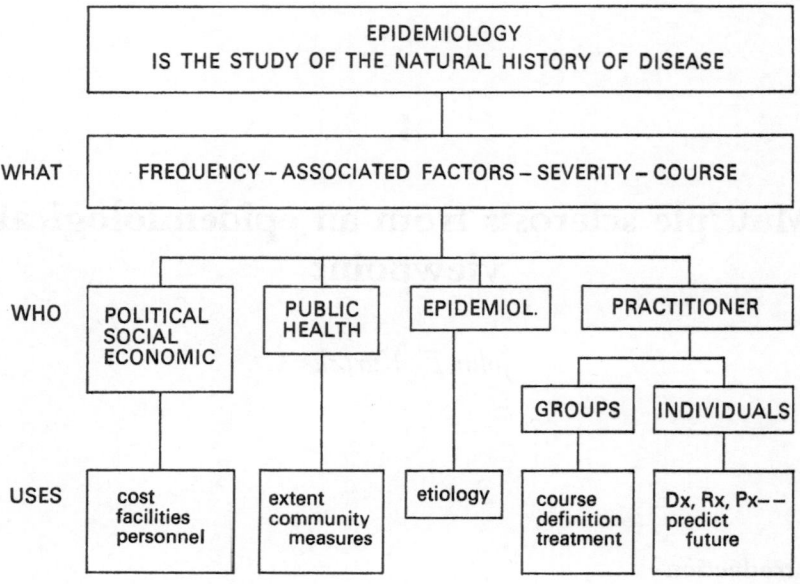

Figure 4.1 Epidemiology: content and uses (from 44)

application to disease of the original roots of the word, as a study ($\lambda o\gamma$- from $\lambda \acute{e}\gamma \epsilon \iota \nu$) of what is upon ($\dot{\epsilon}\pi \acute{\iota}$) the people ($\delta \hat{\eta}\mu o\varsigma$). The term itself, however, is of nineteenth-century origin, and can be traced to fifteenth-century English *epidemy* (an epidemic disease), which arose via old French *ypidime* from Latin *epidemia* and Greek $\dot{\epsilon}\pi \iota \delta \eta \mu \acute{\iota}a$. In fact, at least in the United States, the background of practitioners of the field can often be inferred from their pronunciation of the term. To many infectious disease workers it is epi-demm'-iology, while most others call it epi-deem'-iology.

The present concept then clearly extends beyond epidemics and infections, but it is for the most part still limited to diseases or deviations from health within human populations, and the unit of study is the affected with a given disorder.

As listed in Figure 4.1, the content of such studies is those aspects of a disease or a dysfunction having to do with how often it occurs and in whom; with what characteristics are common to the affected versus their unaffected peers; with how bad is the disorder; and with what happens to the affected in terms of this disorder. In the present discussion we shall for lack of space not consider the last two points, but they are certainly within the province of the field.

Diagnosis

Basic to all epidemiological works—and all of medicine—is the diagnosis of the disorder in view. The condition may be a specific entity like kuru or pneumococcal pneumonia; or a number of manifestations subsumed under one mantle like diabetes or stroke; or a general class of dysfunction like hemiplegia or impaired hearing.

The definition of an individual disease depends upon the presence of a specific set of signs, symptoms and laboratory findings which together separate out the affected from both the normal and those with other disorders. Note that a disease is defined by the behaviour of *groups*, and membership therein for an individual depends on his meeting the specified criteria for the group.

Unless or until one has a specific aetiological cause or pathognomonic signs and symptoms, the diagnosis of a disease is dependent on many factors aside from the skill of the diagnostician. These would include diagnostic fashions and current nomenclature; the frequency of the disease in the area in question as well as the frequency of other disorders with which it may be confused; the availability, specificity and reliability of laboratory tests; and the characteristics of the patient (age, sex, race, occupation, etc.). The diagnostician is a vital factor. Some diseases are self-diagnosed and still others well within the competence of minimally trained health professionals. Others are readily apparent to general practitioners. Many though require the skills of competent specialists, and some demand the full armamentarium of diagnostic tools available only in major centres.

Uses

As stated, the diagnosed case is the raw material of epidemiological data. The uses to which these data may be put are summarized in Figure 4.1. Socioeconomic planners for a community require the knowledge of the burden of illness expected in order to allocate the required facilities (hospitals, clinics, offices, teaching units) and personnel (specialists, other physicians, nurses, technicians, ancillaries). The costs of these services, as well as the economic onus of illness otherwise on the patient and his family, need to be measured in order to acquire the requisite moneys. These statements hold regardless whether one is speaking of a state-controlled or a *laissez-faire* economy. The closer one gets to an accurate estimate of needs the more likely there is to be an appropriate (or at least a rational) allocation of available resources. The softer the data on which such estimates are based though, the more likely are edicts from on high to be erroneous; there is much to be said for the law of supply and demand. Paediatricians do not set up practices in retirement villages, and tuberculosis sanatoria have gone the way of leprosaria in much of the world.

The public health worker requires epidemiological data to determine the baseline experience of his community in order to ascertain changes therein over time, whether increases (including epidemics) or decreases. The projections of these trends are used to estimate future needs versus those of the past and present. The identification of major and especially of increasing health problems signals areas of concern and investigation. Development and employment of environmental control and preventive measures are also in his province.

Even the clinician uses epidemiological methods and information. When he is concerned with groups of patients with a disease, it is with the view to learning more about the illness as such. The search for factors associated with the disorder and for modifications of course (treatment) often provide excellent examples of applied epidemiology. Among 'associated factors' would be laboratory findings which might better define the diagnosis.

On the other hand, when confronted with his individual patient, it is as a consumer that he can use epidemiological data. The patient wants a fortune-teller—he wishes to know what is to become of him with the symptoms at hand. Diagnosis may be assisted by knowledge of local frequency and predilections by age, sex, and other characteristics among the various possibilities entertained. Knowledge of the course permits the physician to determine the need for its alteration by available therapy.

The epidemiologist is most often to be found employed within one of these other categories of users, or as a teacher. But when wearing no other hat, his function is the investigation of disease characteristics among groups of the affected within populations, in order to attain knowledge as to aetiology and methods of disease control and prevention.

Frequency of disease

The basic question, after diagnosis, is how common is a disease. This will first of all refer to a count of the cases of a disease within a given place and time. Then in that place the diagnosed cases may be assorted as to sex and age, and perhaps to other general characteristics such as race or colour, occupation, education, marital status and the like. They may also be assorted along concomitant or antecedent physical or laboratory criteria, including height and weight, other diseases and so on. Both the parts and the whole will then be described according to the source of the material.

CASE SERIES

Much of our information in medicine has arisen from series of cases encountered by individual practitioners, clinics, or hospitals. They still provide the bulk of medical reportage on disease characteristics. At times the modifier 'consecutive' is applied to such; all this means is that no one has deliberately excluded known appropriate individuals from the series. Such series are often subdivided along some of the factors just noted in order to provide frequency distributions—by age-group and sex, for example. A unique subset of the hospital case series is the autopsy series, wherein those instances of the disease which are ascertained at postmortem examination are listed.

RELATIVE FREQUENCIES

Knowing that one has 50 cases of a disease leads to the question, among what? The next step is usually to relate such cases to the rest of the experience of the investigator, where the denominator is all cases (or admissions or autopsies) at his office, clinic or hospital.

INPUT BIAS

Either taken as numerator alone (case series) or versus all admissions (relative frequency), the problem with such material is that one has little assurance that what has been included is at all representative of the affected. And this is of course essential to generalization—which is the purpose of virtually all scientific investigation. An illustration of what is meant by input bias is drawn in Figure 4.2.

Let there be, within the community from which our series arises, a certain number of persons affected with our disease. This group will contain persons of varying severity of illness, age, blood pressure, income and a myriad of other factors. Now let the group be ranked on *each* of these factors separately along a 0–9 scale. For income, for example, patients with little means may go to Dr A because he charges less than Dr B. Or they may present directly to hospital A because it is the city hospital, while hospital B is a private institution. On the other hand, they may borrow the money and go to Dr C who is a specialist. Dr D may be an obstetrician who does careful evaluations and thus ascertains some asymptomatic individuals from among the affected. Or Dr A and B or hospital A and B may be the same person or place, but at different times. One can readily find published instances of series from hospital A pointing out differences from those of hospital B— inferring these are differences in the disease (or the treatment), but with no consideration as to whether the input bias of hospital A differs from that of hospital B.

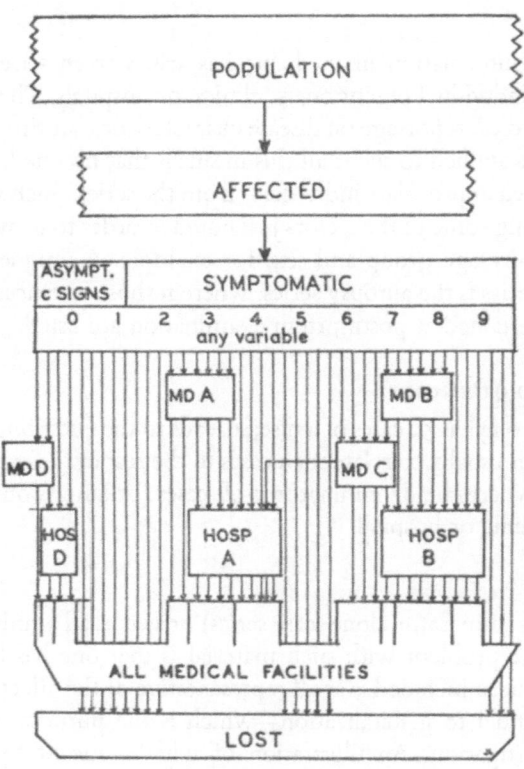

Figure 4.2 Input bias: Variability of factors leading patients to present at different doctors or hospitals, or not at all. The factors represent any given characteristic of the patients, each one to be ranked separately on an arbitrary 0–9 scale

Hospital D may have a special interest in (or a grant for) a given disease. Thus many patients with this disease may be found among their lists of other entities. The presence of two illnesses may influence attendance at any hospital—either positively or negatively. The presence of a third illness may lead to spurious associations between the other two. This last is described as Berkson's fallacy, for its recognition rather than its commission[1].

Input bias is also relevant to hospital case-control comparisons. The factors affecting a patient's presentation for care of one disease may differ markedly from those pertinent to another.

The only way in which one can have any assurance that one's case series *may* be representative of the disease within the community under study then, is to draw the series from the *entirety* of the medical facilities serving that community. The next question would concern generalization from this community at this time to other times or places.

POPULATION-BASED DATA

Figure 4.3 represents a diagram of ascertainment of the diseased within a community. Within the finite resident population, there will be at any one

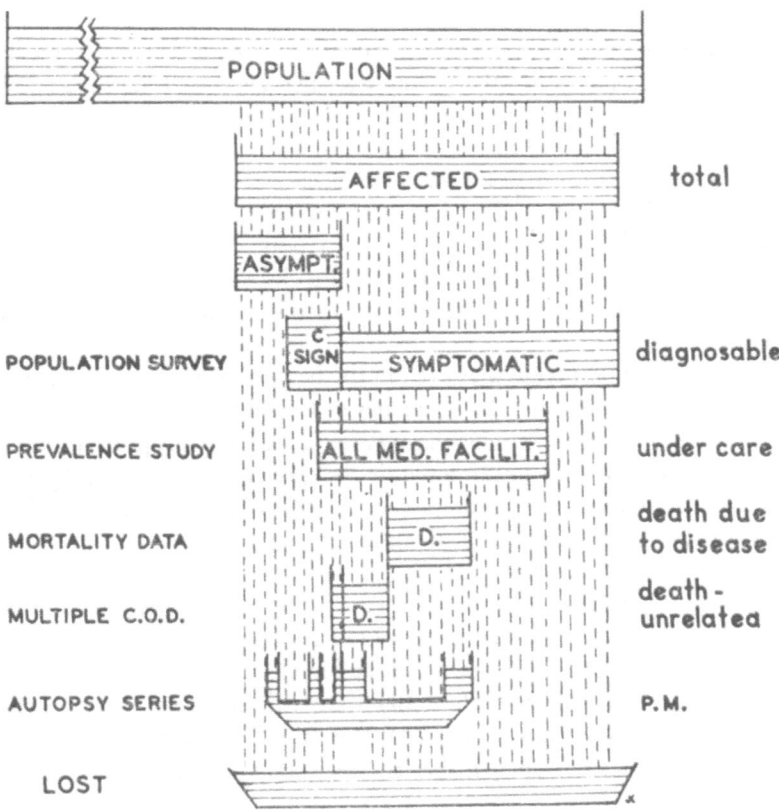

Figure 4.3 Catchment diagram of case ascertainment of disease within a population (from [31])

time a finite number of persons affected with the disease. As is true of almost every illness, some of these will be asymptomatic while a proportion will have symptoms appropriate to the condition. Among the asymptomatic, a subset will have abnormalities discoverable by examination or laboratory methods, and the remainder will then be, to all known criteria, free of disease even though affected.

Now if our ideal diagnostician (being one who never errs) examined the entirety of the population, he would discover all the symptomatic cases and those with the relevant signs although without complaints. If he examined an appropriate sample of the population instead of the total, he could still estimate the numbers expected within the total. Such measures can be and have been taken for common diseases (hypertension, diabetes), but are impractical for rare entities.

One step removed from this true population survey is that which we have noted in the prior section—that is, the ascertainment of all the affected who have come to medical attention. This I have loosely referred to as the 'prevalence study' rather than a 'population survey', because this is in fact how most of the information on the prevalence of neurological diseases has been attained. Note that this demands not only our ideal diagnostician within all the medical facilities serving our population, but also the ideal recording and retrieval system, so that all such listed cases are readily found, and in each instance with all pertinent information completely and accurately at hand.

But here we must accept that even in the best of all worlds, some patients will not be known because they have never presented themselves before our diagnostic eye. There is no assurance either as to their proportions among the affected or as to their position within the spectrum of the disease (see also Figure 4.2). Of course, the more severe the illness though, the more likely would they generally be present themselves.

One step still further removed from complete enumeration is a listing of deaths which the disease has caused. This has many benefits, not the least being the availability of such information for many entities and the unequivocal nature of death. Since we are still in the ideal world, all these cases are correctly allocated; but obviously they will still refer only to those instances where the condition was fatal. And this is for most disorders but a fraction of the affected. There is then the very real question whether the fatal cases represent all cases.

The basic datum for mortality rates is the death certificate, and specifically that item written thereon as the 'underlying cause of death'. On the standard certificate there are also places for 'contributory causes of death' and 'associated conditions'. In selected instances these too can be obtained, and provide another (undefined) fraction of the affected.

We have already mentioned the autopsy series as a subset of hospital data. Even if all autopsies are collected from all the resources of the community (including the medical examiner), they will still represent a very fragmentary portion of the affected. In most areas, far from all of the deceased are subject to postmortem examination (selection bias). Of pertinence to neurology, not all autopsies done include the examination of the brain by neuropathologists, and seldom is the spinal cord included. Aside from that, we must accept that the autopsy series is limited to *some* who die because of the disease, plus *some* who die with the disease known but for other reasons, plus *some* who die with the disease clinically manifest yet undiagnosed, plus *some* in whom the disease would have been impossible to determine during life.

At every step along this pathway then, we must have missed a proportion of the affected. And the further we get from a true survey of the subject population, the larger will be this proportion—and the more undefinable its setting within the range of the illness.

POPULATION-BASED RATES

The proper definition of frequency of disease and delineation of the characteristics of the affected therefore depends upon the measurement of a numerator (the cases) within its true denominator (the population at risk). These ratios, with the addition of the time factor to which they pertain, are referred to as rates. The population-based rates in common use are the *incidence rate*, the *mortality rate*, and the *prevalence 'rate'*. They are all ordinarily expressed in unit-population values. For example, ten cases among a community of 20 000 represents a rate of 50 per 100 000 population or 0·5 per 1000 population.

(*a*) *Incidence rate*—The incidence or attack rate is defined as the number of new cases of the disease beginning in a unit of time within the specified population. This is usually given as an annual incidence rate in cases per 100 000 population per year. The date of onset of clinical symptoms ordinarily decides the time of accession, though occasionally the date of first diagnosis is used.

(*b*) *Mortality rate*—The mortality or death rate refers to the number of deaths with this disease as the underlying cause occurring within a unit time and population, and thus an annual death rate per 100 000 population. The *case fatality ratio* refers to the proportion of the affected who die from the disease. When this is high, as in glioblastoma multiforme, then accurate death rates reflect the disease well. When this is low, as in epilepsy, then death data may be exceedingly biased.

(*c*) *Prevalence 'rate'*—The point prevalence rate is properly a ratio, and refers to the number of the affected at one point in time within the community, again expressed per unit of population. If there is no change in case fatality ratios over time and no change in annual incidence rates (and no migration), then the average annual incidence rate times the average duration of illness in years equals the point prevalence rate.

(d) *Rate resources*—Both incidence and prevalence rates of diseases are derived from surveys for the disease in question as it occurs within circumscribed populations. Mortality rates come from official published sources. Characteristics of the diseased in terms of associated factors, course and treatment should come from the population prevalence studies as well, but much of our current information on these aspects is actually derived from case series from hospitals.

(e) *Types of rates*—When the numerator and the denominator refer to the entirety of a community, then their quotient is a *crude rate, all ages*, for the entity in question. When both terms of the ratio are delimited by age or sex or colour or other criteria, then we are speaking of *age-specific* or *sex-specific* (or whatever) rates. Taking rates within consecutive age-groups from birth to the eldest group for each sex, one has then described the disease according to age-specific and sex-specific rates for the entire community.

Since different communities will differ in their age distributions, the proper comparisons among communities are those for the age- (and sex-) specific rates. Such comparisons become unwieldy when more than a few surveys are considered, and the proper step then is the calculation of *age-adjusted* rates. One method of age-adjustment is to take each age-specific rate and multiply it by a factor representing the proportion of the standard population that this age-group contains. The sum of these individual adjusted figures provides an *age-adjusted rate, all ages*, or a *rate all ages, adjusted to a standard population*. One common standard population is that of the United States for a censal year. This method is important when dealing with common disorders that affect primarily either end of the age-spectrum. It is less indicated when considering rare entities which have no notable age (or sex) predilection. Since it is an average, it still, however, may not reflect adequately those age-specific rate curves which are badly skewed.

Population surveys

In medicine there are three general kinds of population-based surveys, which I have called the *Assyrian*, the *in-law*, and the *spider*.

THE ASSYRIAN

As Byron put it in *The Destruction of Sennacherib*, 'The Assyrian came down like a wolf on the fold.' This is the type common to most population surveys, whose methodology will be outlined below. In brief, it is the deployment of a team of workers throughout a community in order to identify the numerator (cases), and to perform whatever examination, laboratory, and questionnaire procedures had been planned. The entirety of input data is obtained in a short period, often no more than a matter of months depending on the extent and intensity of the project. Thereupon the investigators will follow Longfellow and 'Shall fold their tents, like the Arabs, And as silently steal away'.

This kind of survey has been directed toward the ascertainment of cases within the population by door-to-door inquiry of its entirety or of a representative sample—what I referred to in Figure 4.3 as the (true) population survey. It has also been directed to the ascertainment of cases known to the medical resources of the community without querying the population at large—which I have called the prevalence study. Obviously both, however, are surveys of the population to detect prevalent cases.

The survey population may comprise not only the general populace of a town or county, but may also refer to more restricted groups: employees of a plant, schoolchildren, cloistered nuns, the military, airline pilots, retirement villagers. The choice of such groups depends on the purposes of the study; stroke surveys are more efficient when only the more elderly are studied. All such restrictions, however, may limit the applicability of the results to the general population. For example, the economic status of retirement community residents differs greatly from that of a group receiving old age assistance pensions.

THE IN-LAW

There is a very expensive, albeit important, method for carrying out population surveys, to which I have attached this label. In such instances the survey team moves into a community, screens the residents, and then remains to keep the community under direct surveillance with ongoing or repeated assessments over a prolonged period. In this fashion one can define directly incidence as well as prevalence, and can identify risk factors before the event and assess their impact, as well as provide survival estimates and even treatment or prevention comparisons. Such works demand the full and sustained cooperation of both the inhabitants and the medical care providers of the area. They are also limited to regions expected to have little migration, and perforce are limited to small communities. This last point is important: even after decades the case-material will be small. Further, the goals of the team must also be drastically limited, since a prospective study of all diseases is impossible. And one requires a group of investigators willing to dedicate its professional life to a single study. The greatest limiting factor, though, is the expense of such an undertaking.

In the United States the primary example of this approach has been the cardiovascular and cerebrovascular disease study of Framingham, Massachusetts, where a cohort of some 5000 adults has been followed for almost 20 years.

THE SPIDER

Rather than seeking out the patients, it would be well to devise studies wherein the patients come to the investigator. When one has an excellent medical facility incorporating high quality diagnosis in all areas of medicine and serving a defined community as its sole resource, and where the reporting and retrieval systems permit the collection of complete and accurate data, there is a potential for numerous epidemiological inquiries of first quality.

In the United States the solitary example of such an epidemiological resource is the Mayo Clinic in Rochester, Minnesota. This community of (now) some 50 000 population has the good fortune to be the site of an internationally renowned diagnostic centre whose record system was designed for accessibility for research purposes. The contributions of this centre to virtually all fields of medicine have been outstanding, and this includes a number of incomparable epidemiological surveys. The major drawback is the need to extrapolate to the entire United States from a small all-white midwestern population of limited ethnic and socioeconomic background. Another question is the reason for new residents to immigrate into this town, which may well be medical. We should note that the community itself would be totally unable to finance even a fraction of this centre, whose existence depends upon the massive number of diagnostic referrals handled.

State-oriented medical care systems of quality have the potential to be similar epidemiological resources. Valuable information has thus come to us from Scandinavia and parts of a number of other countries, for selected entities. But this is a resource whose potential is still, for the most part, just that—a potential.

Performance of a population survey

While this is not the place for an investigator's field manual, an example of how such studies are done may be helpful in appreciating the problems.

The steps and a flow diagram for a population survey are drawn in Figure 4.4, adapted from Sartwell[2]. His *preconditions* to performing the survey include: (a) hypothesis or hypotheses to be examined; (b) selection and validation of test procedures; (c) selection and training of survey team; (d) selection of community for study; (e) performance of pilot trial; (f) census of com-

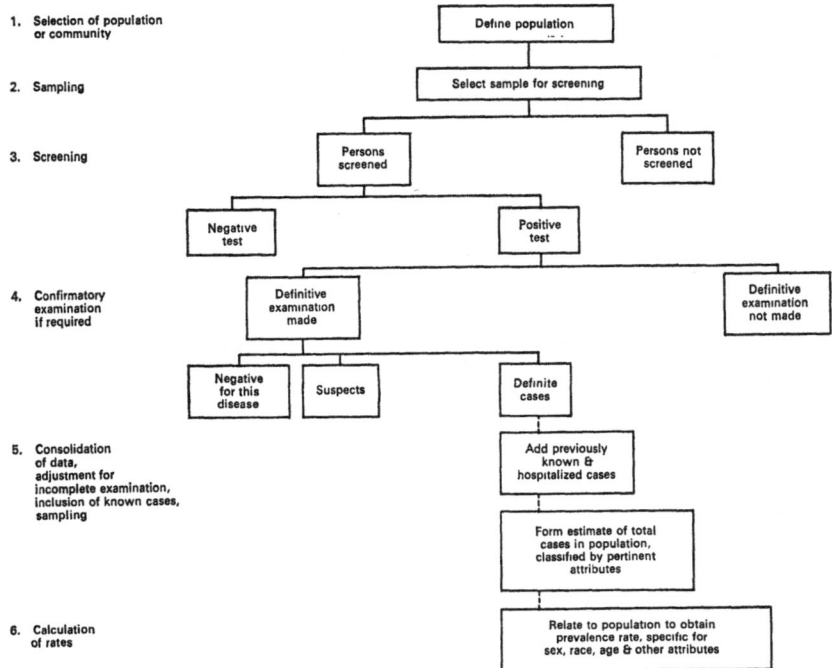

Figure 4.4 Steps in performing a population prevalence survey, adapted from [3]

munity. 'The point I wish to emphasize is that the survey itself is only one of a sequence of steps and is likely to be of limited value if these other steps are neglected.'[2]

For our purposes, the hypothesis will be simply the question: What is the prevalence of Field's disease? Field's disease is a disorder which turns one's left hallux purple and is associated with small ears and elevated blood zirconium levels.

We chose the town of Croydon-upon-the-Fork as our survey site and November 1st, 1975, as prevalence day. This town had a resident population of 43 204 according to the census of April 1st, 1975, and 43 220 on April 1st, 1970. A 10% sample was to be screened for Field's disease. Of the 4320 chosen, 60 refused to remove their shoes and 40 chased the interviewers off the property. There were thus 4220 persons screened.

The screening procedure was observation of the left hallux. Of the 4220, 4180 had a normal-coloured left hallux, 20 had a purple hallux, and 20 had no toes on the left foot. The 40 of the last two groups were referred for definitive examination, but only 30 (18 purple, 12 no-toe) arrived. Among these 30 examined, five with purple toes had normal ears and zirconium levels, as did ten of those with no toes. Two no-toes had elevated zirconium and small ears; since these are not pathognomonic findings they were placed in the 'suspect' group. Also classified as 'suspect' were two of the purple-toed with elevated zirconium and normal ears and two more with small ears and normal zirconium.

Nine cases met all criteria and were diagnosed as definite Field's disease. The prevalence of definite Field's disease was thus 9/4220 or 2·13 per 1000 population. Among the five purple-toed who were otherwise normal there were discovered to be three who had a curious method of testing the temperature of their table wine (a modest local vintage), and were thus false-positives. The other two were added to the 'suspect' list for a total of eight suspects. The prevalence of Field's disease from the field survey was thus raised to (8 + 9)/4220 or 4·03 per 1000, when possible cases were included.

Records of the local practitioners and the county hospital upon review revealed ten instances (eight definite and two possible) of Field's disease not previously known to us among current residents of the town. This is a prevalence of 8/38 984 (43 204 less 4220 screened) for definite cases, and 10/38 984 for the total including possibles. These give rates of 0·21 and 0·26 per 1000. Adding them to the field survey rates, we assert the prevalence of definite Field's disease in this town on prevalence day is 2·34 per 1000 population; and there is a prevalence of 4·29 per 1000 for all cases including the possible ones.

Now at each stage there were some individuals lost to observation. What to think about these, and what questions otherwise should be considered at each step of the survey are noted in Figure 4.5, which is the completed diagram from Sartwell[3], page 22.

Performance of incidence and mortality studies

INCIDENCE DATA

If a community survey is carried out for a long enough period, it will afford a direct measure of annual incidence rates as new cases of the disease are encountered. For short-term surveys, incidence can be estimated only by retrospective reconstruction of the appropriate series. Dangers here include not only all the points already raised above, but also questions as to lost cases because of migration, death or cure before prevalence day. Secular changes in incidence are practically impossible to determine with such material.

Prospective ongoing surveys are not without their problems either. One real point is a question of changing diagnostic criteria over time as medicine

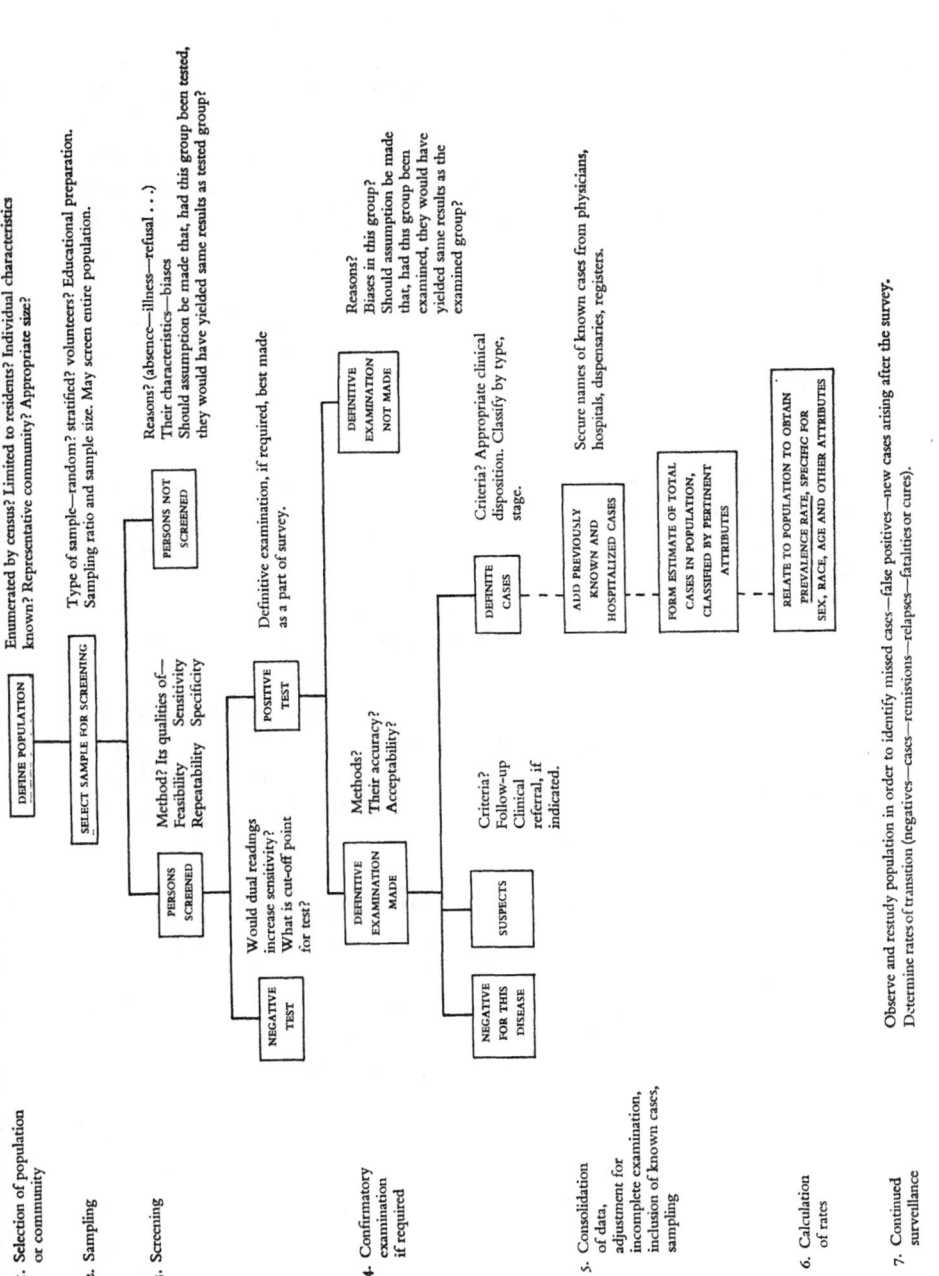

Figure 4.5 Steps and questions in the performance of a population prevalence survey, from [3], with permission from the author

advances. There may also be an almost unconscious loosening of diagnostic standards with time as the examiner keeps observing one 'normal' after another. Another aspect is the interaction of the survey team with the study population. This may lead to effective treatment or preventive measures on occasion, but more often to a heightened awareness of illness in the community with a consequent greater propensity to report. Conversely, it may lead to community resistance to attendance as boredom and lack of benefit to the individual become apparent. All these may alter the incidence recorded.

It is possible of course to measure mortality rates from population surveys in a manner analogous to the incidence rates. But the usual death data are not derived from such works.

MORTALITY DATA

The (underlying) cause of death on the official death certificate required in all civilized countries is coded according to a three- or four-digit number which represents a specific diagnosis within the International Statistical Classification of Diseases, Injuries, and Causes of Death—the ISC[4]. In the United States a slightly altered version known as the ICDA is used[5]. The ISC is revised every 10 years, and the changes in the current (eighth) revision were major ones.

Deaths and death rates for a large number of individual entities so coded are published annually by the governments of many countries. For many of these disorders the data are available by age, sex, race or colour, and geographical subdivisions of the country. When the causes of death are available in such detail, international comparisons of death rates by cause can be readily made after age-adjusting the rates to a single standard.

The great advantages of these materials are their current availability across time and space for many conditions in which we have an interest. Geographical distributions are especially attractive, since most of the population studies available are of necessity 'spot surveys' which may tell us little about the areas that were not investigated. Most often, too, the numbers are larger by magnitudes than our prevalence studies can provide.

The principal disadvantage is the question of diagnostic accuracy. Of secondary importance are questions on coding practices including the choice of the underlying cause of death. There are also the generally minor problems as to demographic errors in both the numerator and denominator (age and residence in particular). And not every disease is coded, nor are they always defined in an optimal fashion. For example, ISC code 348 is motor neurone disease and 348·0 is amyotrophic lateral sclerosis. But primary lateral sclerosis is also code 348·0. The categories for cerebrovascular disease are quite poor.

Still, for disorders which have their own specific code (and in particular a three-digit code which is all that is obligatory under international rules), which have a high case-fatality ratio and short survival, and which are readily diagnosed by the average practitioner—the death data provide a valuable resource.

In a few countries routinely, and in several others on occasion, there is available a similar categorization of the deaths listed as contributory causes or associated conditions. The sum of this grouping and those classed as underlying would provide the data for total deaths with this disorder noted on the death certificates.

Risk

'The basic premise of epidemiology is that disease does not occur randomly but in patterns which reflect the operation of the underlying causes . . . that knowledge of these patterns is not only of predictive value with respect to future disease occurrence, but also constitutes a major key to understanding causation. . . .'[6]. The 'patterns' mentioned are those which comprise the 'risk factors' for a disease.

In simple terms, risk may be defined as the chances (likelihood, probability) of an occurrence. For example, the risk of death from bronchogenic carcinoma within the general population in a single year is the annual death rate from bronchogenic carcinoma. The risk of acquiring the disorder is similarly the annual incidence rate. The cumulative risk from birth of acquiring bronchogenic carcinoma would be the sum of the single-year age-specific incidence rates after adjustment for expected survival.

The risk of bronchogenic carcinoma varies greatly with age, as we know. Thus age is a *risk factor* for bronchogenic carcinoma. We generally consider only the positive (deleterious) factors as related to risk, while their converse would be 'protective' factors; strictly, of course, anything which alters risk could be thought of as a risk factor regardless of its direction. Every conceivable characteristic of macroclimate (the environment) and of the microclimate (the individual) is a potential risk factor for any and all diseases.

The principal risk factors considered routinely for diseases are age, sex, race, time and geography. Spatiotemporal clustering may provide clues to aetiology, as may marked age predilection. In many illnesses one can demonstrate differential risk between the sexes, but seldom does this lead us very far unless the difference is striking (Duchenne dystrophy, for example). Residence may extend to birthplace, and studies of migration patterns between areas of different risk may be useful clues to cause. Age of the parent may also be meaningful; there is a striking correlation between maternal age and the risk of Down's syndrome. Racial predilections are found among a number of conditions, and understood in a few.

But generally these basic factors have their principal value as items which need to be accounted for when we search for other risk factors as causes or precipitants of illness. We would believe these other factors to be important as potential causes or precipitants when the risk in their presence exceeds that in their absence regardless of age, sex, race, and geography. Among those of potential importance but not often of aetiological value would be marital and socioeconomic status, and occupation. Factors related to geography (climate, urbanization, pollution, insolation, altitude, precipitation, forestation, crops) need often be considered.

Among the microclimatic factors often investigated are blood pressure; smoking and alcohol habits; medications; prior illnesses, operations and exposures; and laboratory measurements, the last limited thus far only by the state of the art.

Risk factors may be discovered either haphazardly or by design; they may support or reject a hypothesis, or provide the basis for new ones. But the more consistent, and especially the more specific the factors delineated, the more likely are they to include (or lead to) the cause(s) of the disease.

RELATIVE RISK

So far we have been speaking of an excess of disease over that expected, which requires a knowledge of the incidence rate. If the incidence of a disease is 4 per 100 000 population a year among individuals without factor X, and 8 per 100 000 for those with factor X, then for factor X the relative risk is 2.

When one does not have available true incidence rates, one can still compare the frequency of disease occurrence between two groups which differ only in terms of this factor. In this case, if twice as many with the factor develop the disease as those without, then again the relative risk is 2.

Retrospective comparisons can also be made, and if a group of affected differs from a group of matched controls on a given factor, this is then a measure of risk. Relative risk in such case-control comparisons is defined as ad/bc in the following table, adapted from MacMahon[7]:

factor	case	control
+	a	b
−	c	d
total	a+c	b+d

It is the quotient of 'hits' over 'misses' in this circumstance.

The relative risk in general then is the *ratio* of the rate in the 'exposed' to the rate in the 'standard' ('unexposed'). The higher this ratio, the more likely is this factor to be directly related to the cause or precipitation of the disease in question.

ATTRIBUTABLE RISK

The *excess* of the rate in those 'exposed' to a factor over the rate in the 'standard' not exposed to the factor is a measure of the disease risk attributable to the factor. This is the amount by which the disease would be reduced in frequency were the factor not present (by treatment or prevention). Another example from MacMahon[7] may clarify these types of risk. This lists the risk of death from bronchogenic carcinoma and from coronary thrombosis according to smoking habits.

C.O.D.	death rate per 100 000		attributable	relative
	non-smoker	*heavy smoker*	*risk*	*risk*
bronchogenic carcinoma	7	166	159	23·7
coronary thrombosis	422	599	177	1·4

Comments

I hope the paragraphs above provide some understanding of what is subsumed under epidemiology. We have considered only a few facets of the discipline, little more than a brief elaboration of some of the basics. The problems inherent in obtaining useful data should have emerged to some degree, as well as their relations to the work of the 'pure' clinician or the basic scientist dealing with human disease.

We have not at all touched upon the statistical handling of data—not for lack of importance but rather for lack of space. While calculations of rates are but simple arithmetic given the requisite data, tests for associations, significance of differences, and many other manipulations are far from simple —not so much in terms of their performance perhaps, but rather in their applicability and their interpretation. Big differences with big numbers are usually meaningful—unless there is also big bias. Small differences with big numbers are ordinarily not of biological importance regardless of statistical significance. With small numbers only big differences will test out as significant; when they do not attain this level, *no* inference—positive or negative—is really warranted.

Most of what we have covered is *descriptive epidemiology*. With considerations of risk factors we get into *analytic epidemiology*, which is the attempt to explain the patterns of disease found. There is also an *experimental epidemiology* wherein one tests the hypothesis in view in a direct fashion. This is seldom possible, and most of our epidemiological inferences must rest upon observation of the experiments of nature. The limits of potential risk factors in any disease are those of our own imagination, and even the strongest and most consistent findings may be artefactual, or, if real, epiphenomena.

Still, we must live and work in the world we have. The clinician does not leave a comatose patient unattended merely because the history is incomplete. After doing what evaluation is possible, he is forced to act on the basis of his presumptive diagnosis.

If multiple sclerosis is our comatose patient, where do we now stand, epidemiologically, in terms of our diagnosis?

Multiple sclerosis

The disease

Other chapters are devoted to the proper descriptions of this fascinating illness. There are two aspects that might be in order here though, of which the first is diagnosis. The diagnosis of MS is clinical. Seldom in any series— whether epidemiological or not—has one proved this at autopsy in any appreciable proportion of cases. Further considerations of diagnosis are in Fog's chapter (2).

But the clinical diagnosis is always one of gradation. Regardless of what categories are used, some patients are more likely cases of MS than others. My preference is to delete from epidemiological comparisons those classed as 'possible' or 'unlikely' MS, and to limit attention to 'probable' and 'definite' or 'clinically definite' cases. *Within* these better categories, published series are quite uniform in clinical characteristics, age, sex and course, regardless of the source (save perhaps from the Orient). The 'possibles' are too heterogeneous for inclusion. Those who favour their inclusion make the valid point that thereby not only are some true cases not excluded, but also they are frequently the milder ones. This is true, and they are especially mild if they are not MS. My brief for the stricter limitations is that even with the possibles we do not have all MS. As alluded to elsewhere, subclinical deficits are definable in most patients with the disease, lesions are doubtless present before symptoms in probably all the patients, and in some persons the illness never attains a clinically manifest state. The question is whether MS is a lily-pad or an iceberg in terms of the diagnostic water-line, and this we do not know. Certainly if it is an iceberg, missing the few MS among the admixtures categorized as 'possibles' would have little influence.

IS MS ONE DISEASE?

The question without an answer is whether MS is (principally) a single disease of a single aetiology, or a syndrome of varied causation but with similar clinical and pathological features. My faith lies with the former, since elucidation of cause in one group would then have applicability elsewhere. The more features an entity has in common the more likely is it to be a single entity. Most would agree that pathological and clinical similarities are insufficient, and perhaps would maintain this view as well when age at onset, sex and course are added.

We have one bit of information that might support the single-disease concept.

For some years we have been studying a series of cases whose first diagnosis of MS was made in US Army hospitals during the Second World War. Based upon all records available to 1962, we reassessed their diagnoses. Of the 762 cases the Army called MS, we reclassified 527 as 'definite' (476) or 'probable' (51) MS, and considered 146 as 'not-MS—other diseases'[8]. Of these, 234/527 MS and 101/146 not-MS had been first diagnosed as MS during their first bout of illness for which they were then hospitalized in the Army[9]. The neurological deficits of these groups at onset examination are compared in Table 4.1. Even for the groups it is difficult to decide which

Table 4.1 Percentage frequency of neurologic involvement according to functional systems at examination at entry to United States Army hospitals in the Second World War for onset bout of 'MS' for men later reclassified as MS and not-MS[9]

Functional system	MS	not-MS
	(percentage with signs)	
Pyramidal	88·4	63·2
Cerebellar	76·7	67·1
Brain stem	73·2	83·8
Sensory	54·5	34·3
Visual	23·1	31·7
Bowel and bladder	19·4	16·7
Cerebral (total, includes mood)	20·2	18·9
Cerebral (mentation)	1·5	8·1
Miscellaneous	15·1	17·7
(N)	(234)	(101)

should be the MS; there were somewhat fewer with pyramidal and sensory signs and somewhat more with mentation impairment among the not-MS, but the differences are certainly not great.

Conversely, in our epidemiological case-control comparisons of these *same* patients, there were striking differences found for the MS which were not seen among the not-MS[10]. One example is presented in Table 4.2.

Table 4.2 Case-control ratios for socioeconomic status at induction for 'MS' cases in United States Army in the Second World War, for men later reclassified as MS and not MS[10]

Socioeconomic	Case-control ratios	
status score*	MS	not-MS
0–69	0·69	1·06
70–109	0·81	0·82
110–149	1·35	1·13
150–200	1·61	0·94
Total	1·00	0·98
(N)	(369)	(108)

* Sum of scales for occupational status and education

In this context then, those we had called 'MS' behaved as a group distinct from their matched controls on a number of factors, as if they represented one disease, while those we had called 'not-MS' were not differentiated from their own controls on these same factors, as if they represented a syndrome—a heterogeneity of diseases (as they did).

We should point out though that the same factors which differentiated the 'true' MS from controls were found (though somewhat weaker) when the comparisons were made with the entire group of cases—MS, not-MS, possibles and unknowns. This should give some assurance to findings from 'dirty' material. So long as a group is perhaps 2/3 or 3/4 'pure' and the contaminants are heterogeneous, any differentiating factors found are likely to be valid. On the other hand, the greater the 'noise' in the system the less the reliance that can be placed on *negative* findings (lack of associations). My preference for excluding 'possible MS' from studies rests in the realization that even our 'clinically definite MS' are *not* always MS.

MS by age and sex

For some orientation to the epidemiological material, I shall present figures representing incidence, prevalence and mortality rates from Denmark. In my view these data represent the best information available, and I use them as the model for MS in a high-frequency area of the world.

PREVALENCE

The prevalence data are those of the nationwide MS registry of Hyllested[11] as of October 1949 (Figure 4.6). The 'definite' plus 'probable' cases numbered 2481, and their configuration (both sexes combined) differed very little from the crude averages of the age-specific rates including 'possibles' which are drawn for each sex in Figure 4.6. Note the clear maximum in the 40–49 age group, where the rate among females is some 180 per 100 000 and that for males is almost 140.

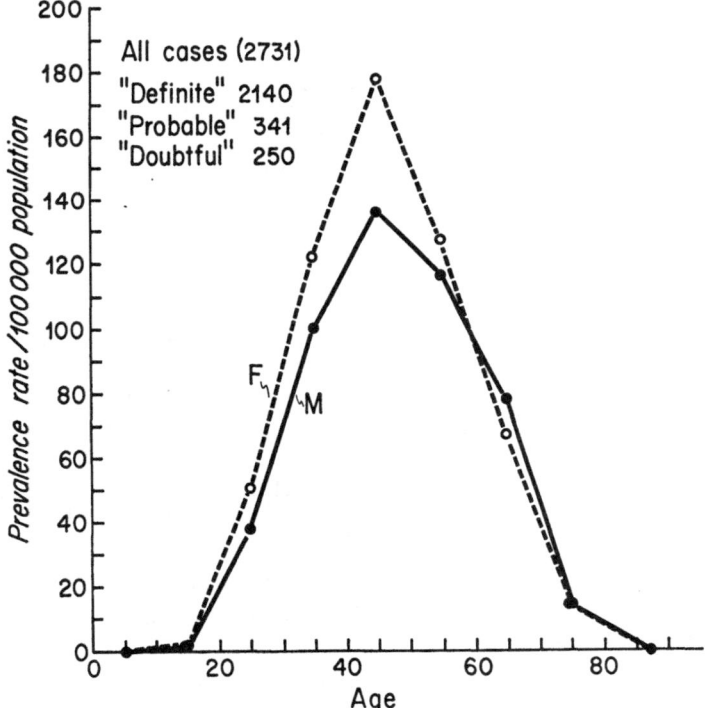

Figure 4.6 Age and sex specific prevalence rates per 100 000 population for multiple sclerosis in Denmark from data of Hyllested[11] (from [31])

With this almost symmetrical and central curve, the differences among age distributions found for native populations of most of the world would have little influence on the rates. Thus for most purposes, age-adjustment of MS prevalence rates is unnecessary.

INCIDENCE

By taking distributions at onset by age and sex for the Danish prevalent cases of definite and probable MS as of 1949, the population distribution of Denmark for 1940, and the average number of incident cases for 1939–45 (128·86 per year), it was possible to reconstruct age- and sex-specific annual incidence rates for MS[12]. These rates are drawn in Figure 4.7, and demon-

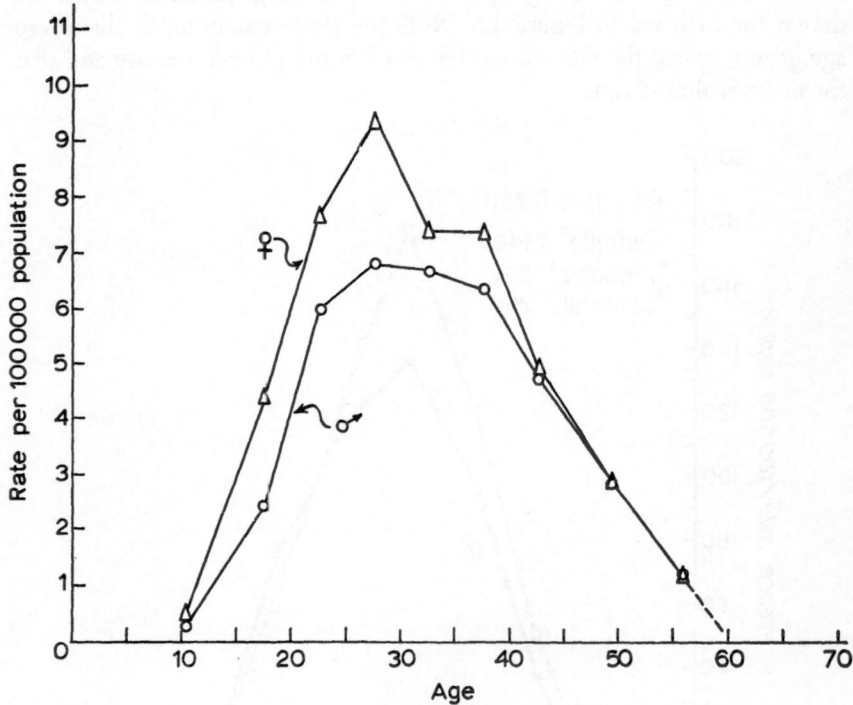

Figure 4.7 Average annual age and sex-specific incidence rates per 100 000 population for 'definite' + 'probable' multiple sclerosis in Denmark calculated from the prevalence series of Hyllested[11] (from [25a])

strate the female excess in the young and the maximal incidence at age 25–29. The annual incidence rate, all ages, is calculated as 3·35 per 100 000 population (3·00 male and 3·69 female). Here too the configurations do not suggest the need for age-adjustment in the usual material.

MORTALITY

Death rates for MS for the years 1963–68 are drawn in Figure 4.8[13]. The rates for MS as the underlying cause of death are represented by the lower

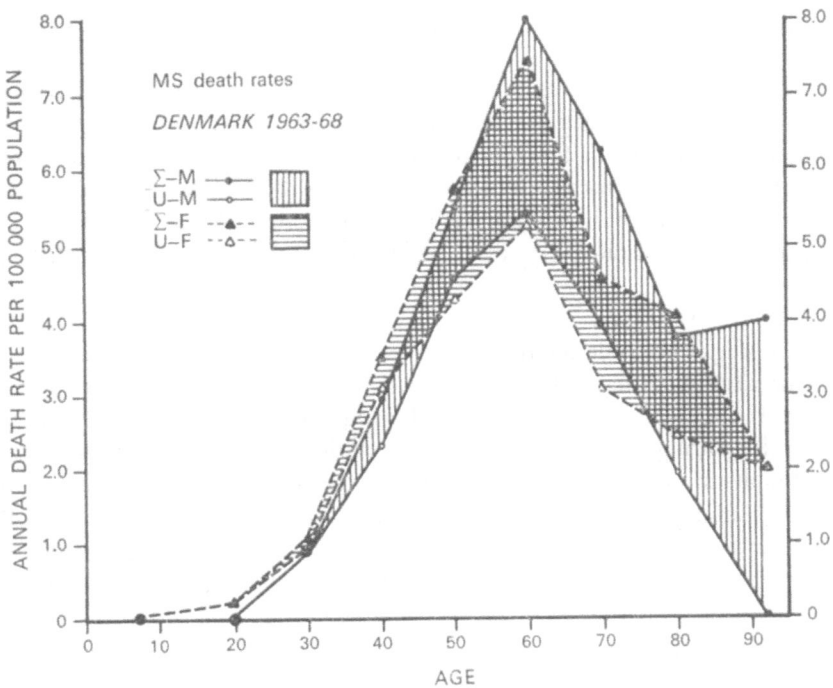

Figure 4.8 Average annual age and sex-specific mortality rates per 100 000 population for multiple sclerosis in Denmark as the underlying cause of death and as total deaths. Shaded portion represents the contributions from deaths coded as contributory cause or associated conditions (from [13])

lines with open symbols, while those for all deaths with MS listed on the certificate are defined by the upper lines with solid symbols. The shaded portions are the contributions to the total death rate for MS when this disease was listed as a contributory cause or associated condition at death.

Comparison with the incidence rate curves shows a fair degree of similarity of shape and, for total deaths, of height, save that the one is about 30 years beyond the other. The age at death showing the maximal rates is the 55–64 age-group, regardless of type of cause or sex. The area under the total death-rate curve is not greatly less than that of the incidence-rate curve, suggesting rather complete ascertainment of MS deaths in Denmark.

This death-rate curve is *not* typical of that from all countries. In the United States the underlying cause death-rates are almost plateaued beyond age 45 with perhaps a slight maximum near age 70, while adding the secondary causes produces in males (but not in females) a much sharper maximum, again about age 70. Configuration of the curves for MS deaths in Norway is intermediate between those of Denmark and the United States[13].

Although the age-specific death-rate curve for Denmark is still rather symmetrical, it is shifted considerably toward the right along the age spectrum. Adjustment for age then might well be thought indicated for comparisons of death-rates in MS. For no source though, whether incidence, prevalence or mortality, would it appear necessary to consider the sexes separately, even though they do demonstrate a female predilection in MS.

CUMULATIVE RISK

There might be some interest in an answer to the question of what one's chances are of getting multiple sclerosis. For an individual born in Denmark, there is about one chance in 500 of having this disease diagnosed (appropriately) during his lifetime. By means of the age-specific incidence rates and tables of normal survival in Denmark, the cumulative probability from birth (cumulative risk) is calculated at 0·002, somewhat less in males (0·0018) and more in females (0·0022). After birth, the lifetime risk does not begin to drop appreciably until about age 25. The full data will be published shortly[14].

Geographical distribution

There is a massive literature on the geographical distribution of multiple sclerosis, and no attempt whatsoever will be made to review either the specific material or its development. I will try to provide a bare minimum on death distributions, and as summary a statement as possible on the morbidity data. This though is the epidemiological information which constitutes the basic 'facts' on MS, upon which all hypotheses need to be built.

MORTALITY RATES

A very useful contribution was the paper by Goldberg and Kurland[15], presenting death-rates for a number of neurological diseases from all the countries which were able to provide the required data. For most lands the deaths were those for 5 years within the 1951–58 period, and all the rates were age adjusted to the 1950 population of the United States. All rates referred to diseases coded as the underlying cause of death.

These death-rates from multiple sclerosis are drawn in Figure 4.9 from the data of Goldberg and Kurland, but reorganized according to geography.

Note that the rates in most of western Europe are in the order of 2 per 100 000 per year or higher. The northernmost lands are close to 1 per 100 000, as are Canada, US whites, and New Zealand. Deaths from the disease would then appear overall to be notably less common in the latter countries. The

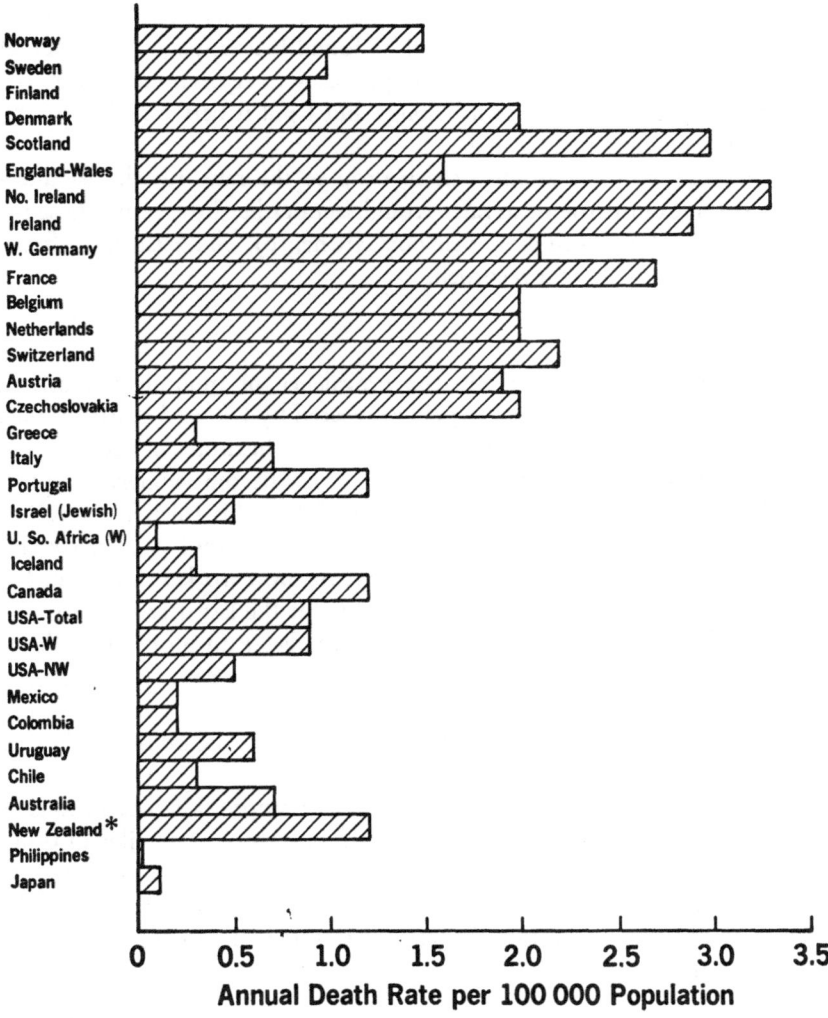

Annual Death Rate per 100 000 Population

*Excludes Maori

Figure 4.9 Average annual mortality rates per 100 000 population for multiple sclerosis from various countries, 1951–58, adjusted for age to the 1950 US population. Redrawn from data of Goldberg and Kurland[15]

inclusion of Portugal in this 'middle' grouping may be questioned. There are no morbidity data for Portugal. In Spain the crude death-rate from MS for 1951–57 was recorded at 1·9 per 100 000[16], but this is clearly an over-estimate, as deaths from cerebral arteriosclerosis were included. Whether this holds true for the Portuguese rate as well is conjectural.

The rate from Iceland (0·3) is low, but would be based on only three deaths in the 5 years considered; Iceland will be found below, page 112, to be of high frequency for MS. Iceland should probably have been included in the Scandinavian countries, where it belongs, but I put it between Europe and the Americas, where it is located.

Within Europe there seems a sharp drop to the rates for the Mediterranean basin. South American rates would seem rather low, as are those for US non-whites (of whom more than 90% are negro). The Asian and African rates are clearly the lowest recorded.

PREVALENCE STUDIES

Community surveys to ascertain the prevalence of multiple sclerosis in varied parts of the world were largely pioneered by Leonard Kurland, then of the US Public Health Service at the National Institutes of Health. The methodology he set down in the early 1950s has become widely accepted, and almost all of the better quality surveys follow his rules. If Hirsch of Germany may be called the father of geographical pathology, perhaps Dr Kurland is the father of neuroepidemiology. As most workers know, he has been continuing his work at the Mayo Clinic for the last decade or so.

Before the Second World War, there were *almost* no proper prevalence surveys for MS. Since the war they have been burgeoning, and I have recently tried to put some order into these studies, which now number somewhere near 170—probably more than those of all other neurological diseases combined[17, 18].

When first reviewed some years ago, it was my impression that prevalence rates for multiple sclerosis divided the world into three areas, like all Gaul, comprising high, medium, and low prevalence regions[19]. This impression was based on the less than 50 works then available, and was contrary to the prevailing opinion of a rather smooth relationship of MS frequency with geographical latitude.

(a) *Prevalence by latitude*—The prevalence studies available for western Europe are summarized in Figure 4.10, as a correlation of the rates with north latitude. The numbers refer to specific surveys described elsewhere[17, 18]. The solid circles are what I have considered Class A studies, as representing proper surveys with well-defined and comparable methodology and diagnostic standards. Those I rated Class B (open circles) are good surveys but have reason(s) why they are not fully comparable to those of Class A. Surveys denoted by diamonds are Class C. These have obvious defects which make them likely to be unreliable, and they should not be taken at face value. Open boxes are Class E surveys, which represent an *estimate* of the

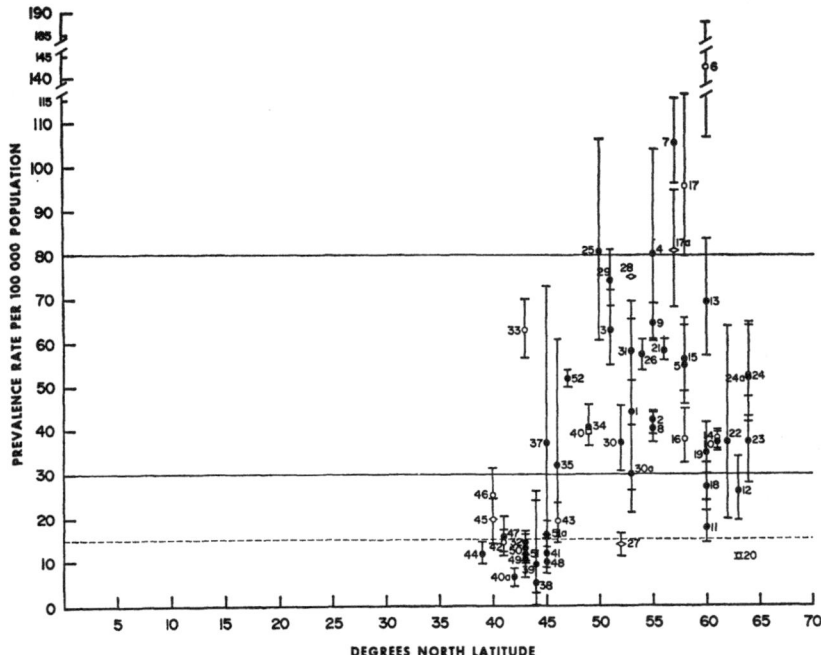

Figure 4.10 Prevalence rates per 100 000 population for probable multiple sclerosis in western Europe, correlated with geographical latitude. Numbers identify the specific survey in Kurtzke[17, 18]. Solid circles represent Class A studies, open circles Class B, diamonds Class C, and squares Class E. Vertical bars define 95% confidence intervals of the rates (from Kurtzke[17])

prevalence from the ratios of MS to ALS cases in series from hospitals. Relative frequencies from hospitals appear in a later section below.

The vertical bars define the 95% confidence intervals for each rate. What this means is that, if the cited rate arose from a random sample of its parent universe, the 'true' rate for this universe would be found to lie within this interval 19 times out of 20. Therefore it might be better were the bar to be taken to represent the likely prevalence for the community rather than the locus of the symbol, which was the actual rate as measured. At least, one should not pay too much attention to the precise digits, nor to minor differences among them.

It seems to me that MS in western Europe is distributed according to latitude within two clusters: a high-frequency zone with prevalence of some 30–80 per 100 000 population (or more) extending from about 43° to 65° north latitude; and a medium-frequency zone with prevalence of some 5–25 per 100 000, and mostly 10–15, from about 38° to 46°.

Similar data for eastern Europe are drawn in Figure 4.11. Note the relative paucity of good quality studies. There still seems to me to be a disposition of the rates into the same two frequency zones; high from about 45° to 65°

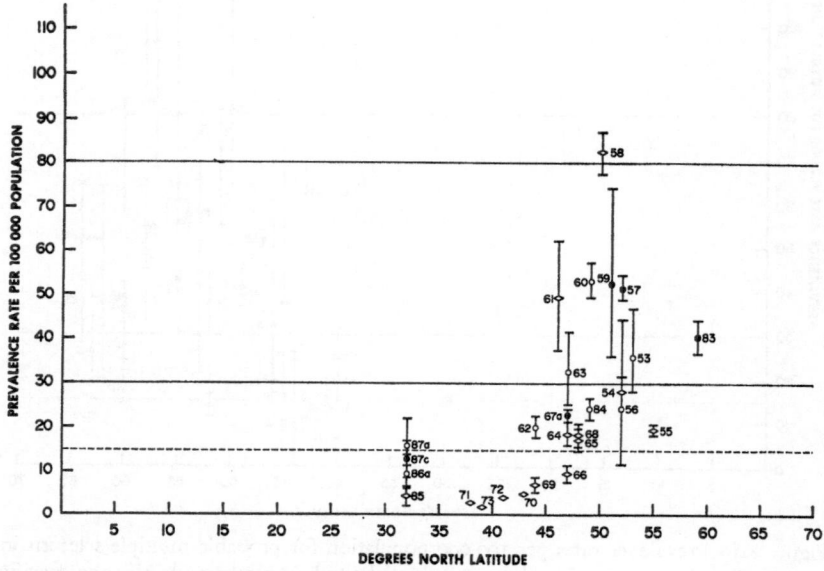

Figure 4.11 Prevalence rates per 100 000 population for probable multiple sclerosis in eastern Europe and Israel, correlated with geographical latitude, as in Figure 4.10 (from [17])

and medium from 32° to perhaps 50° or so. Certainly though in eastern Europe, latitude alone does not serve fully to separate the two risk areas.

The mortality data for Europe (Figure 4.9) had also indicated a decrease in the south versus the north. Survey number 40a in Figure 4.10 is from Spain and 41–51a are from Italy. The Scandinavian rates (numbers 10–24a) need more elaboration, but there there is support in nationwide prevalence studies for the lower death rates reported, as will be mentioned below. Iceland has numbers 23–24a and is clearly high, despite the mortality rate.

Prevalence surveys from the Americas are denoted in Figure 4.12. Here we see all three risk zones: high frequency from 37° to 52°, medium frequency from 30° to 33°, and low frequency (prevalence less than 5 per 100 000) from 12° to 19° and from 63° to 67° north latitude. The conterminous United States and southern Canada are represented by all the surveys from 88–119a, except for numbers 106 (Greenland), 109 (Jamaica), 113 (Alaska), 117 (Netherland Antilles), and 118 (Mexico City). The prevalence

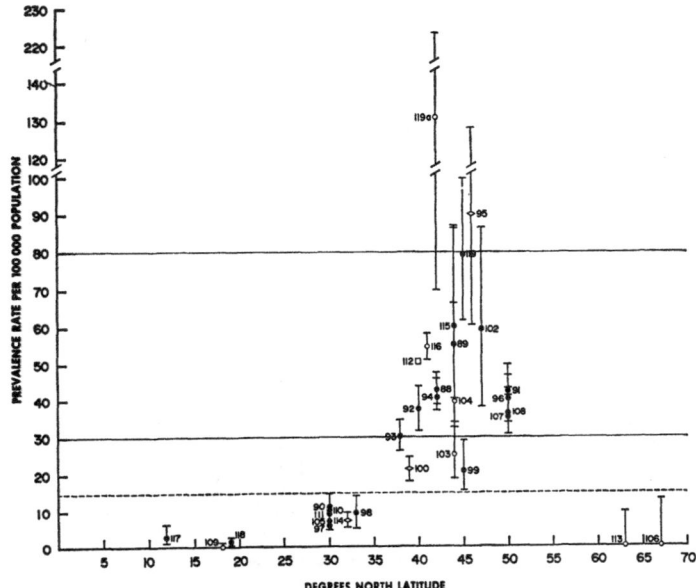

Figure 4.12 Prevalence rates per 100 000 population for probable multiple sclerosis in the Americas, correlated with geographical latitude, as in Figure 4.10 (from Kurtzke [17])

rates for the northern United States and southern Canada are quite similar to the high-frequency rates of western Europe. The lower death-rate for the United States would thus reflect the inclusion of two separate risk areas. By inference then, northern Canada may also be low, but there are no data. The few rates available for Latin America support their even lower death rates, but we have absolutely no population-based information from South America, where some of the death-rates were rather high.

Thus, within *parts* of the United States and Canada, the reported prevalence is as high as in western Europe, while the remainder of the rates in these lands match those of the Mediterranean basin.

Australia–New Zealand comprise principally a high frequency zone for 44–34° south latitude, and a medium frequency region for 33–15° south (Figure 4.13). The recorded rates which are considered high though are toward the lower end of this range.

Rates from Asia and the Pacific in the northern hemisphere are all low, except that Hawaii (numbers 145, 146) is likely to be in the medium zone (Figure 4.14). These study sites extend from 8° to 47° north latitude. In the southern hemisphere with surveys from 30° to 6° south, all rates from Asia and Africa are also low, except for English-speaking native-born whites of

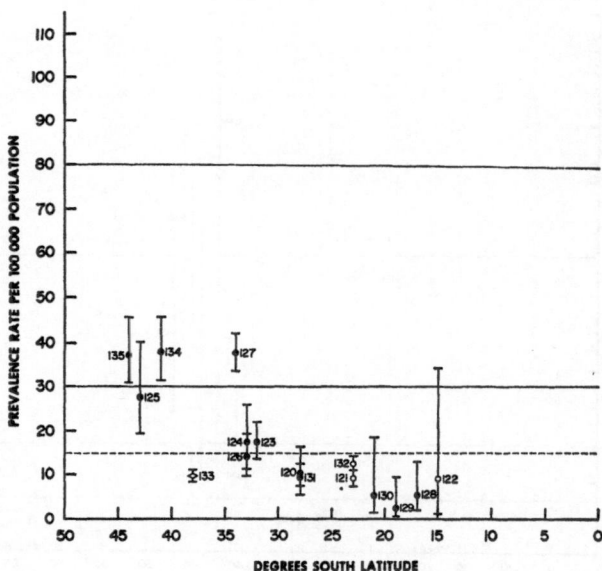

Figure 4.13 Prevalence rates per 100 000 population for probable multiple sclerosis in Australia and New Zealand, correlated with geographical latitude, as in Figure 4.10 (from Kurtzke [17])

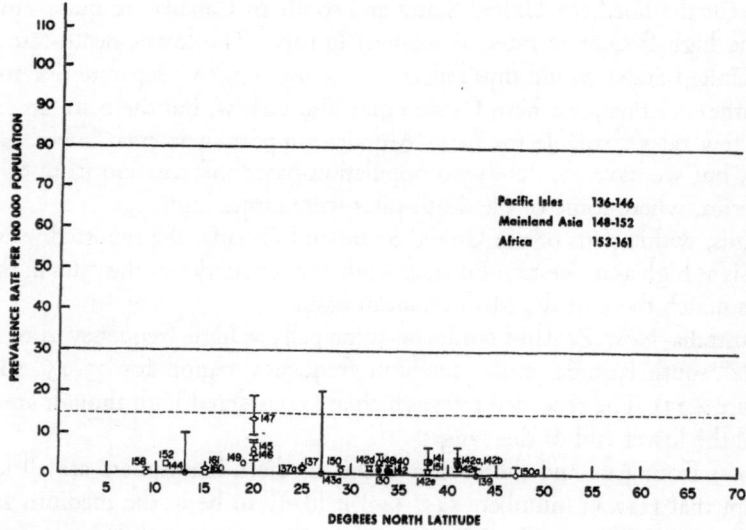

Figure 4.14 Prevalence rates per 100 000 population for probable multiple sclerosis in Asia and Africa (northern hemisphere), correlated with geographical latitude, as in Figure 4.10 (from Kurtzke [17])

South Africa (number 156), as seen in Figure 4.15. These rates would support the death data of Figure 4.9.

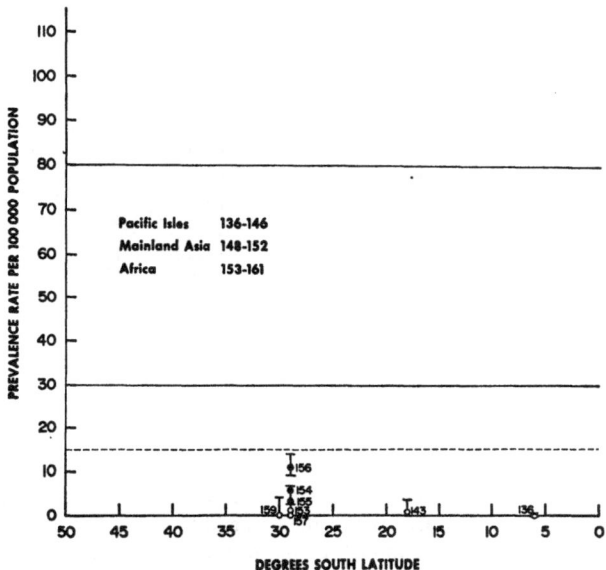

Figure 4.15 Prevalence rates per 100 000 population for probable multiple sclerosis in Asia and Africa (southern hemisphere) correlated with geographical latitude, as in Figure 4.10 (from Kurtzke [17])

(b) *Prevalence by longitude and latitude*—While there seems to be then a reasonably clear separation into three zones of MS, latitude alone appears to be an insufficient criterion both in Europe and America; and in Asia and the Pacific, latitude does not seem to be a factor at all.

Figure 4.16 represents an attempt to describe the rates in Europe by both latitude and longitude. Parallels of latitude, with open numbers, run diagonally upward from left to right, while meridians of longitude, with solid numbers, run diagonally downward. The prevalence surveys are again denoted according to quality with the same symbols, and designated by the same numbers as in Figures 4.10 and 4.11. The prevalence rates themselves are measured by the height of the vertical bars, and the locus of each study is at the foot of each bar.

The areas of special interest are the grids between 50° and 40° north latitude and 0° and 20° east longitude. There is a sharp drop in MS prevalence within these grids, along an arc that extends from about 50° N, 20° E,

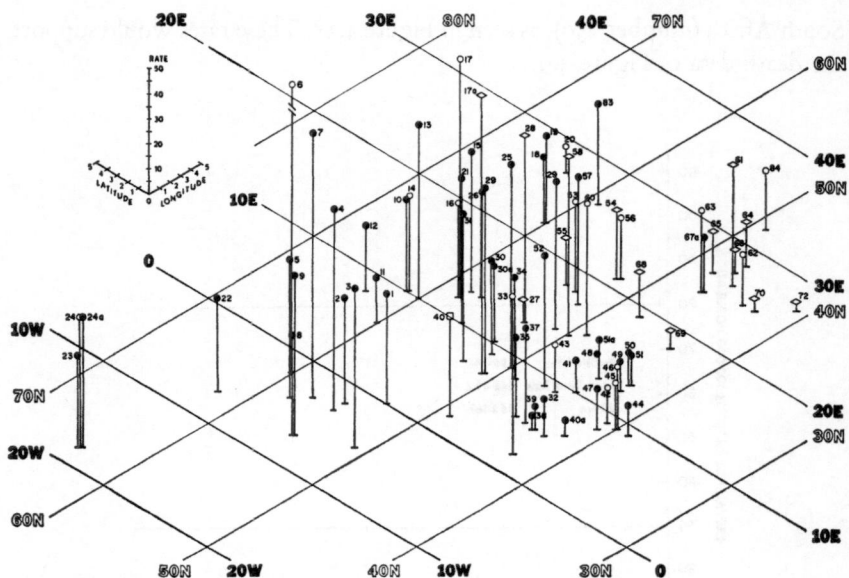

Figure 4.16 Prevalence rates per 100 000 population for probable multiple sclerosis in Europe, correlated with geographical latitude and longitude. Symbols are as in Figure 4.10. Locus of each study is at the base of the bar, and the height of the bar is the prevalence rate with the scale in the top left corner of the figure (from Kurtzke [18])

through some 47° N, 10° E and 45° N, 5° E, toward about 40° N, 0° E. The division eastward is not clearly defined, and *may* extend well north of 50° N, 30° E.

To either side of this dividing line, most of the rates are of similar magnitude within their own region: high to the north and distinctly lower to the south.

We can simplify the presentation considerably if we accept prevalence rates of 30–80 per 100 0000 population (or more) as representing *high-frequency MS*, those of 5–25 as *medium-frequency*, and those under 5 per 100 000 as *low-frequency MS*. We can further group the studies into 'good' (Class A, B, E) and 'poor' surveys, the latter including not only Class C but also several relative frequencies (percentages) from hospitals within the USSR.

In this manner we can define the frequency of multiple sclerosis for Europe and Africa in one figure (Figure 4.17). Note the western European cluster of high rates surrounded on three sides by medium rates (and on the fourth by water). The sparse African and southwestern Asian rates are low, save for Israel and the one ethnic group of South Africa, which are medium.

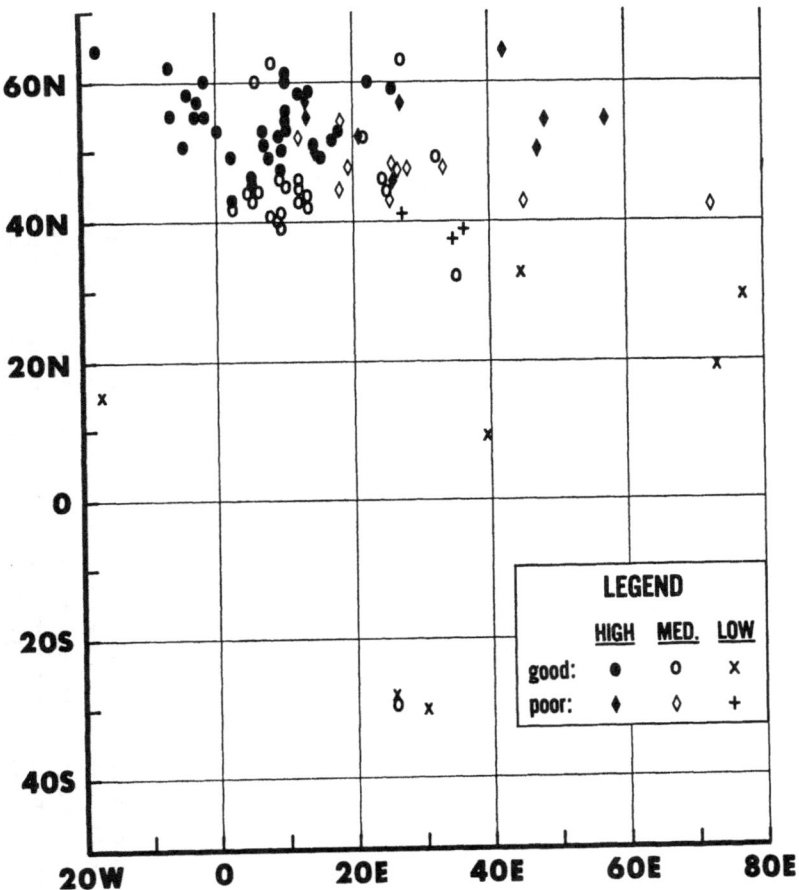

Figure 4.17 MS frequency by latitude and longitude in Europe and Africa. Ovals and xs represent 'good' studies (Class A, B, E), and vertical diamonds and +s 'poor' studies (Class C, %). Solid symbols are high frequency MS survey sites, open symbols are medium frequency, and xs and +s are low frequency as defined by prevalence rate ranges. Only one study per site is plotted (from Kurtzke[18])

More geographical orientation is provided by plotting the surveys for Europe directly on the map (Figure 4.18). Here solid squares represent *all* high-frequency surveys regardless of quality, and open (actually shaded) squares represent all medium ones. The triangles reflect rates which may be medium or low, but are likely to be medium.

The heavily shaded part of the map defines the high-frequency MS zone of Europe, and the dotted portion defines the medium-frequency MS band.

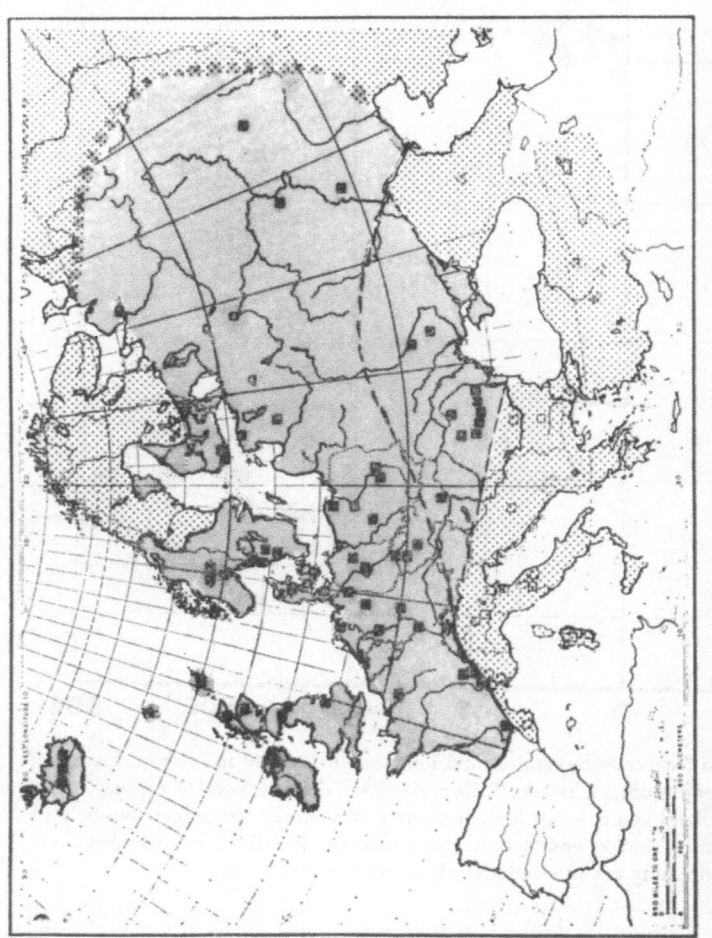

Figure 4.18 MS prevalence bands of Europe with survey sites spotted on the map. Heavy shading represents high frequency MS (prevalence 30 or more per 100 000); dotted shading medium frequency MS (prevalence 5 to 25); no European area is low (prevalence 0–4). Solid squares are high frequency rates, open squares medium frequency, and triangles likely but not surely medium frequency. Dashed line may be the proper dividing line between high and medium, but data are insufficient for definition. Surveys are listed regardless of quality.

Within the heavily shaded portion the dashed line may be the actual separa-tion of high- from medium-risk areas, but the data are inconclusive[18]. It may be seen from prior figures that many of the open squares in the shaded part are in fact Class C studies.

Not too apparent on the southwestern coast of Norway (dotted) are two open squares which reflect good surveys. The configuration for the remainder of Scandinavia will be documented below. The eastward (and northern) extension of the high-risk zone across the USSR is poorly defined, as in fact is the further eastward delimitation of its medium-risk area.

In the same fashion as in Figure 4.17, we can describe MS distribution in the Americas (Figure 4.19). Again the high-frequency zone is bounded by a

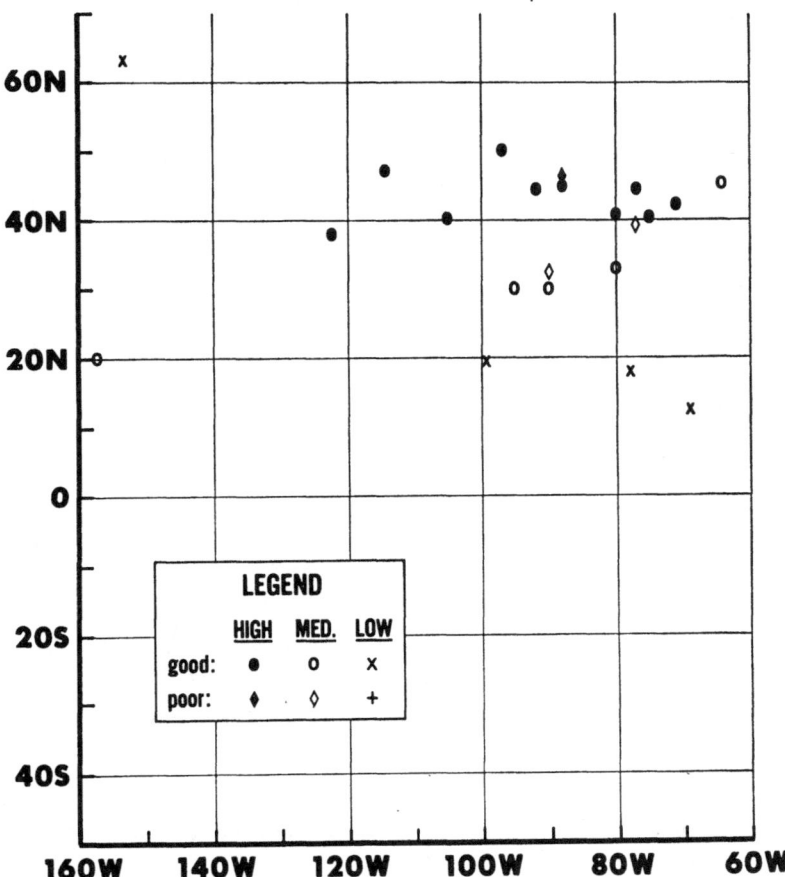

Figure 4.19 MS frequency by latitude and longitude in the Americas, as in Figure 4.17 (from Kurtzke[18])

medium-frequency area (or water), which in turn gives way to a low-risk zone. Note too how many fewer studies than in Figure 4.12 there are when only one per survey site is plotted.

The rates from Asia are spotted in like manner in Figure 4.20. The high-risk 'band' is New Zealand, southern Australia—and ocean. To the top left is

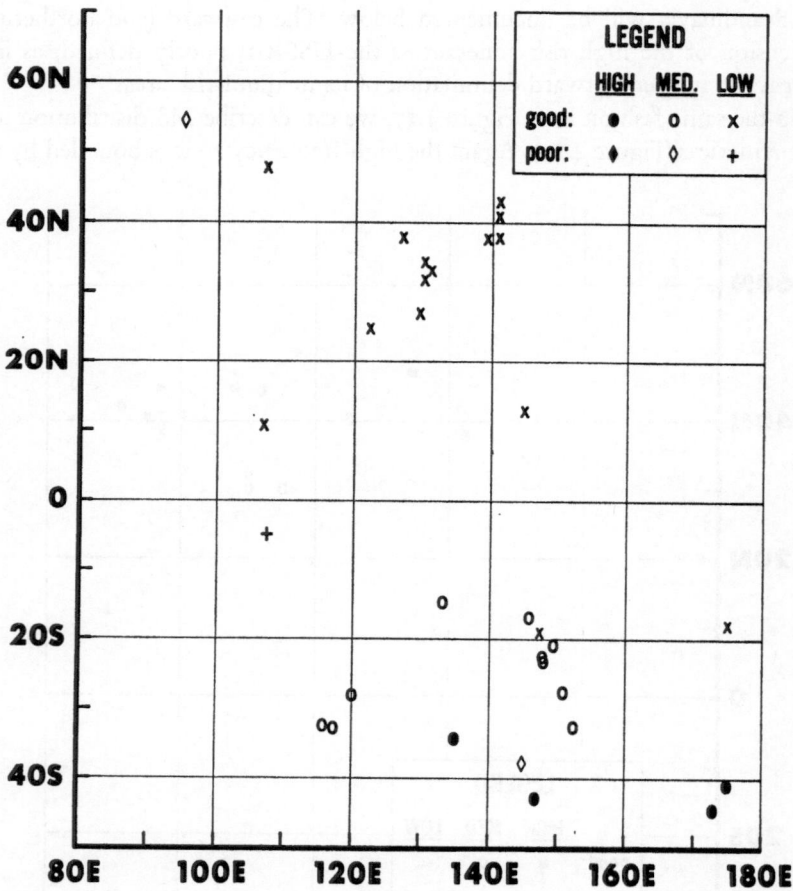

Figure 4.20 MS frequency by latitude and longitude in Asia, as in Figure 4.17 (from Kurtzke[18])

what may be the eastern limit of the Eurasian medium-frequency zone. All other medium-frequencies are from Australia, and the remainder of Asia is low.

(c) *Clustering*—When the entirety of a single country is surveyed at a single time by a single team, then it is possible to describe the geographical distribution across the land in some detail. Such surveys have been accomplished for Norway, Denmark, Sweden, Switzerland, Northern Ireland, northern Scotland, the Netherlands, Iceland and Finland. Repeated surveys covering different generations of patients (and doctors) have been accomplished for Norway, Denmark and Switzerland.

While the distribution within Northern Ireland was uniform and that within the Netherlands and Iceland rather equivocal, in all other countries surveyed there were very highly significant deviations from homogeneity, and the high-rate areas tended to be contiguous, forming clusters or foci. The differences in the rates between the highest and lowest regions were in the order of 6-fold on the average, and thus the variations would seem of biological as well as statistical significance[20, 21]. Essentially the same clusters were found when small geographical units rather than the large counties were used as the units for testing[22]. In Denmark the clustering was across middle Jutland on to Fyn, the island next to mid-Jutland; in Switzerland the concentration was in the northwestern part of the country. The MS distributions were not related to availability of medical facilities, including hospitals, hospital beds and admissions, all physicians, and neural specialists[23].

Not only was there clustering of MS, but in the lands resurveyed a generation apart, there was a very strong correlation between the early and the later distributions, with coefficients of correlation of about 0·8[24, 25]. In Figure 4.21 the rates by county from each survey are correlated for the three countries with such data: Denmark, Switzerland, and Norway. Each county rate is expressed as its percentage of its own national (mean) prevalence rate at each survey.

With this evidence of stability over time, it was thought appropriate to compare studies from neighbouring countries to determine whether any broader pattern might be apparent. In this fashion, the high-frequency MS areas appeared to describe one single *Fennoscandian focus*[25, 26b]. With the smallest test-units available, this focus extended from the waist and southeastern mountain plains of Norway eastward across the inland lake area of southern Sweden, then across the Bay of Bothnia to southwestern Finland, and then back to Sweden in the region of Umeå (Figure 4.22).

(*d*) *Comments*—This clustering, as well as the broader geographical distributions already considered, mean to me that the occurrence of MS is intrinsically related to geography, and therefore that MS is an acquired, exogenous, *environmental* disease.

While perhaps agreeing with the final phrase as not unlikely, eminent authorities have not been overly impressed with this evidence for clustering in MS. Acheson[27] thought the Fennoscandian focus to be 'much more

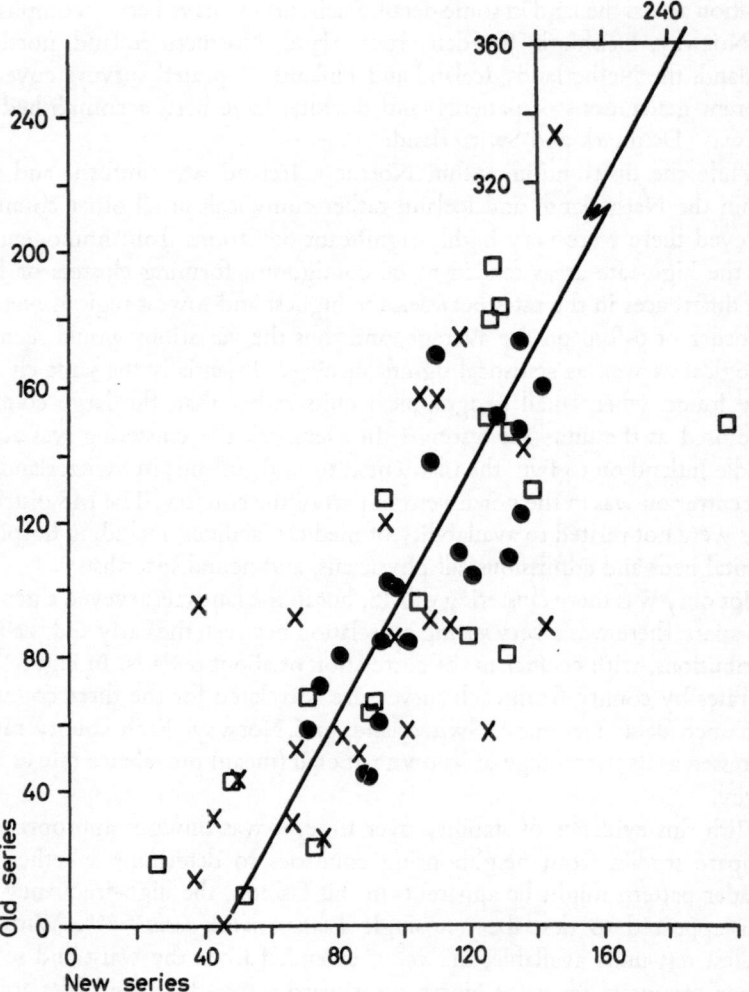

Figure 4.21 Correlation of the distributions of MS by county between old series and new series of prevalence surveys of three countries, each covering different generations of patients: Denmark (solid circles); Switzerland (xs); Norway (open squares). Each county rate is expressed as the percentage of its respective national (mean) rate (from Kurtzke[25])

problematical'; and Kurland[28] stated that 'convincing proof of focalization must await the recognition of some meaningful pattern', by which he meant a biological explanation for the clusters. And this is most definitely *not* available to date.

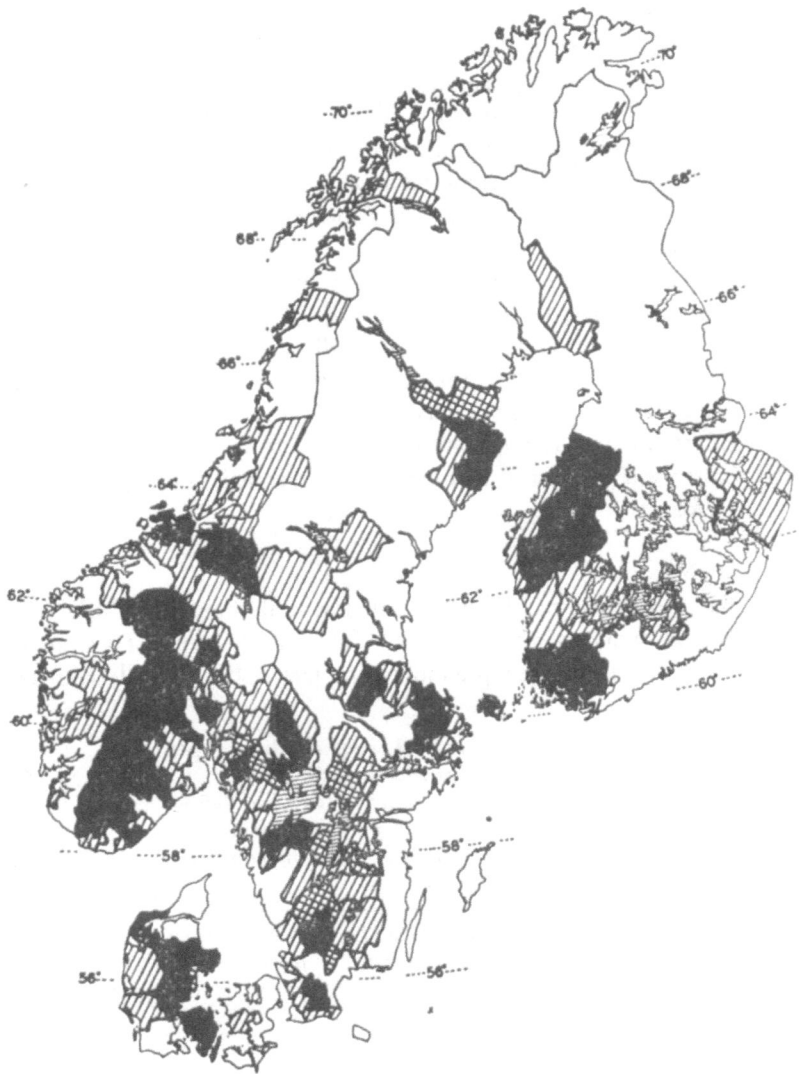

Figure 4.22 Distribution of MS in Fennoscandia. Areas significantly above their respective national means ($\chi_a^2 > 4\cdot0$) are in solid black; those high of dubious significance
(χ_a^2 $2\cdot0$–$4\cdot0$) are cross-hatched; those insignificantly high ($\chi_a^2 < 2\cdot0$) are diagonal-lined;
those below the national mean are unshaded. Unit boundaries are omitted. Data represent
cumulative death rates within 104 small units of Norway (1951–65); prevalence rates
from hospital cases within 106 small units of Sweden (1925–34); disability prevalence
rates within 20 hospital districts of Finland (1964); and childhood prevalence rates within
23 counties for the national series of Denmark (1949). Fine horizontal shading represents
lakes in Sweden and Finland (from Kurtzke[25])

The incorporation of two zones of MS frequency in Scandinavia would be a likely explanation for the lower death-rates recorded in Figure 4.9 versus their southern neighbours, just as in the United States. Also, as in the United States, the zones would be high and medium. No area of high prevalence for MS has been found appreciably above 65° north latitude. But latitude—as stated above—is far from a sufficient criterion. At 40° north latitude, for example, MS is of high frequency in America, of medium frequency in Europe, and of low frequency in Asia.

In closing this section on prevalence, the curious may wonder why no attention has been paid to incidence rates by geography, since incidence is generally a more meaningful reflection of disease than is prevalence. The reasons, aside from the fact that for MS the prevalence rates are certainly the more stable, are (a) a paucity of such studies; (b) rates from several include persons affected before residence in the survey site which in turn is a diagnostic centre; and (c) most of them are in fact reconstructions derived from prevalence data.

MIGRATION

So far, most of what has been presented would meet with little major argument from workers in the field, aside from the clustering. There are still some who prefer latitude as a predominating factor, but virtually all neuro-

Table 4.3 **Average annual crude death rates per 100 000 population for MS according to birthplaces of foreign-born whites who died in the United States, 1959–61, compared with reported rates for natives of the same countries, 1951–58**[29]

Country of origin	Immigrant rates (United States)	Native rates for country of origin
Ireland	2·9	2·8
Germany	1·6	2·3*
Czechoslovakia	1·5†	2·1
Austria	2·3	2·2
Norway	1·7†	1·7
Canada	1·6	1·0
Sweden	1·7†	1·2
Italy	1·0	0·7
Mexico	0·5†	0·1

* West Germany
† Rate based on less than 20 but more than five deaths in three years

epidemiologists I know are quite agreed that geography is intrinsic to MS, and that MS is most likely an environmental disease. We now enter another aspect wherein many agree on the overall impressions, but differ in interpretations—and wherein the data themselves pose a number of problems. This is migration.

In Table 4.3 are crude death-rates for MS among immigrants to the United States, versus the crude rates for natives of their country of origin[29]. It appears from their similarities that MS patients carry with them the risk of their birthplace—but most of the rates deal with high to high migration sites. Table 4.4 summarizes material on prevalence rates (all ages) among immigrants to and from different MS risk areas[30, 31]. The specific studies are cited in the aforementioned references. The rates are those regardless of age at immigration and of time of clinical onset of MS in reference to migration.

In broad terms, the immigrants do tend to retain the MS risk of their birthplace. 'Risk' is defined according to the same three frequency zones previously discussed. The evidence for risk retention is better for immigrants from high-risk areas to low than is the reverse, where there are in fact almost no data.

Table 4.4 Prevalence rates per 100 000 population for probable MS among native-born and immigrants (modified from [30])

Immigration site according to its own MS risk	Native born	Prevalence rates among Immigrants from risk areas		
		High	Medium	Low
High				
S. Australia	38	37	4	—
Medium				
Perth, W. Aust.	40*	87*	—	—
Perth, W. Aust.	14	22	—	—
W. Australia	10	31	—	—
Queensland	9	15	—	—
Israel	9†	——19†——		6†
Israel (crude rates)	4	33	8	3
Low				
South Africa	6‡	48	15	—
Neth. Antilles	3	59	—	—
Hawaii	5	——35——		—

* Age-specific rate, 40–49 years
† Age-adjusted to 1960 US population
‡ Rate of 3 for Afrikaners and 11 for English-speaking whites

Two points are worth noting. First, in no survey is the rate for immigrants born in high-frequency areas *higher* than that expected of their homelands. This is important when we come to interpretations. Secondly, the migrants to Australia—all but one group from high risk countries—appear to have appreciably lower rates than expected for their homeland. This though is explicable by Australian immigration laws dealing with the disabled; few of these MS migrants would be likely to have had clinical onset—or at least diagnosis—before immigration. In the South African study to be discussed below, about half the European immigrants were symptomatic before their move. Were this to apply to Australia, then the immigrant rates there could perhaps be doubled.

The Israeli data should be considered from the age-adjusted rates, since their several populations have strikingly different age compositions. The European immigrants too include many survivors of the concentration camps of the Second World War, who are a very select group. It *may* be that the Afro-Asian immigrants (low risk) to Israel (medium risk) have an increased frequency over that of their birthplace, but it is really too early to be sure.

Other data on low to high areas are sparse. Dassel[32] recorded three instances of MS among immigrants from Indonesia to Holland. Their onsets were at ages 17, 23, and 25 years, and took place respectively 7, 9, and 8 years after their arrival in the Netherlands. They are probably whites of Dutch origin, but neither this nor the population at risk was provided. Regardless, three cases out of what is likely to be a small migrant group looks impressive.

We have discovered three instances of exacerbating–remitting MS among a series of some 3400 children who were born in Vietnam of Vietnamese mothers and French fathers, and who came to France under the age of 20. At interview in 1975, 80% were age 20–39. The three patients each had clinical onset about 15 years after immigration, which for them was under the age of ten. Their crude prevalence rate for MS was 89 per 100 000, with a 95% confidence interval of 18–260. Since the group is still at risk for MS, adjusting this rate for age would be misleading. The age-specific prevalence rate was 169 per 100000 age 20–29 (confidence interval 35–494). It appears then that these half-Oriental Asians have a significantly higher rate than had they stayed home, but whether it is really as high as expected in France is not known at present[33]. Further evidence on migration appears with considerations of age.

(a) *Age of migration*—If one grants there is to some degree a retention of birthplace risk in MS for migrants from high to low-frequency areas, the next question would be whether this is dependent on age. If this risk is acquired at or near birth (or is innate), then birthplace alone and time of birth would be the critical point.

In the United States, death-rates for MS are distributed so that the states to the north of 37° north latitude have twice the rates of those to the south. One should see the mirror image of this distribution for those who exchange risk areas (between north and south) between birth and death, if birth is the

Table 4.5 Migration in multiple sclerosis: ratios* of death rates for residence at birth and death in high and low MS risk areas of Norway and United States[29]

Place of death	Place of birth			
	US (1959–61)		Norway (1951–65)	
	High	Low	High	Low
High	1·00*	0·68	1·00*	0·57
Low	0·87	0·46	0·59	0·44

* High/High = 1·00

critical time. In fact though, one sees almost an *obliteration* of the north–south difference when such migrants are considered, as illustrated in Table 4.5. In the US the ratios of Table 4.5 are also the actual death-rates. Similar data

Table 4.6 Multiple sclerosis: mean annual death rates according to birthplace, California and Washington, ten years to 1964*

Group	Death rate†	
	California	Washington
US white, born in state	0·9 (0·8–1·0)	1·5 (1·2–1·8)
US migrants from north‡	0·8 (0·7–0·9)	1·3 (1·1–1·5)
US migrants from south§	0·4 (0·4–0·5)	0·5 (0·3–1·0)

* Recalculated data of Detels, R., et al.: *J. Chronic Dis.*, **25**, 3, 1972[31]

† Per 100 000 population, adjusted to age and sex (95% confidence interval)

‡ New England, West North Central, East North Central, Pacific, Middle Atlantic census regions

§ East South Central, West South Central, South Atlantic census regions

are also found for Norway. Regardless of direction, those who change risk areas no longer differ significantly as to their MS death-rates.

However the death-rate for US southern-born MS who had died in the north (0·68) was significantly higher than that for the southern-born who died in the south (0·46). Thus it would also appear that moving north does increase the risk of MS.

Our US data were limited to seven of the nine US census regions which lie in the eastern two-thirds of the country, since the Mountain and Pacific regions extend from Canada to Mexico. Detels et al.[34] provide additional information for the west coast (Table 4.6). Here the small numbers of southern migrants show no significant difference when they move north, but the northern migrants to California have a significantly lower death-rate than those who moved to Washington. Similar findings are seen for the prevalence study that Detels (personal communication) has been conducting there.

Table 4.7 Residence by tier in United States at birth, at induction and in service, expressed as case-control ratios, for MS patients in the United States Army in the Second World War[29]

| Tier | Time of residence | | |
	Birth	Induction	In service*
Northern	1·45	1·38	1·03
Middle	0·86	0·86	0·99
Southern	0·75	0·80	1·07
Total	1·01	1·00	1·03
No. of residences	373	388	578
P	<0·01	<0·01	>0·10

* Residences in service prior to clinical onset only

Therefore, the critical time for risk acquisition in MS is well after birth regardless of birthplace. In Table 4.7 are case-control ratios for residences among our US Army series of 'definite + probable MS'[10, 29]. The very clear difference in MS risk (as defined by the ratios) that was present for residence at birth or at entry into service had totally disappeared in the rather short interval between entry and clinical onset. We cannot differentiate between birth and induction residences since they were the same place for about 85% of the men. The inference here is that the critical age in risk of MS is well before age 20 or so.

From ages of maximal clustering of MS in Denmark and several other features, it was 'tentatively concluded that the actual onset of MS appears to take place on the average between the ages of 10 and 15 years, and that there is probably a "latent" or "incubation" period of some 20 years before the onset of clinical symptomatology'[35] Included in this assessment was an ingenious approach to the problem by Poskanzer and his colleagues[36]. They considered

Table 4.8 Childhood onset and 'incubation' in multiple sclerosis: common exposure periods in 16 sibling-pairs with MS in Northumberland–Durham (adapted from [36])

Mean age at clinical onset	Mean of individual average ages of common exposure	Mean total years of common residence	Mean years of 'incubation'
33·8	12·9*	19·9*	20·5
33·8	12·2†	18·3†	21·3

* To end of common residence or clinical onset of second case if earlier

† To end of common residence or clinical onset of first case if earlier

that, for siblings both of whom had MS, any common exposure would likely have occurred while they were living together (Table 4.8). The period of cohabitation before onset averaged almost 20 years, and the mean age of such common exposure was 12 or 13 years of age, with a mean 'incubation' period then of some 20 years. The mean *minimal* exposure time was six years

Table 4.9 MS prevalence rates, all ages, per 100 000 immigrants in 1960 according to age at immigration (AAI) for northern European immigrants to Republic of South Africa (modified from [38])

AAI	UK	all
0–14	12·8	12·9
15–19	66·1	81·1
20–24	31·8	31·3
25–29	59·4	58·4
(20–29)	(45·7)	(44·9)
30–39	58·2	52·4
40–49	57·7	62·4
50+	70·5	80·8
N	65	114

to the first case and 16 years to the second[35]. About all these means though the range was considerable.

In one study at least, we were able to define a very specific age that was critical for the risk of MS, and this concerned a survey of European immigrants to South Africa[37]. For such immigrants, the MS prevalence rate, adjusted to a population of all ages, is provided in Table 4.9 according to age at immigration[38]. For immigration under age 15 there is the same medium prevalence rate as for the native-born English-speaking South Africans[39]. But for all older age groups, the prevalence is about what one would expect from their high-risk homelands. This change is sharp, as seen from Figure 4.23, where each MS immigrant is represented by his own horizontal bar. The height of the bar on the y axis reflects his age at immigration, and the length of the bar denotes the number of years between immigration and clinical onset. The diagonal is the average age of clinical onset for the entire

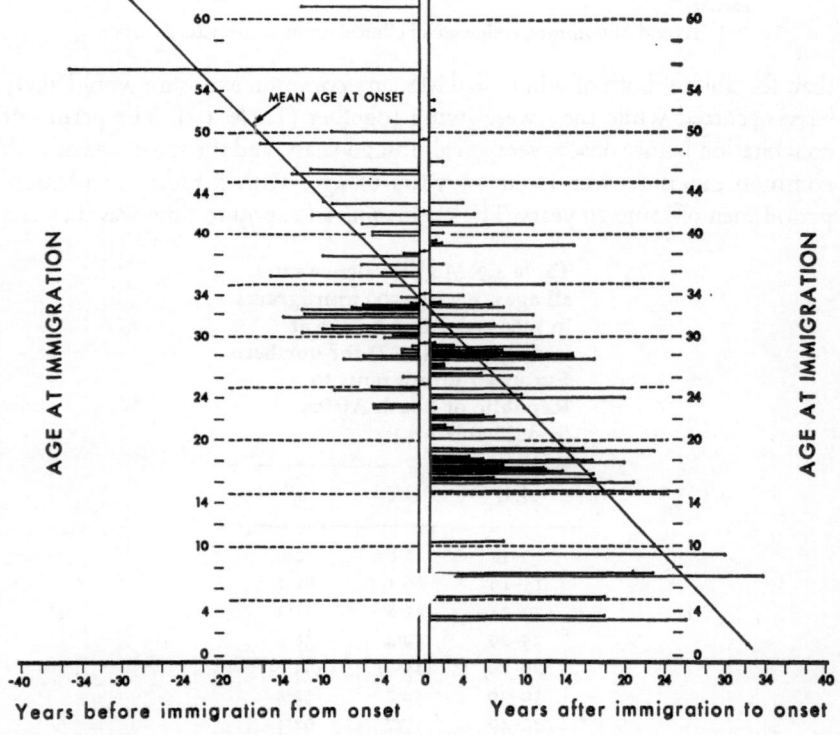

Figure 4.23 Age at immigration (y axis) and years from immigration to clinical onset (x axis) for each of 114 northern European immigrants to South Africa ascertained as multiple sclerosis in 1960 prevalence survey (from Kurtzke[30])

group. It is clear that there were very few immigrants who developed MS if they arrived under age 15, as opposed to the large number who arrived beyond age 15. In this series then, age 15 was critical for the acquisition of MS among those who came from high-risk areas.

Two alternative explanations for this age selectivity have been put forth. The first is that arrival before age 15 in a low-frequency area protects one from MS. The other is that by age 15, one has already acquired the disease in high-risk areas, and his residence thereafter is irrelevant to its clinical expression. To define which of these is correct could well give us the answer as to what indeed is this disease we call multiple sclerosis. I believe that for those born in high-risk areas the disease is acquired near the age of puberty, and geography thereafter plays no role. What the *limits* of susceptibility are, such as for migrants *to* high-risk regions, is not yet clear. Nor is it clear—despite all the above—that the age of acquisition *or* the 'incubation' period is so sharply delimited. But disease onset well before clinical manifestations does seem highly likely.

Predilections for MS

FAMILIAL FREQUENCY

For a number of years it has been well known that more cases of MS appeared within families than one might expect, and not all of them could be attributed to inclusion of the heredofamilial ataxias. The frequency of multiple cases in families within published series is in the order of 6% with a range of 2 to 17%. Among these series the frequency of MS among sibs and parents was about 1 and 0·5% respectively. When these last are corrected for birth rates and likely survival, we can estimate the prevalence to be in the order of 400 per 100000 for siblings and 200 per 100000 for parents. If one ignored the selection bias of most of the series, these rates would be about eight and four times the expectations for the general population in areas considered[40].

Within Hyllested's[11] national prevalence survey of Denmark, there had been 152 familial cases among 2731 MS. The living familial MS at prevalence day included 44 sibs and 10 parents. The prevalence rate for sibs was 362 per 100000 (44/12 146) and for parents 183 (10/5460), being respectively six and three times the concurrent prevalence of 64 per 100000 for the general population. Thus it is likely that there is truly an increased risk of MS among siblings of the affected; some reservations may still be made as to their parents, though a modest excess does seem probable for them as well.

The explanation for the increase again brings up the nature–nurture controversy. As to the genetic aspects, the proponents point to either multifactorial (polygenic) inheritance or autosomal recessive inheritance with reduced penetrance. Unbiased data on twins, which might settle this point, are unavailable. They further indicate the rarity of conjugal MS (which seems to be about that for the general population) as an argument favouring a genetic influence. This last argument though is not valid if childhood onset and long latency are the fact. My own view has been that a genetic factor is *unnecessary* to consider in seeking an explanation for the cause (not that there cannot be one), which cause to me lies in the environment.

The recent evidence that, especially in northwestern Europe and the United States, there may be immune response genes associated with MS has re-awakened the controversy. Jersild *et al.*[41] have recently reviewed the data. The major histocompatibility system determinants (MHS) in man are the HLA-A, B and C serum antigens and the lymphocyte-defined (HLA-D) cell antigens. In these lands, HLA-A3 and HLA-A7 are about twice as common in MS as in controls, with several others of their HLA-A and HLA-B series also high. HLA-A3 is usually linked with HLA-B7, and the latter is thought the major factor in MS.

With the mixed lymphocyte culture (MLC) method (HLA-D), the HLA-DW2 determinant (linked in half the population with the HLA-A3, HLA-A7 haplotype) was found to be some five times as frequent among MS as among controls (though with small numbers). Somewhere between $\frac{1}{2}$ and $\frac{3}{4}$ of MS cases were found to carry HLA-DW2 as opposed to perhaps one-fifth of normals.

Whether these determinants (or the HLAs which are low) are linked to an 'MS susceptibility' (or an 'MS resistance') gene is being actively pursued. Further discussions on this fascinating topic are elsewhere in this volume (Chapter 2). This is an area which has stimulated those involved not only in the genetic but also in the immunological aspects of MS—including the therapeutic.

We should recall though that no one pattern is unique to MS, and in different parts of the world very different 'immune response genes' may be found associated with this disease. I do not believe that the evidence so far warrants any erasures in the previous sections of this chapter.

RACE AND COLOUR

While the histocompatibility antigens may still be deemed *sub judice* as to the individual, they should also perhaps be considered as well in terms of 'macrogenetics' or 'population genetics'.

As recently as 1970, there was 'uncertainty as to selection by race'[28], independent of geography for MS. Within the Army series noted above, negroes were about half as frequent among the MS as service-wide proportions would suggest, regardless of birthplace or induction residence[10].

We have recently been investigating a much larger series of all US veterans who are 'service-connected' for MS. Service-connection requires evidence of symptomatology of MS either during military service or within seven years of discharge from service. Thus, for Second World War veterans, we have in essence a ten-year-incidence material of nationwide composition. These cases we have matched with *military* controls (before they were ill.) The original matching provided 5318 pairs of cases and controls, with over 4200 from the Second World War, some 900 from the Korean War, and over 200 from both wars[42]. The full paper is still in preparation, but Table 4.10 shows case-control ratios for the major sex and race groups. There is a

Table 4.10 Multiple sclerosis: case-control ratios by sex and race according to tier of residence at induction, for veterans of the Second World War* (from [42])

Sex and race	Total	North	Middle	South
		Tier of induction		
Total (ratios)	1·00	1·38	1·01	0·53
White female	1·91	2·71	1·94	0·78
White male	1·04	1·38	1·04	0·57
Black male	0·40	0·55 –	0·50	0·29
Other male	0·29	0·27†	0·11†	0·33
Total (case/control)	4401/4391	1924/1395	1857/1834	620/1162
White female	162/85	84/31	60/31	18/23
White male	4097/3943	1819/1322	1736/1677	542/944
Black male	120/303	17/31	58/116	45/156
Other male	17/59	3/11	1/9	13/39

* Includes those who also served in Korean conflict
† Unstable due to small numbers (case + control < 20)

clear excess of females among the whites and a clear deficit of black males, regardless of geography. The ratios for black males are about the same as we had previously found with the much smaller sample and without matched controls.

Further detail on the 'other' males, those who were neither white nor black, is provided in Table 4.11. The apparent deficit for Mexican-Americans (6/10) is more likely a reflection of geography than of race. On the other hand, while the numbers are too small for confidence, they *suggest* a paucity of MS cases among Amerindians (3/8) and Japanese-Americans (2/4) regardless of birthplace.

Table 4.11 Multiple sclerosis: case control ratios for
'other' males (neither white nor black) by birthplace
and race, for veterans of the Second World War,
and/or Korean War (from [42])

Birthplace and race	Ratio	Case/control
Conterminous US	0·48	11/23* (N 6/12 S 5/11)†
Amerindian	0·38	3/8 (N 3/6 S 0/2)
Mexican-Sp. Am.	0·60	6/10 (N 1/1 S 5/9)
Japanese	0·50	2/4 (N 2/4 S 0/0)
(All white male)	(1·04)	— (N 1·2 S 0·6)
Mexico, Central Am.		
Mexican-Sp. Am.	0·00	0/5
Puerto Rico		
Puerto Rican	0·38	6/16
Hawaii		
Japanese	0·00	0/10
other	0·00	0/5
China		
Chinese	0·00	0/4
Philippines, SE Asia		
Filipino	0·00	0/9
other	0·00	0/1

   * One Filipino control included
   † Ratios of cases to controls for those born in northern
and middle states (N) or in southern states (S)

The low ratios for all servicemen born outside the conterminous United
States may reflect either race or geography, or both. To explore this further
we looked at all foreign-born servicemen regardless of race (Table 4.12). In
Latin America including Puerto Rico, there is no evident difference by race,
but a significant deficit by geography. In Hawaii the deficit is among
Japanese (0/10) and perhaps the Polynesians (0/5), while the single white case
has a single control. In the rest of the Orient there is a significant difference
for Filipinos as well. In these case-control comparisons, the smallest number
which excludes a ratio of 1·0 at the 95% level is 0/6.

From these data, there arises the real possibility of at least a relative protection against MS for Orientals, irrespective of geography. It is said, by the
way, that Japanese have little or no HLA-A3 antigens.

Detel's group in California was unable to find a single case of MS among
12 000 Japanese-Americans in Seattle, Washington, where the native white
prevalence rate was 69 per 100 000. The 95% confidence limit on the rate of

Table 4.12 Multiple sclerosis: case–control ratios according to race and birthplace in selected regions, United States veterans of the Second World War and/or Korean War (from [42])

Region	Ratio	Total	Case/control White	Black	Other
Mexico, Central America	0·14	2/14	1/9	1/–	–/5
Puerto Rico	0·42	14/33	6/14	2/3	6/16
Hawaii	0·06	1/16	1/1	–/–	–/15
Japan, Korea	—	4/–	4/–	–/–	–/–
China	0·00	–/4	–/–	–/–	–/4
Philippines, Southeast Asia	0·00	–/12	–/2	–/–	–/10

0 would be 31 per 100000. There were 8/84000 Japanese-Americans born in Los Angeles for a crude prevalence of 10 per 100 000, significantly lower than the native white rate of 22[43]. The numbers cited here are modified from the abstract based on further data from this group (Detels, personal communication). There is therefore support for their thesis that MS is rare in Japanese-Americans. Detels found no cases of MS among 20000 Japanese immigrants to Seattle or 4000 to Los Angeles.

COMMENT

Thus there is growing evidence for racial predilection in MS. Negroes in the United States have less than half the risk of whites, regardless of geography, and this may be true as well for Amerindians. Japanese from the continental US and Hawaii, and Filipinos from the Philippines are also relatively 'immune', as would be the Bantu of South Africa. *MS, therefore, is the white man's burden.*

Looking back on the geography, we may see that all high-risk areas for MS—and indeed all medium-risk areas as well—are in Europe or in European colonies (like the United States). It would seem then that MS is the *western European disease*, which has been spread to other parts of the world.

'Further work is necessary to see if one can define better the nature and the timing of the spread from Europe to other lands. Unfortunately early information on MS frequency is largely anecdotal. There is some evidence, though, that the distribution of MS in the United States has changed in this century. There is also evidence that the clustering of MS seen in Scandinavia and Switzerland has become less pronounced over time, further suggesting diffusion of the disease[25]. There is also the curious difference in risk between the two groups of native whites of South Africa that requires exploration, but that *could* indicate the establishment of MS as a reasonably common disorder in that land within the past few decades'[18].

Where within Europe the disease originated is sheer conjecture, even should one accept the above. Were I forced to speculate (and not to document), I *might* hazard the guess that MS *could* have originated in Scandinavia, possibly in southern Norway; when, however, is even more tenuous.

Quo vadimus?

Where then are we going in this disease? More precisely, can epidemiology really help define its cause(s)?

The prevailing opinion about MS for much of this century up to the 1950s had been that MS was some sort of allergic (or hypersensitivity, or autoimmune) disease. Thus a bevy of workers have dedicated their lives to EAE (experimental allergic encephalomyelitis). Very few neurologists then thought seriously about an infectious origin, and virologists thought not at all of the disease.

I think it is safe to say that the attention of virologists to MS has been the direct result of the epidemiological studies. Whether this has been a step forward or back remains for the future, but I do believe that the evidence is persuasive that we *are* dealing with an acquired, exogenous, environmental disease, whose acquisition is long before clinical onset in the normal situation. For natives of high-risk areas this acquisition seems to be at adolescence, and one's geographical locale thereafter seems irrelevant.

Aside from the postulate of some unknown protective factor in low-risk areas, two conflicting interpretations to this last exist, as we mentioned above. They are: (a) moving to low-risk areas before adolescence is protection from the disease because it is thereafter acquired as a subclinical illness in low-risk areas; and (b) moving thus is protection because one is too young to have acquired it by then in one's native land. The former demands the disease agent to be rife where it is clinically absent, and the analogy has been with paralytic versus non-paralytic poliomyelitis. The latter requires the disease agent to be located in the same place whether it causes clinical or subclinical involvement.

My vote is for the latter. All the evidence suggests early acquisition—but acquisition well after birth—and the polio analogy demands heavy exposure virtually from birth. I could not fit this concept in with a critical age in adolescence. Further, where naive (unexposed) groups move to endemic areas of illness, they are supposed to be affected much more often than had they stayed in their sporadic-epidemic environments—such as the armed forces in North Africa in the Second World War with their polio epidemics.

This is why attention was drawn above to the somewhat *lower* rates in migrants to low-risk areas than their homeland provides, even though they were distinctly higher than expected for their new land. This was most clear with death-rates.

More importantly, according to this 'subtle' hypothesis (as Acheson called it), migrants from low-risk areas are already protected by having been exposed from birth. *Unless* one demands 'constant exposure from birth to age X' in order to be protected, then any move at age X must be free of increased risk of MS.

There is I think considerable evidence from the death data and modest evidence from the morbidity work that migrants moving from low to high-risk areas *do* indeed increase their chances of having MS. While there are still t's to cross and i's to dot, I therefore continue to favour the 'simple' hypothesis of Acheson—that the cause of the disease is to be found where the disease is seen.

Much more needs to be done in migration studies though; high to low needs more definition as to whether age 15 is truly 'critical'. Alter[45,46] too has suggested this age for Israel and Hawaii, but his numbers were so small as to permit a comparison of immigrants only above and below the age of 15. For migrants over, say, age 30, their appearance in a place may be more the result than the cause of the disease. This was why I paid so much attention to the 15–24 immigration ages in South Africa, and especially those of 15–19. Here there is virtually no basis for migration to be influenced by the disease, and the difference from those below age 15 was marked—and was exactly at 15.

As stated earlier, for migrants the true population at risk according to age at survey and age at migration and age at clinical onset can be very difficult to define, and the choice of denominator—or the type of rate required (incidence, prevalence, death, cumulative risk)—can get very involved. The desired denominator is generally not available from routine sources. In the South African study we had the opportunity also to compare the MS with a population sample surveyed as to radio listening habits, and their immigration patterns did confirm our findings of a paucity of MS among those immigrating below age 15. But with one study we are far from concluding that this precise age is either unique or universal.

As to low-to-high movement and age, there are almost no data. From studies too early (and too small) to be definite, the increased risk seems to begin with moves in the first or second decade of life (our Vietnamese, the Indonesian, for example). Where it ends we don't know.

In addition, migrant studies now must also take into account the confounding effects of the likely racial predilections discussed above.

IS MS AN INFECTION?

There is not space to review other epidemiological evidence on characteristics of MS patients. Many relationships have been posed. Beebe et al.[10] found a positive association with MS for urbanization, education and socioeconomic status independent of geography. There is other evidence as well of a relation with population density. Alter[47] correlated MS distributions positively with sanitary levels and, with the polio analogy, favoured investigating the water in areas of low frequency MS to find the cause. Poskanzer[48] reported histories of tonsillectomy in excess among MS patients versus spouse or nearest sibling. The huge literature on viral and other antibodies, and in particular measles, will not be considered here. The excess for measles at least has been generally acknowledged—and generally discounted as of direct aetiological significance.

But the principal question remains, if MS is an acquired disease, is it toxin, deficiency, or infection? The epidemiological evidence would be explained most *simply* by an infection. And with the advent of the 'slow viruses', a model does exist for an infection persisting for years with little evidence in the neuraxis and with a long incubation.

If this is an infection, there should be evidence that it is a transmittable illness—in the laboratory or in the populace. The former is not at hand as this is written, though flurries of interest continue to arise as one agent or another is proposed, and from reliable groups.

In the population, one can take transmissibility as *one* explanation for what seems to me to be the dispersion of this disease from Europe. Were that the fact, one would need to posit a toxic or infectious basis as being too rapid for genetic change and too varied for deficiencies. But even an enthusiast would agree such an interpretation is premature.

Good evidence for transmissibility would be the description of epidemics of MS. While pockets of cases have been described occasionally, most either do not hold up, or the numbers are so small that chance cannot be rejected as their explanation. I am not speaking here to the clustering I noted above; this of itself—even if accepted—is hardly evidence for transmissibility, though certainly compatible with that idea.

I think though that we *have* encountered a genuine epidemic of MS.

Hyllested and I have been studying MS in the Faeroes, a small group of formerly Danish islands lying between Norway and Iceland. A preliminary report dealing with our 1974 survey has now been published[49]. Our later visit in 1975, and current investigations on five or six more deaths, may alter the numbers somewhat, but I believe the main outline still seems valid.

In essence, all of 21 native cases of MS now known to us as of 1975 to have occurred in the Faeroes had their clinical onset between 1943 and 1960, save one whose onset was in 1962 after four years in Denmark, and one with onset in 1970. The 19 'native' cases of 1943–60 to me comprise an epidemic, with a sudden appearance *and* a sudden *disappearance* of the disease.

As to a likely cause of the epidemic, the only unusual occurrence in the Faeroes in recent times that we could discover was their occupation in the Second World War by British forces for five years from April 1940. They numbered some 8000 men, or almost one Briton for every three Faeroese. Locations of the cases and the British stations on the islands during the war were identical for most of the MS, and direct social contact with the troops was admitted by most of the patients or their surviving relatives.

If this holds up, I think we do have strong evidence that—at least on the Faeroes—MS is a transmittable disease. Further speculation would be premature, but I think this is a very exciting area for our continued investigations.

References

1. Colton, T. (1974). *Statistics in Medicine*, pp. 305 and 372 (Boston: Little, Brown and Co.)
2. Sartwell, P. E. (1968). Desiderata in population studies. In P. H. Bennett and P. H. N. Wood (eds.). *Population Studies of the Rheumatic Diseases* (International Congress Series No. 148), pp. 3–13 (New York: Excerpta Medica Foundation)
3. Sartwell, P. E. (ed.) (1973). *Maxcy-Rosenau Preventive Medicine and Public Health*, 10th edition, pp. 22 and 1189 (New York: Appleton-Century-Crofts)
4. World Health Organization (1967, 1969). *Manual of the International Statistical Classification of Diseases, Injuries and Causes of Death*, 1965 revision, Vol. 1, Vol. 2 (Geneva: World Health Organization)
5. National Center for Health Statistics (1968). *Eighth Revision International Classification of Diseases, Adapted for Use in the United States*, Vol. 1 Tabular List, Vol. 2 Alphabetical Index (PHS Publ. No. 1693) (Washington: US Government Printing Office)
6. Fox, J. P., Hall, C. E. and Elveback, L. R. (1970). *Epidemiology. Man and Disease*, pp. 185 and 339 (London: Macmillan)
7. MacMahon, B. (1967). Epidemiologic methods. In D. W. Clark and B. MacMahon (eds.). *Preventive Medicine*, pp. 81–104 (Boston: Little, Brown and Co.)
8. Nagler, B., Beebe, G. W., Kurtzke, J. F., Kurland, L. T., Auth, T. L. and Nefzger, M. D. (1966). Studies on the natural history of multiple sclerosis. 1. Design and diagnosis. *Acta Neurol. Scand.*, **42**, suppl. 19, 141

9. Kurtzke, J. F., Beebe, G. W., Nagler, B., Auth, T. L., Kurland, L. T. and Nefzger, M. D. (1968). Studies on the natural history of multiple sclerosis. 4. Clinical features of the onset bout. *Acta Neurol. Scand.*, **44,** 467

10. Beebe, G. W., Kurtzke, J. F., Kurland, L. T., Auth, T. L. and Nagler, B. (1967). Studies on the natural history of multiple sclerosis. 3. Epidemiologic analysis of the Army experience in World War II. *Neurology*, **17,** 1

11. Hyllested, K. (1956). *Disseminated Sclerosis in Denmark. Prevalence and Geographical Distribution*, pp. 147 + atlases (Copenhagen: J. Jørgensen and Co.)

12. Kurtzke, J. F. and Hamtoft, H. (1976). Multiple sclerosis and Hodgkin's disease in Denmark. *Acta Neurol. Scand.*, **53,** 358

13. Kurtzke, J. F. (1972). Multiple sclerosis death rates from underlying cause and total deaths. *Acta Neurol. Scand.*, **48,** 148

14. Kurtzke, J. F. (1976). On the risk of multiple sclerosis in Denmark. (In preparation)

15. Goldberg, I. D. and Kurland, L. T. (1962). Mortality in 33 countries from diseases of the nervous system. *World Neurol.*, **3,** 444

16. Dominguez Carmona, M. (1961). Esclerosis en placas. Epidemiología en España. *Rev. Sanid. Hig. Públ. (Madr.)*, **35,** 113

17. Kurtzke, J. F. (1975). A reassessment of the distribution of multiple sclerosis. Part 1. *Acta Neurol. Scand.*, **51,** 110

18. Kurtzke, J. F. (1975). A reassessment of the distribution of multiple sclerosis. Part 2. *Acta Neurol. Scand.*, **51,** 137

19. Kurtzke, J. F. (1964). General features of the prevalence of multiple sclerosis. *J. Indian Med. Prof.*, **11,** 4896.

20. Kurtzke, J. F. (1966). An evaluation of the geographic distribution of multiple sclerosis. *Acta Neurol. Scand.*, **42** suppl. 19, 91

21. Kurtzke, J. F. (1967). Further considerations on the geographic distribution of multiple sclerosis. *Acta Neurol. Scand.*, **43,** 283

22. Kurtzke, J. F. (1967). On the fine structure of the distribution of multiple sclerosis. *Acta Neurol. Scand.*, **43,** 257

23. Kurtzke, J. F. (1965). Medical facilities and the prevalence of multiple sclerosis. *Acta Neurol. Scand.*, **41,** 561

24. Kurtzke, J. F. (1969). Some epidemiologic features compatible with an infectious origin for multiple sclerosis. *Add. Int. Arch. Allergy*, **36,** 59

25. Kurtzke, J. F. (1974). Further features of the Fennoscandian focus of multiple sclerosis. *Acta Neurol. Scand.*, **50,** 478

26a. Kurtzke, J. F. (1968). Multiple sclerosis and infection from an epidemiologic aspect. *Neurology*, **18** (2), 170

26b. Kurtzke, J. F. (1968). A Fennoscandian focus of multiple sclerosis. *Neurology*, **18** (1), 16

27. Acheson, E. D. (1972). The epidemiology of multiple sclerosis. In D. McAlpine, C. E. Lumsden and E. D. Acheson, (eds.). *Multiple Sclerosis. A Reappraisal*, 2nd edition, pp. 3–80 (Baltimore: Williams and Wilkins)

28. Kurland, L. T. (1970). The epidemiologic characteristics of multiple sclerosis. In P. J. Vinken and G. W. Bruyn (eds.). *Multiple Sclerosis and Other Demyelinating Diseases*, pp. 63–84 (Amsterdam: North-Holland)

29. Kurtzke, J. F., Kurland, L. T. and Goldberg, I. D. (1971). Mortality and migration in multiple sclerosis. *Neurology*, **21**, 1186

30. Kurtzke, J. F. (1972). Migration and latency in multiple sclerosis. In E. J. Field, T. M. Bell and P. R. Carnegie (eds.). *Multiple Sclerosis Progress in Research*, pp. 208–228 (Amsterdam: North-Holland)

31. Kurtzke, J. F. and Kurland, L. T. (1973). The epidemiology of neurologic disease. In A. B. Baker and L. H. Baker (eds.). *Clinical Neurology*, Vol. 3, pp. 1–80 (Hagerstown, Maryland: Harper and Row)

32. Dassel, H. (1972). Discussion on the epidemiology of MS. In E. J. Field, T. M. Bell and P. R. Carnegie (eds.). *Multiple Sclerosis. Progress in Research*, pp. 241–242 (Amsterdam: North-Holland)

33. Kurtzke, J. F. and Bui, Q. H. (1976). Multiple sclerosis in a migrant population. 2. Prevalence among half-white Orientals. (In preparation)

34. Detels, R., Brody, J. A. and Edgar, A. H. (1972). Multiple sclerosis among American Japanese and Chinese migrants to California and Washington. *J. Chronic Dis.*, **25**, 3

35. Kurtzke, J. F. (1965). On the time of onset in multiple sclerosis. *Acta Neurol. Scand.*, **41**, 140

36. Schapira, K., Poskanzer, D. C. and Miller, H. (1963): Familial and conjugal multiple sclerosis. *Brain*, **86**, 315

37. Dean, G. and Kurtzke, J. F. (1971). On the risk of multiple sclerosis according to age at immigration to South Africa. *Br. Med. J.*, **3**, 725

38. Kurtzke, J. F., Dean, G. and Botha, D. P. J. (1970). A method of estimating the age at immigration of white immigrants to South Africa, with an example of its importance. *S. Afr. Med. J.*, **44**, 663

39. Dean, G. (1967). Annual incidence, prevalence, and mortality of multiple sclerosis in white South-African-born and in white immigrants to South Africa. *Br. Med. J.*, **2**, 724

40. Kurtzke, J. F. (1965). Familial incidence and geography in multiple sclerosis. *Acta Neurol. Scand.*, **41**, 127

41. Jersild, C., Dupont, B., Fog, T., Platz, P. J. and Svejgaard, A. (1975). Histocompatibility determinants in multiple sclerosis. *Transplant. Rev.*, **22**, 148

42. Kurtzke, J. F., Beebe, G. W. and Norman, J. E., Jr. (1975). Epidemiology of multiple sclerosis in the United States: Preliminary data. *Neurology*, **25**, 356

43. Detels, R., Visscher, B., Coulson, A. and Malmgren, R. (1975). Evidence for lower susceptibility to multiple sclerosis among Japanese. *Neurology*, **25**, 357

44. Kurtzke, J. F. (1974). Neurologic needs of the community. In J. F. Kurtzke (ed.). *Neuroepidemiology. American Academy of Neurology Special Course*, pp. 61–65 + tape cassette (Minneapolis: Education Marketing Corp.)

45. Alter, M., Leibowitz, U. and Speer, J. (1966). Risk of multiple sclerosis related to age at immigration to Israel. *Arch. Neurol.*, **15**, 234

46. Alter, M. and Okihiro, M. (1971). When is multiple sclerosis acquired? *Neurology*, **21**, 1030

47. Alter, M. (1972). The distribution of multiple sclerosis and environmental sanitation. In U. Leibowitz (ed.). *Progress in Multiple Sclerosis. Research and Treatment*, pp. 99–131 (New York: Academic Press)
48. Poskanzer, D. C. (1965). Tonsillectomy and multiple sclerosis. *Lancet*, **ii**, 1264
49. Kurtzke, J. F. and Hyllested, K. (1975). Multiple sclerosis. An epidemic disease in the Faeroes. *Trans. Am. Neurol. Assoc.*, **100**, 213

5

A multiple sclerosis-associated virus: past, present and future*

R. I. Carp, G. S. Merz, P. A. Merz and P. C. Licursi

Introduction

The search for the cause of multiple sclerosis (MS) was initially wide in scope and has only recently begun to centre upon virus. Over the past few years our laboratory has accumulated convincing evidence of a high degree of association of a small virus-like agent with MS. In this report, we will give the rationale of our approaches, summarize our results and provide a brief discussion of the salient points raised by the data.

Our studies on MS began in 1971 when we attempted to settle the question raised by reports in the early 1960s from the laboratories of Palsson[1] and Field[2]. In these early studies CNS disease occurred in sheep and mice following inoculation with MS autopsy material. The disease had neither the clinical nor the histopathological features of MS. Instead it was indistinguishable from scrapie, a slow, degenerative encephalopathy that occurs naturally in sheep and experimentally in mice[3]. According to the first report, sheep inoculated with the MS material developed scrapie-like disease several years later. The disease was successfully transmitted from sheep to sheep with a shorter incubation period than in the human-to-sheep inoculation. In the second report[2], mice inoculated with MS material were clinically normal when sacrificed 8 months later. Their brains were then placed in formalin for pathology studies. Later, acting on a report that scrapie agent is extremely

* This work was supported in part by Grants 723 B-2 and RG 979 A-5 from the National Multiple Sclerosis Society.

resistant to inactivation by formalin, the formalinized brains were homogenized and the homogenates were inoculated into mice. Between 13 and 17 months later the inoculated mice were sacrificed and some showed pathology typical of scrapie. After the third serial passage in mice, clinical scrapie developed in 5 to 6 months. Although the possibility of contamination of the sheep and/or mice with scrapie seems unlikely since test animals were maintained in areas free of scrapie, the question of contamination of the inoculum at some point has never been resolved. Furthermore, the significance of these results is clouded by the fact that despite numerous attempts these findings have not been duplicated.*

Based on work we have reported elsewhere[4,5], we can suggest an explanation of these anomalous results which can be generalized into a novel but potentially important concept. One can view pathogenesis as a sequence of discrete events that begins at the subcellular or cellular level, and culminates in functional disintegration at the level of organs or organ systems. It is the last stage that generates the clinical disease state. It is self-evident that the failure to complete any of the preceding events could block the overall process and prevent the development of clinical disease. It is possible, however, that events occurring before the block might lead to alterations in the host that: (1) would not be debilitating, (2) would persist indefinitely, perhaps for the life of the host, and (3) would leave the animal in a 'primed' state for the resumption of the process if ever the block were somehow removed or bypassed.

The above assumptions could explain what might be a real but sporadic transmission of a disease from MS to healthy sheep and/or mice. One need only assume that all transmission attempts were successful in that something (a virus?) was transmitted to the test host but that the culmination of the pathological processes was somehow prevented or aborted. Those few cases in which disease was observed would then represent rare instances in which the block had been bypassed.

It was with this concept in mind that we began a search for 'preblock' alterations in mice inoculated with MS autopsy material. We were looking specifically for alterations similar to those known to occur in the early, preclinical period of scrapie disease. These changes included alterations in brain enzyme activities[6], differences in water and food consumption[7] and alterations in the protein patterns seen in the electropherograms of mouse

* Editor's note: Unknown to Palsson, Pattison and Field (1965), transfer of the Newcastle material into new containers for transport purposes took place in a laboratory intermediate between Newcastle and Reykjavik, in which scrapie work was active. The association of scrapie with MS has been withdrawn (see Chapter 9), on the basis that scrapie sheep do not give MS results with the laboratory tests developed.

cerebrospinal fluid (CSF)[8]. In addition to the above, we tested several routine parameters including leukocyte differentials in the peripheral blood. The most striking finding was a 2-to-3-fold decrease in the percentages of circulating polymorphonuclear neutrophils (PMN)[4,5]. This was found in mice inoculated with either scrapie or MS brain homogenates, whereas mice inoculated with normal mouse or human brain homogenates had PMN percentages similar to those found for uninoculated mice[4,5]. These results will be discussed in detail in a subsequent section, but as an introductory point it should be mentioned that the agent causing the decrease in PMN could be passed from mouse to mouse and replicated in mice. For this reason, we were interested in determining if this agent would replicate in a spontaneously transformed mouse tissue culture cell-line termed PAM. During the course of this work we observed that MS material caused a reduction in cell yield as compared to the yield obtained for non-MS treated or control PAM cell cultures[9-12]. These data will also be discussed in detail in the Results section. Also, in keeping with the original objective of our work, the effects of scrapie material on both the PMN percentage in mice[5] and the yield of PAM cells[13] were analysed and these results are outlined.

Results

THE PMN DECREASE

In our initial work, mice injected either intracerebrally (IC) or intraperitoneally (IP) with a pool of three brain homogenates, developed a decrease in the per cent of circulating PMN that was detected as early as two weeks, and persisted for at least 16 months. During this period no other histopathological or clinical change was observed. Counts of the total number of PMN and lymphocytes established that the reduction was due to a real decrease in the number of PMN, as opposed to an apparent decrease engendered by an increase in the number of lymphocytes or other white cell types. The agent causing the decrease replicated in mice and was readily passed from mouse to mouse. The agent was present at titres of $10^{11}/g$ to $10^{12}/g$ in the human MS brain pool and at similar titres in the brains of inoculated mice. Based on millipore filtration, the diameter of the agent was between 25 and 50 nm.

These results constitute the first evidence to indicate clearly the existence of an MS-associated virus. Figure 5.1 gives a picture of the distribution of the PMN percentage among MS and control-inoculated mice. Although there is some overlap of the control distributions with the MS, the difference is clear. Based on these data, we established a PMN percentage of 10 as the

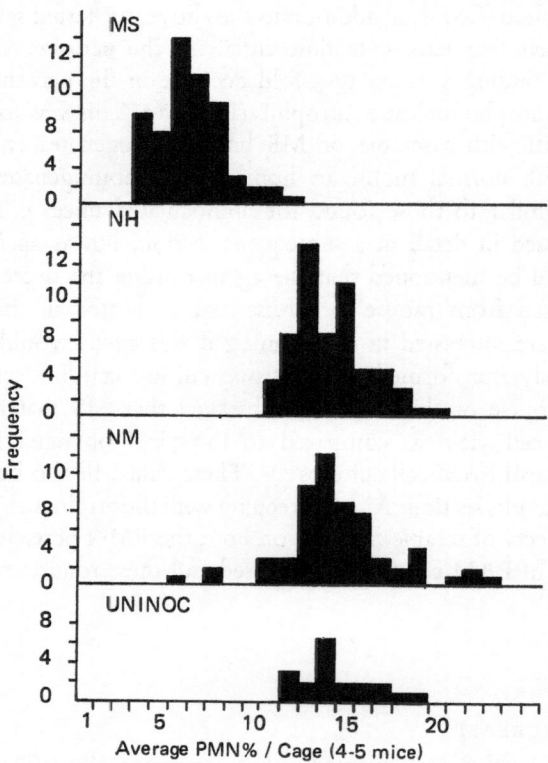

Figure 5.1 Frequency distribution of average PMN percentage of four or five mice. MS = multiple sclerosis; NH = normal human; NM = normal mouse; Uninoc = uninoculated

basis for deciding whether a sample is positive (PMN % $\leqslant$ 10) or negative (PMN % > 10).

ASSOCIATION OF THE PMN AGENT WITH MS TISSUES

Our next step was to determine the extent to which the agent/virus was (1) present in MS tissue samples, and (2) specific for MS disease. Table 5.1 shows the distribution and description of the diseases that were tested in this phase of the work, Table 5.2 shows the distribution of tissues among the sample collection.

After testing samples both directly by inoculation into mice and indirectly by blind passage from mouse to mouse, we arrived at the following conclusions:

(1) The average PMN percentage of mice inoculated with MS material

Table 5.1 Diseases represented in sample collection

Disease class	Disease or MS status	Number of cases	Number of samples
Healthy		24	28
Total		24	28
Non-CNS			
	Vaginal herpes	1	1
	Cirrhosis	1	2
	Pneumonia	1	1
	Arteriosclerosis	1	1
	Pancreatitis	1	1
	Melanoma	1	1
	Liver necrosis	1	1
	Lumbosacral strain	1	1
	Lumbar radiculitis	1	1
	CVA	3	3
	No diagnosis	1	1
Total		13	14
CNS			
	Encephalopathy	1	1
	Bechat's syndrome	1	1
	SSPE	8	9
	Epilepsy	1	1
	Demyelination	1	2
	Spongy degeneration	1	2
	Myoclonic lipidosis	1	1
	Huntington's chorea	3	5
	Parkinson's disease	5	6
	Cerebral palsy	1	1
	Spinal cerebral degeneration	2	2
	Alcoholic cerebral degeneration	1	1
	EAE (rat)	9	9
	Presenile dementia	1	1
Total		36	42
MS			
	Autopsy	10	14
	No information	21	21
	Retrobulbar neuritis (RBN)	4	8
	Stage I–III	5	7
	Stage IV–VI	5	10
	Serial bleeds	2	8
Total		47	68

Table 5·2 Distribution of tissues among the disease classes

Tissue (152)*	MS (68)	CNS (42)	Non-CNS (14)	Healthy (28)
		Class of disease		
Brain (17)	8	3	6	0
CSF (39)	26	4	2	7
Serum (86)	28	33	4	21
Spleen (6)	3	1	2	0
Lymph gland (1)	1	0	0	0
Kidney (3)	2	1	0	0

* Number in parentheses is the total number in each tissue of class or disease.

was lower than that for mice inoculated with healthy, CNS or non-CNS material.

(2) If the criteria for detecting the presence of the PMN factor includes the capacity to cause the PMN drop on mouse passage, as it should with an infectious agent, then 73% of MS samples were positive and only 20% of CNS and other non-MS samples were positive.

(3) A significant number of MS samples that were negative on primary inoculation were positive on mouse-to-mouse passage, while the reverse trend was observed with the CNS samples.

(4) Multiple samples from one individual were usually all positive or all negative.

(5) In human material, the agent has been found in every type of tissue examined. These include brain, spleen, kidney, lymph gland, serum and CSF.

Our results with the PMN factor have recently been confirmed[14,15] in virtually every detail. In addition, these workers made a number of additional findings: (1) the PMN decrease was induced in a number of other mouse strains, and in several different species, including guinea-pig, rat and hamster, (2) a neutralizing antibody to the PMN factor was found in a number of MS patients and in close contacts of patients, such as relatives, nurses and doctors, and in blood samples from East Africans. In contrast, sera from a sampling of the normal population in the United States showed that virtually none contained neutralizing antibody.

Two other studies, each encompassing a small series of experiments employing comparatively few mice, failed to confirm our basic findings[16,17]. One group, however, did find a statistically significant change in the leukocyte distribution in mouse bone marrow induced by MS inoculation[17]. Failure with this test can often be related to problems with the physiological and/or medical status of the mice, and careful control of these parameters is critical. This will be discussed in detail in a subsequent section.

Reduction in PMN percentages in scrapie-inoculated mice

The experiments with scrapie in mice were initiated at the same time as the MS studies. A decrease in the percentage of PMN in the peripheral blood of mice appeared three days after IC inoculation with scrapie mouse brain homogenate[5]; IP inoculation was also effective in causing a decrease in PMN percentage. Mice inoculated IC or IP with normal mouse brain had PMN percentages similar to those found for uninoculated mice. This difference between normal and scrapie-inoculated mice continued throughout the preclinical phase of the disease. In the clinical phase of the disease, the percentage of PMN was either higher or lower than that found in normals. The factor causing the decrease in PMN percentages was found in the filtrates from 220, 100 and 50 nm filters, but not in the filtrates from a 25 nm filter. In addition to two genetically different scrapie mouse brain isolates, homogenates of mouse spleen, sheep brain and sheep spleen from scrapie-affected animals caused a decrease in per cent PMN, whereas the corresponding normal tissue homogenates did not. We have also shown that the titre of the agent causing the reduction in PMN is approximately 10^6 times greater than the infectivity titre of scrapie[18]. The PMN agent replicated in mice that never showed signs of scrapie, i.e. mice inoculated with approximately 6×10^{-4} LD_{50} units of scrapie. Nine weeks after inoculation with 100 units of PMN agent (but no scrapie) mouse brain contained 10^{11} units of PMN agent. Inoculation of mice with 10^{11} units of PMN agent, which had been produced in the absence of scrapie infectious units, failed to cause scrapie disease[18]. Thus, the scrapie infectious unit and the PMN agent are separable, although the PMN agent is always found in conjunction with scrapie disease.

Dickinson et al.[19] have shown a reduction in PMN percentages in C57BL mice following inoculation with six different scrapie agents that had been passaged and characterized in mice. Furthermore, these authors reported that six sources of scrapie from sheep and two from goats ('scratching' and 'drowsy' types) caused a significant reduction in PMN percentages.

ASSESSMENT OF THE PMN TEST FOR MS-ASSOCIATED VIRUS

In spite of the success in establishing that there is undoubtedly a virus-like agent associated with MS tissues, the PMN test has some severe limitations and shortcomings[14–16,19]. First, the health of the mice is critical. We have had numerous recent mouse shipments from many various suppliers which, on the day of arrival, had severe chronic interstitial pneumonitis or chronic bronchitis. These mice were completely asymptomatic, with no increase in mortality. The only overt manifestations of the disease were a reduced level of circulating PMN, increased variability in lymphocyte and the PMN counts, and on occasion, a slight increase in the number of immature lymphocytes. Inoculation of these mice with MS material failed to produce any noticeable effect, since the PMN counts were so low and variable prior to inoculation. The results obtained when we tested these mice were similar to those reported by Brown and Gajdusek[16] in several of their experiments.

On other occasions we had rounds of a disease of unknown origin and aetiology. This 'plague' was characterized by (1) an increased number of immature lymphocytes, and (2) abnormally high variation in PMN percentages among the mice. Compared to healthy mice the mean PMN percentage among mice inoculated with MS brain pool was elevated slightly and was indistinguishable from those inoculated with normal brain pool. More telling, however, was the increase of 2- to 2·5-fold in the standard deviations of the PMN values for mice inoculated with both MS and normal brain pools over that obtained using healthy mice.

Third, because of the normal responses to trauma (increased circulating PMN) and various husbandry factors, a number of other parameters should be carefully controlled. These include the following:

(1) Repeated bleeding of the same mouse at intervals of less than two weeks should be avoided.

(2) Ear snipping and all other procedures that result in tissue damage should be avoided.

(3) Always bleed mice at the same time of day and ensure that noise and disturbance are kept to a minimum.

(4) If fighting occurs in a cage, the attendant wounds and infections will obviously render the PMN values of mice in that cage worthless. For this reason, we routinely use female mice, which are considerably less aggressive than males.

Quite aside from these considerations, there is also the problem of the distributions of the MS and control PMN percentages overlapping, and our criteria for whether a sample is positive or negative is therefore somewhat arbitrary. This is particularly vexing when it comes to interpreting the significance of negative MS samples and, more importantly, positive non-MS samples. When all the above are considered, the PMN test becomes unwieldy and unworkable for further work, such as characterization of the agent, etc. It was with these considerations in mind that we began searching for a more facile test for the MS-associated virus.

MS–INDUCED DECREASE IN TOTAL CELL YIELD OF PAM CELL CULTURES

Our search began with an attempt to determine whether the MS-associated virus could replicate in cells *in vitro*. MS tissue was applied to PAM cells, a spontaneously transformed mouse cell-line derived from mouse embryo fibroblasts of CFW random-bred mice. Our original intent was simply to inoculate mice with PAM cell culture samples 16-18 passages after treatment with MS material and look for a PMN reduction. To our surpirse, there was a direct response to MS tissues; a decrease in the total cell yield. Reductions in cell yield were noted as early as the second passage after treatment. The effect was produced by eight of eight MS brain homogenates and three of three MS spleen homogenates; the samples were from ten different cases[9]. The reduction in total cell yields was not observed among PAM cultures treated with non-MS homogenates (six brain and two spleen) from eight control individuals. Five of the MS-inoculated cultures were maintained for 18 subcultivations, and the reduced cell yields persisted throughout (Figure 5.2). The agent responsible for the reduction was present in the cell-free

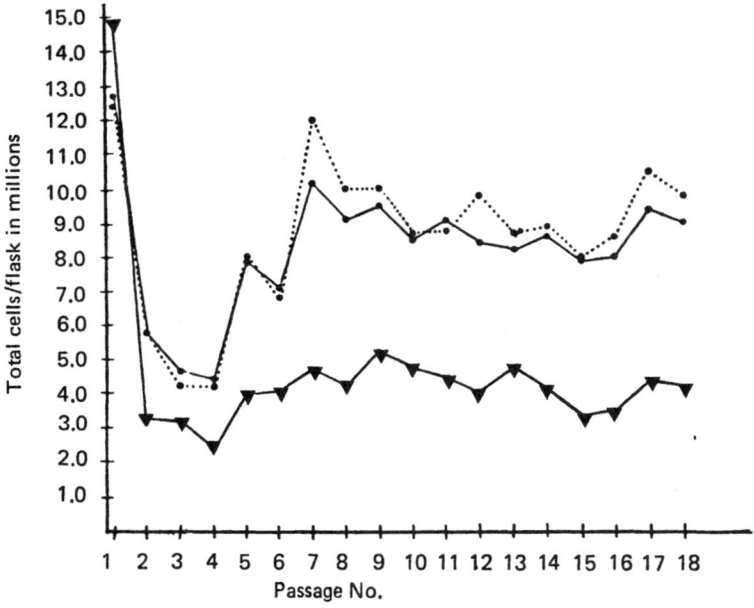

Figure 5.2 Total cell yield per flask as a function of culture passage number ●——
averaged cell yield of four non-MS treated cultures; ▼—— average cell yield of five
MS-treated cultures; ●- - - - cell yield of medium-treated culture

lysates (prepared by repeated freezing and thawing) from all of the five MS cultures at passage 18, in that treatment of fresh PAM cells with these lysates led to a reduction in PAM cell yields. Inoculation of the lysates into mice caused a reduction in PMN implying the presence of the PMN agent (Table 5.3). Calculation of the dilution effect (at least 10^{18}-fold) that had occurred by the end of the passage series implies that the agent(s) causing the decreased

Table 5.3 Effect of MS-treated PAM cell lysates on PAM cell cultures and polymorphonuclear neutrophil percentages in mice

	Cell yield/flask $\times$ 10^{-6}		
Treatment at passage 0	At passage 18 after exposure	Among PAM cultures exposed to lysates prepared from passage 18 cells	PMN percentage in mice inoculated with passage 18 lysates
N–1	8·5	10·6	16·0[a] (1·34)
N–2	8·7	11·4	15·6 (1·21)
N–3	9·7	10·0	15·6 (0·51)
N–4	9·2	11·6	17·0 (1·30)
Average (SE)[b]	9·0[c] (0·3)	10·9[d] (0·4)	15·8[e] (0·38)
MS–1	4·1	5·3	6·0 (0·43)
MS–2	4·5	5·6	4·2 (0·58)
MS–3	3·8	4·8	2·4 (0·51)
MS–4	4·5	6·0	5·2 (1·44)
MS–5	4·0	5·8	5·2 (0·97)
Average (SE)	4·2[c] (0·15)	5·5[d] (0·21)	4·6[e] (0·62)

[a] Average (SE) for groups of five mice
[b] SE standard error
[c] P of no difference (t test) $\ll$ 0·001
[d] P of no difference (t test) $\ll$ 0·001
[e] P of no difference (t test) $\ll$ 0·001

PAM cell yield and the PMN decrease in mice had replicated *in vitro*. Filtration of a pool of five MS brain homogenates through graded pore size millipore filters revealed that the PAM agent is between 25 and 50 nm in diameter.

ASSOCIATION OF THE PAM AGENT WITH MS TISSUES

Once again, the question of association with and specificity for MS became crucial. A collection of 71 MS and 45 non-MS samples, composed of unpassed and mouse-passed material was applied to PAM cultures in eight separate experiments. Because the yields of PAM cell cultures vary somewhat in a concordant fashion with time and subcultivation, each experiment contained an untreated PAM culture as a control, in addition to MS and non-MS treated cultures. All yields were expressed as the percentage of this untreated control. Whereas the non-MS distribution is unimodal, it appears that the distribution of MS yields is bimodal, with one group distributed similarly to the non-MS and one that is distributed on a much lower range (Figure 5.3). Based on these observations, we have adopted the following convention: all yields (calculated as a percentage of control) less than 80% are considered as a positive response, whereas all yields equal to or greater than 80% are considered as no response.

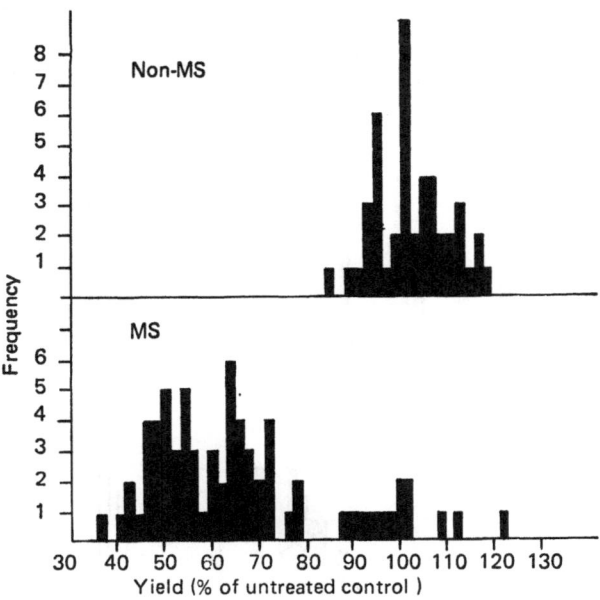

Figure 5.3 Frequency distribution of PAM cell yields as a percentage of yields for untreated controls

Of the PAM cultures treated with MS material, 80% (58) showed a reduction in cell yield (compared with untreated controls) of at least 20% by the third passage after inoculation. The MS samples were from 40 different MS cases, and a total of 36 cases yielded at least one positive sample. The agent responsible for the decrase was not limited to brain and spleen tissue, but also was found in serum, plasma, CSF, kidney and lymph node of MS patients. Positive samples were present at every stage of the disease.

The non-MS category included 12 samples from healthy individuals, 13 assorted non-CNS disease samples, and the following CNS disease samples: five subacute sclerosing panencephalitis, three Huntington's chorea, two Parkinson's disease, six amytrophic lateral sclerosis, one stroke, one encephalopathy and one epilepsy.

At this point, 48 of the MS and 32 of the non-MS treated PAM cultures were serially passaged through a total of 16 or 17 passages. Yields were determined at passages 3, 4, 5 and 10 through 16 or 17, expressed as a percentage of the untreated control culture and averaged. All of the averaged cell yields for MS cultures except one were less than 80% of the untreated control, while the averaged cell yield for the non-MS cultures was between 85 and 125% of the controls (Figure 5.4A).

It should be emphasized that the cell yields for MS samples at any single

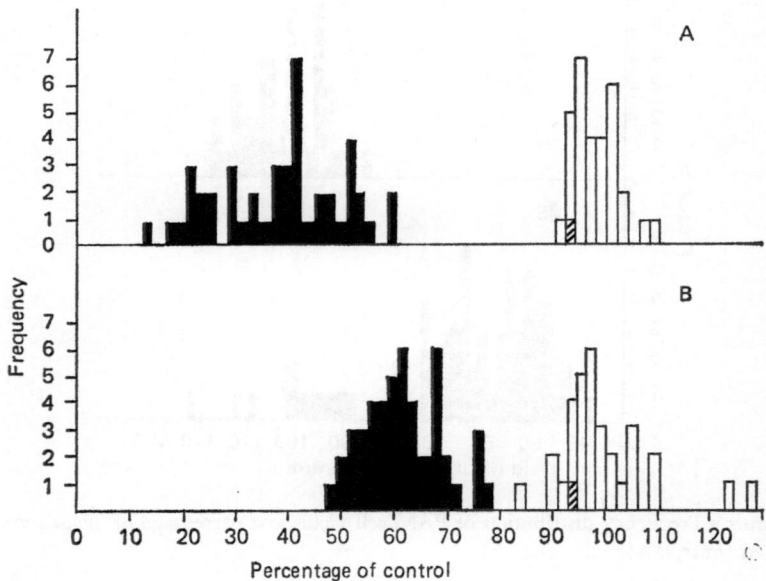

Figure 5.4 A: Frequency distribution of the average per cent cell yields from passage 3 to 5, and 10 to 16 or 17; per cent cell yields were averaged for each MS and each non-MS treated sample. Solid bars=MS samples; open bars=non-MS samples; cross-hatched bars=MS sample in non-MS range.

B: Frequency distribution of the per cent cell yields at the 3rd passage after treatment with cell-free lysates of passage 16 or 17 of MS and non-MS treated cultures. Designation of bars is the same as in Figure 5.4A passage are occasionally greater than 80% of control. The key point is the average of the values obtained over a series of passages. For example, in the experiment noted above in which values for passage 3 were analysed, 20% of 71 samples had values higher than 80% of control. Virtually all of these 'negative' samples were found to be positive for the PAM cell effect when yields were averaged over an additional extended series of passages. Likewise, at any given passage a few non-MS samples have values less than 80% of control. However, over a series of passages the average yield values for all non-MS treated cultures were greater than 80% of control values.

Although the decreased PAM cell yields persisted at least through the 17th passage, there remained the question of whether the decreased yield was a consequence of the continuing presence of the agent or an initial alteration that persisted even after the causative agent had disappeared. To answer this question, 46 of the MS-treated PAM cultures at the final passage were frozen and thawed three times. These cell-free lysates were then used to infect fresh PAM cultures. The per cent yields at passage 3 have been arranged in a histogram (Figure 5.4B). All of the MS-treated cultures exhibited a decreased yield at the 3rd passage except one, the same sample which had failed to cause a decrease from passage 3 to 17, following the primary treatment. Combining the 46 MS samples tested in this experiment with the five tested previously, the results show that 50 of 51 MS samples contained a small, self-replicating virus. By contrast, none of 36 non-MS samples appeared to contain a similar agent.

Filtration experiments established that for 43 of 45 samples (cell-free lysates from passage 16 or 17) tested, the size of the agent present in late passage MS-treated PAM cells is between 50 and 25 nm. This is consistent with the size found for the agent in a pool of five MS brain homogenates[9]. The establishment of the size of the agent in PAM cells, many passages after treatment, is significant for several reasons. PAM cells contain C-type particles[10], and the MS-induced effect on cell yield might be mediated through an initially induced modification of the C-type particles, and their subsequent interaction with PAM cells. The replicating agent present in PAM cells 16 or 17 passages after treatment might then be this modified C-type particle. This interpretation appears to be extremely unlikely, in that the size of the causative agent in late passage cell-free lysates is much less than the size of C-type particles. Finally, the size of this virus also differentiates it from the paramyxoviruses that have been isolated from MS material on rare occasions[20,21].

Recently, Smith et al.[22] showed that MS-treated PAM cells (and only PAM cells) produced an antigen which reacted in radioimmunoassay with approximately 30% of MS sera. Furthermore, they showed that some MS sera contained an agent which replicated in PAM cells and, in this manner, produced the antigen used in the radioimmunoassay test.

ENHANCED HAEMAGGLUTINATION (HA) BY MS-TREATED PAM CELLS

When mixed together, rhesus monkey RBCs and PAM cells undergo what macroscopically appears to be HA (microscopic examination suggests that mechanisms other than classic HA are operating)[23]. After 33 tests performed at different times under somewhat different conditions, we found the following:

(1) In any single test, MS PAM cell titres were invariably equal to, or higher than, those of control PAM cells exposed to non-MS tissues. The titre difference was as great as 32-fold in some cases.

(2) In 11 of the tests, the MS PAM cells had HA titres of 1:64 or higher, whereas in none of 33 tests did the normal controls exceed 1:32.

(3) In 85% of the tests, HA titres of MS cultures were higher than control titres.

These results are important for three reasons: (a) it may prove to be an additional way to quantitate the MS-associated virus, (b) it provides additional evidence that MS-treated PAM cells are different from non-MS treated cells; (c) it gives a facile means to search for antibody, which might be directed against either the MS-associated virus or antigenic changes induced in cells treated with the virus.

REDUCTION IN THE TOTAL CELL YIELD OF PAM CELLS INDUCED BY SCRAPIE MATERIAL

Exposure of PAM cells to brain homogenates from mice infected with scrapie caused a decrease in total cell yield, which persisted from the 2nd or 3rd passage to the 18th passage after treatment[13]. The effect was elicited by each of the eight independent scrapie isolates tested. Lysates prepared from cultures 16 passages after treatment with scrapie caused the decrease when applied to fresh PAM cultures. Mice inoculated with 14th and 18th passage lysates developed a reduced percentage of PMN by five weeks, and scrapie disease by six to nine months after inoculation. Based on the total dilution from treatment of the PAM cultures with scrapie material to the preparation of the lysates, we conclude that the agent(s) responsible for the reduced PAM cell yield, the decreased per cent PMN and the induction of scrapie disease had replicated in the PAM cells. By filtration, the diameter of the agent causing the reduction in cell yield was estimated to be between 25 and 50 nm.

Discussion

The idea that virus plays a significant role in the aetiology of MS was founded primarily on two early findings: (1) epidemiological studies that were consistent with viral aetiology[24], and (2) immunological surveys showing that MS patients had higher measles antibody titres than matched controls[25]. From these studies plus others the search for an infectious agent in MS has taken the following routes:

(1) *Animals:* The search has been aimed at obtaining an animal model system in which an MS-like disease would occur.

(2) *Tissue culture:* Here, early unfruitful efforts at finding classical *in vitro* viral infections with attendant CPE etc. have given way to more sophisticated, indirect approaches such as co-cultivation and cell fusion with cells known to be susceptible to a presumed MS virus (primarily members of the paramyxovirus group)[20,21].

(3) *Electronmicroscopy:* The examination of thin sections has also largely been geared toward a search for paramyxovirus particles and/or nucleocapsids[26].

(4) *Immunology:* Here the approach has been to search for antibody against presumed MS virus in sera and CSF of MS patients. Again, the emphasis has been on the paramyxovirus group[25].

Consideration of these approaches and their results so far provide us with the following current picture:

(1) Despite the success of passaging kuru and Jacob-Creutzfeldt into experimental animals and producing a similar disease[27], efforts with MS have not yielded an animal model system.

(2) The techniques of co-cultivation and cell fusion led to the isolation of measles virus from a number of SSPE cases[28], and the initial successes with studies on MS in which a measles virus was isolated from one case and a parainfluenza virus from two cases[20,21]. However, extensive studies since then, involving many MS samples, have failed to yield additional virus isolates[29,30].

(3) With electronmicroscopy, tubular structures were seen which were similar in size and appearance to paramyxovirus nucleocapsids[26]. However, extensive work in this area has shown that similar structures are seen in inflammatory conditions in which an infectious agent is not incriminated[31]. Furthermore, some researchers claim that the structures seen in MS differ in appearance from paramyxovirus nucleocapsids[32]. Attempts to label these tubules/nucleocapsids with measles and parainfluenza 1 virus antisera, using

the immunoperoxidase method, have failed[32]. The only other report in the press is of coronavirus-like particles in MS brain[33]. However, the particles were seen in only one brain out of the 12 examined.

(4) In a number of immunological surveys, sera from affected persons have been tested for antibody against a wide range of known viruses in the hope of detecting increased antibody titres against a given virus. This has yielded the important finding that MS patients exhibit an increased antibody titre, both in serum and CSF, against a number of viruses, most strikingly measles[25,34]. The relationship of the elevated antibody titres to the aetiology of MS is questionable on several grounds: (a) the increase in antibody titre is not restricted to a single virus. This suggests that either there are multiple causes of MS, or the antibody increases are related to a more general change in immunological reactivity[34]; (b) attempts to absorb the oligoclonal IgG bands found in MS CSF[35] with measles virus failed[36]; (c) the increases in antibody titres against measles virus may not be correlated with MS disease per se, but rather with the HLA types which predominate in the MS population[37].

By contrast, our approach has involved a search for virus 'footprints', rather than disease or CPE. We did not expect to get disease in our test animals, but rather examined MS-infected mice for subclinical changes in physiological and biochemical parameters. Nor did we expect to find overt virus-induced changes, such as CPE, in our MS-treated tissue culture systems. Instead, we have looked for subtle changes in cell growth and surface characteristics. Using these approaches, we have accumulated some compelling evidence for MS-associated virus. This evidence includes the following key points:

(1) There is a small virus-like agent in MS tissues which causes a reduction in the percentage of circulating PMN[4]. This work has recently been confirmed and extended to include evidence of neutralizing antibodies[14,15]. Unfortunately, this system is unreliable, in view of difficulties we and others have had in obtaining suitably healthy and/or responsive mice.

(2) MS tissues harbour a small virus-like agent which causes a reduction in PAM cell yields[9,10]. To date this virus has been found in 50 of 51 MS samples examined. The sample collection included serum, plasma and CSF, in addition to brain and other solid tissues. Recently, it has been shown that MS-treated PAM cells produced an antigen which reacted in a radioimmunoassay with approximately 30% of MS sera[22].

(3) MS-treated PAM cells showed an increased ability to haemagglutinate rhesus red blood cells[23].

It is interesting to compare the results that we have obtained for scrapie and for MS. Material from each disease causes a decrease in PMN in mice and a reduction in PAM cell yields[4,5,9-13]. The PMN agent from each disease replicates in mice and in treated PAM cells. The PAM cell agent from each disease replicates in PAM cells. The characteristics of the changes in mice and in PAM cells are quite similar. Thus, the time of appearance and the extent of the reduction in PMN percentages and of the reduction in PAM cell yields is quite similar following inoculation with material from the two diseases. The diameter of the PMN and PAM cell virus(es) in both diseases was 25–50 nm by millipore filtration analysis. The only difference in the responses induced by MS and scrapie material is that scrapie contains an infectious agent which causes disease in mice. The interrelationship of the viruses causing the various effects noted poses many interesting questions. Are the PMN and PAM cell effects in MS produced by the same virus or by two different viruses? The same question applies to the effects induced by scrapie tissue. In scrapie, the disease-producing agent is separable from the virus(es) causing PAM cell reduction and PMN percentage reduction. Is there a disease-producing agent in MS material which is separable from the PMN and PAM cell virus(es)? What is the relationship between the PMN and PAM cell virus(es) found in MS and those found in scrapie? Can the PMN and PAM cell virus(es) in MS interfere with the disease-producing agent of scrapie? The questions abound. Certainly, a key approach to a number of these questions is the study of the cross-reactivity of the MS PMN neutralizing antibody described by Henle et al.[15]

One aspect of the PMN and PAM cell work should be stressed. This is a blood-borne virus. For the PMN virus, Henle et al.[15] have demonstrated virus activity in the serum. In our original work, PMN virus was found in two of two MS sera examined[4] and in subsequent unpublished data we have found PMN activity in approximately 70% of 28 sera. In our PAM cell work, all 30 MS sera and plasma samples tested were shown to contain virus, and Smith et al.[22] have reported an agent in MS serum that replicated in PAM cells.

The presence of the PMN and PAM virus(es) in serum and plasma from MS patients has a number of important implications. First, presence in the blood means the virus(es) should be found in most organs, and in fact, our results show that, in addition to brain, the agent(s) is found in spleen, kidney and lymph gland. Second, the fact that the agents are blood-borne suggests the possibility of circulating antigen (agent)–antibody complexes. In the case of the PMN agent, there is such evidence[15]. Third, the fact that the virus(es) is present in easily obtained body fluids increases the possibility that a test for its presence could be used as a diagnostic aid. Should the MS-associated virus(es) prove to be the cause of MS, then its presence in blood has some additional important consequences. The possibility that MS could be transmitted by transfusion should be considered, and a retrospective study of this has been initiated[38]. In this study, an attempt will be made to determine the MS status of individuals who received transfusions with blood supplied by MS patients in either the clinical or preclinical phase of disease. The presence of causative agent in serum would also permit vectors to play a role in transmission. Could the geographical incidence of MS disease be related to specific vectors? Is the high incidence of antibodies to the PMN agent in the general population in Africa[15] related to extensive spread of the virus in the young by the high population density of various insect vectors or of a specific vector?

Changes in the proportion of various leukocyte types are usually related to responses to new antigenic stimuli. An alternative possibility is that a virus could act directly and specifically upon one or more of the leukocyte subtypes or precursor cells, thereby affecting the proportion and/or the responsiveness of the various cell types. In mice it would appear that the MS-associated virus acts directly upon mature leukocytes or their precursors, since the reduction in PMN percentage occurs very rapidly. In humans with MS, PMN levels remain normal, but there is evidence of a change in the proportion of T and B cells.[39] It is possible that the change seen in the proportion of leukocyte types in MS is the result of the direct action of the MS-associated virus, and that this in turn leads to the altered immune potential described for MS patients[25,34,40–42]. In this manner, it is possible that the modulation of the disease process which is characteristic of MS is related to perturbations in the interaction between MS-associated virus and leukocytes. Certainly, if the PMN and PAM cell effects are induced by the causative agent of MS, then the fact that it is present in blood and may act upon leukocyte cell types will add entire new dimensions to the studies of diagnosis, pathogenesis and transmission of this disease.

To conclude, our findings represent the strongest evidence thus far for an MS-associated virus. This discovery raises the hope that this virus is the causative agent of MS disease. Along with this hope, however, comes the frustrating problem of establishing such a causal relationship. The resolution of the question of causality requires progress in several areas. We must improve the means of quantitating the virus so that we can continue its much-needed purification and characterization. We must develop immunological probes which would furnish the means to investigate the distribution of the virus at the population, individual and cellular levels. We must determine the biochemical and morphological characteristics of the virus, so that it can be related to known virus groups. With these capabilities, we should then be able to establish firmly the role of this virus in MS.

Acknowledgements

The authors wish to thank Drs Helen Warner and Richard Kascsak for their helpful criticism of the manuscript.

References

1. Palsson, P. A., Pattison, I. H. and Field, E. J. (1965). Transmission experiments with multiple sclerosis. In: NINDB Monograph No. 2, Slow, latent and temperate virus infections. Eds. D. C. Gajdusek, C. J. Gibbs and M. Alpers. Pp. 49–54

2. Field, E. J. (1966). Transmission experiments with multiple sclerosis: an interim report. *Br. Med. J.*, **2**, 564

3. Chandler, R. L. (1963). Experimental scrapie in the mouse. *Res. Vet. Sci.*, **4**, 276

4. Carp, R. I., Licursi, P. C., Merz, P. A. and Merz, G. S. (1972). Decreased percentage of polymorphonuclear neutrophils in mouse peripheral blood after inoculation of material from multiple sclerosis patients. *J. Exp. Med.*, **136**, 618

5. Licursi, P. C., Merz, P. A., Merz, G. S. and Carp, R. I. (1972). Scrapie-induced changes in the percentages of polymorphonuclear neutrophils in mouse peripheral blood. *Infect. Immun.*, **6**, 370

6. Hunter, G. D. (1972). Scrapie, a prototype slow infection. *J. Infect. Dis.*, **125**, 427

7. Outram, G. W. (1972). Changes in drinking and feeding habits of mice with experimental scrapie. *J. Comp. Pathol.*, **82**, 415

8. Merz, P. A., Merz, G. S. and Carp, R. I. (1973). Higher frequency of a protein band in the cerebrospinal fluid from scrapie mice. *Res. Vet. Sci.*, **14**, 392

9. Carp, R. I., Merz, G. S. and Licursi, P. C. (1974). Reduced cell yields of mouse cell line cultures after exposure to homogenates of multiple sclerosis tissues. *Infect. Immun.*, **9**, 1011

10. Carp, R. I., Licursi, P. C. and Merz, G. S. (1975). Multiple sclerosis induced reduction in the yield of a mouse cell-line. *Infect. Immun.*, **11**, 737

11. Carp, R. I., Merz, G. S. and Licursi, P. C. (1975). A non-cytopathic infectious agent associated with MS material. *Neurology*, **25**, 492

12. Carp, R. I., Merz, G. S. and Licursi, P. C. (1976). A small virus-like agent found in association with multiple sclerosis material. *Neurology*, **26**, 6 (2), 70

13. Carp, R. I., Merz, G. S. and Licursi, P. C. (1976). Scrapie *in vitro*: Agent replication and reduced cell yield. *Infect. Immun.*, **14**, 163

14. Koldovsky, U., Koldovsky, P., Henle, G., Henle, W., Ackermann, R. and Haase, G. (1975). Multiple sclerosis-associated agent: Transmission to animals and some properties of the agent. *Infect. Immun.*, **12**, 1355

15. Henle, G., Koldovsky, U., Koldovsky, P., Henle, W., Ackermann, R. and Haase, G. (1975). Multiple sclerosis-associated agent: Neutralization of the agent by human sera. *Infect. Immun.*, **12**, 1367

16. Brown, P. and Gadjusek, D. C. (1974). No mouse PMN leukocyte depression after inoculation with brain tissue from multiple sclerosis or spongiform encephalopathies. *Nature* (London), **247**, 217

17. McNeill, T. A., Killen, M. and Trudgett, A. (1974). Mouse granulocyte precursors and multiple sclerosis. *Nature (London)*, **249**, 778

18. Carp, R. I., Merz, P. A., Licursi, P. C. and Merz, G. S. (1973). Replication of the factor in scrapie material that causes a decrease in polymorphonuclear neutrophils *J. Infect. Dis.*, **128**, 256

19. Dickinson, A. G., Taylor, D. M. and Fraser, H. (1974). Depression of polymorph counts by various scrapie agents. *Nature (London)*, **248**, 510

20. ter Meulen, V., Koprowski, H., Iwasaki, Y., Kackell, Y. M. and Muller, D. (1972). Fusion of cultured multiple sclerosis brain cells with indicator cells: Presence of nucleocapsids and virions and isolation of parainfluenza-type virus. *Lancet*, **ii**, 1

21. Field, E. J., Cowshall, S., Narang, H. K. and Bell, T. M. (1972). Viruses in multiple sclerosis? *Lancet*, **ii**, 280

22. Smith, K. O., Gehle, W. D., Madden, D. L. and Fucillo, D. A. (1976). Viral and cellular antibodies in multiple sclerosis (MS) and normal subjects' sera. *Ann. Meet. Am. Soc. Microbiol. Abstr.*, p. 254

23. Warner, H. B., Carp, R. I. and Narducci, R. (1976). Haemagglutination-like responses in multiple sclerosis-treated cells. *Lancet*, **i**, 688

24. Leibowitz, U. (1971). Multiple sclerosis: Progress in epidemiologic and experimental research: A review. *J. Neurol. Sci.*, **12**, 307

25. Adams, J. M. and Imagawa, D. T. (1962). Measles antibodies in multiple sclerosis. *Proc. Soc. Exp. Biol. Med.*, **111**, 562

26. Prineas, J. (1972). Paramyxovirus-like particles associated with acute demyelination in chronic relapsing multiple sclerosis. *Science*, **178**, 760

27. Gibbs, Jr., C. J. and Gajudsek, D. C. (1973). Experimental subacute spongiform virus encephalopathies in primates and other laboratory animals. *Science*, **182**, 67

28. Horta-Barbosa, L., Fuccillo, D. A., Sever, J. L. and Zeman, W. (1969). Subacute sclerosing panencephalitis: Isolation of measles virus from a brain biopsy. *Nature (London)*, **221**, 974

29. Barbosa, L. H. and Hamilton, R. (1973). Virological studies with multiple sclerosis brain tissues. *Lancet*, **i**, 1415

30. Ammitzboll, T., Offner, H., Clausen, J., Kobayasi, T., Asboe-Hansen, G., Hyllested, K. and Fog, T. (1976). Lysolecithin fusion of cells from multiple sclerosis patients with vero cells. *Acta Neurol. Scand.*, **53**, 137

31. Lampert, F. and Lampert, P. (1975). Multiple sclerosis. Morphologic evidence of intranuclear paramyoxvirus or altered chromatin fibers? *Arch. Neurol.*, **32**, 425

32. Dubois-Dalcq, M., Schumacher, G. and Sever, J. L. (1973). Acute multiple sclerosis: Electronmicroscopic evidence for and against a viral agent in the plaques. *Lancet*, **ii**, 1408

33. Tanaka, R., Iwasaki, Y. and Koprowski, H. (1976). Intracisternal virus-like particles in brain of a multiple sclerosis patient. *J. Neurol. Sci.*, **28**, 121

34. Norrby, E., Link, H., Olsson, J., Panelius, M., Salmi, A. and Vandvik, B. (1974).

Comparison of antibodies against different viruses in cerebrospinal fluid and serum samples from patients with multiple sclerosis. *Infect. Immun.*, **10**, 688

35. Link, H. (1972). Oligoclonal immunoglobulin G in multiple sclerosis brains. *J. Neurol. Sci.*, **16**, 103

36. Norrby, E. and Vandvik, B. (1974). The relationship between measles virus-specific antibodies and oligoclonal IgG in the cerebrospinal fluid (CSF) in patients with subacute sclerosing panencephalitis (SSPE) and multiple sclerosis (MS). *Med. Microbiol. Immunol.*, **160**, 233

37. Paty, D. W., Furesz, J., Boucher, D. W., Rand, C. G. and Stiller, C. R. (1976). Measles antibodies as related to HLA types in multiple sclerosis. *Neurology*, **26**, 651

38. Zander, H. (1975). Transmission of multiple sclerosis by blood transfusion? *J. Neurol. Sci.*, **24**, 505

39. Oger, J. F., Arnason, B. G. W., Wray, S. H. and Kistler, J. P. (1975). A study of B and T cells in multiple sclerosis. *Neurology*, **25**, 444

40. Utermohlen, V. and Zabriskie, J. B. (1973). A suppression of cellular immunity in patients with multiple sclerosis. *J. Exp. Med.*, **138**, 1591

41. Lamoureux, G., Giard, N., Jolicœur, R., Toughlian, V. and Desrosiers, M. (1976). Immunological features in multiple sclerosis. *Br. Med. J.*, **1**, 183

42. Levy, N. L., Auerbach, P. S. and Hayes, E. C. (1976). A blood test for multiple sclerosis based on the adherence of lymphocytes to measles-infected cells. *N. Engl. J. Med.*, **294**, 1423

6

Proteins and enzymes of myelin

P. R. Carnegie and N. R. Sims

Introduction

Current views on the structure of membranes assume that the genetic control over their structure and assembly is asserted via the protein components and that the nature and alignment of lipids depends on the amino acid sequence of the proteins. Demyelination may result from a defective myelin protein or damage to part of the protein framework which could result in unstable binding of the lipids. Whether the demyelination observed in multiple sclerosis is a result of a primary attack on the myelin sheath or secondary to an attack on the oligodendrocyte is an unresolved question. In this chapter we will describe the proteins and enzymes of myelin and discuss their possible involvement in multiple sclerosis.

Relationship between myelin and oligodendroglial cell

Myelin is considered to be synthetized by the oligodendrocyte but it is possible that the axon contributes some of the higher molecular weight proteins found in myelin[1,2]. The relationship of the oligodendrocyte to the axon and myelin sheath is shown diagrammatically in Figures 6.1 and 6.2. Some unidentified signal from the axon stimulates oligodendrocyte processes to wrap around the axon. The molecular mechanism for this is not understood. Burton and Agrawal[3] consider that the myelin proteins are synthetized as a group and that there are probably three phases, synthesis of proteins by the oligodendrocyte, organization of myelin precursors, and finally formation of compact myelin (Figure 6.1). If the precursors are not required they may be degraded and the amino acids re-utilized. It is possible that myelin is not derived from the oligodendrocyte plasma membrane but is a specially constructed set of membranes formed within an enclosure[4]. This appears

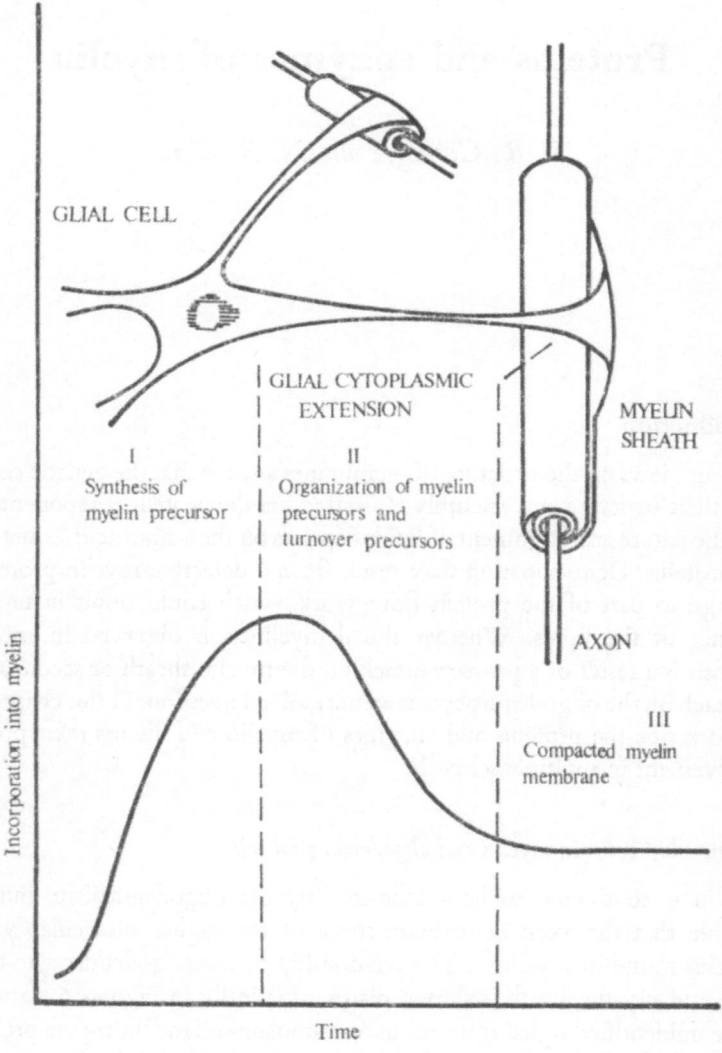

Figure 6.1 Schematic oligodendroglial cell, its cytoplasmic extension, and the myelin sheath. The curve indicates hypothetical time relationship of the incorporation (I), the turnover (II) and the stable (III) phases with the glial cell-myelin sheath 'anatomy' (from Burton and Agrawal[3])

likely as myelin has a quite different content of proteins, enzymes and lipids when compared to the oligodendrocyte plasma membrane[5].

With regard to diseases which lead to damage to myelin, it is necessary to consider the role of the oligodendrocyte. In some genetic disorders such as the leukodystrophies[6] essential enzymes are not produced by the oligodendrocyte and myelin fails to develop. In demyelination induced by toxic agents such as triethyltin, marked changes in the metabolism of myelin protein occur[7]. In multiple sclerosis where there is not a generalized, but a local, attack on myelin, factors such as the permeability of the blood brain barrier must be considered in relation to the infiltration of possible pathogenic antibodies[8], which could damage the oligodendrocyte in some regions of the brain but not in others. Selective degradation of oligodendrocytes has been observed in tissue cultures of brain explants when sera from patients with multiple sclerosis were added to them[9].

Often it is assumed that electrophysiological results obtained on the role of myelin in the peripheral nervous system (PNS) can be utilized when considering central nervous system (CNS) myelin. We wonder how valid such an extrapolation can be since there are considerable biochemical differences between the two types of myelin[10]. The Schwann cells in the PNS maintain myelin on only one axon, whereas in the CNS one oligodendrocyte supports several myelin sheaths. The protein composition of PNS myelin is quite different[10], the main protein being a glycoprotein, not a proteolipid protein. The ratio of basic proteins varies from nerve to nerve, and the content of enzymes typical of CNS myelin is much lower. This review will be limited to a consideration of CNS myelin.

Criteria for myelin proteins

Before a protein can be designated a component of myelin it is necessary that it is clearly shown to be associated with myelin firstly by subcellular fractionation and secondly by developmental studies[3,11]. Although myelin has a much simpler composition and smaller number of proteins than other membranes, recent studies have indicated the existence of several enzymes. In subcellular fractionations myelin is usually defined as the membranous material which floats between a layer of 0·32 M and 0·8 M sucrose. On recentrifugation of this material on a continuous gradient, between 0·60 and 0·85 M sucrose, a broad zone is obtained indicating heterogeneity in density[12]. This heterogeneity is reflected in differing ratios of various protein components; for example in spinal cord myelin the ratio of proteolipid protein to basic protein is approximately 1:1 and represents 80% of the total protein, and the high molecular weight proteins are present in much smaller amounts and predominantly in the denser zones[10]. The relationship of myelin to the axon is shown diagrammatically in Figure 6.2. In the isolation of myelin, during homogenization, sedimentation and washing, the myelinated axons

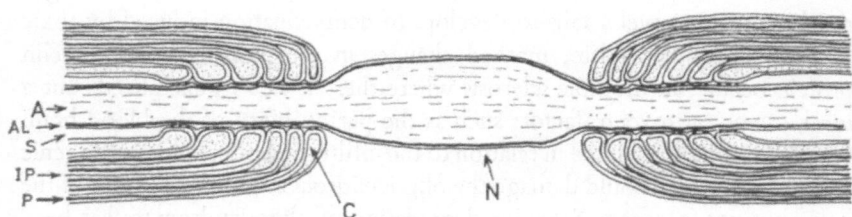

Figure 6.2 Relationship between axon (A) and myelin at a nodal region (N) in the central nervous system. Some of the minor proteins and enzymes could be derived from the axolemma (AL) which is separated from the myelin lamellae by the periaxonal space (S). The lamellae exhibit a characteristic periodicity in the electronmicroscope with the period line (P) thought to have originated from the cytoplasmic surface (C) and the intraperiod line (IP) from the external surface of the oligodendrocyte

are broken off from the oligodendroglial and neuronal cell bodies, and the soluble axonal components are removed. Under isotonic conditions the axolemma remains with the myelin fraction but after osmotic shock it can be separated from myelin[11]. However, it is probable that some of the myelin components of high molecular weight could be derived from the axolemma. These axonal remnants should not be considered as 'contaminants', for it is likely that in sections of the axon which become myelinated there are components which 'signal' the need for myelination and which are likely to be absent in non-myelinated regions.

The second criterion for a myelin component is an association with myelin during development. The period of rapid myelination varies, and in different species during this time an increase in myelinated axons can readily be demonstrated in the electronmicroscope[13]. During the same period certain myelin lipids (cerebroside for example) are accumulated in the brain and the enzymes involved with their synthesis increase in activity. Thus for a protein or enzyme to be designated a component of myelin, its time of appearance in the brain and rate of accumulation should be closely associated with the phase of myelination as determined by microscopy and incorporation of lipids associated with myelin.

Further support for a protein being a myelin component may come from examination of the central nervous system of mutant mice which exhibit defective myelination. Two such mutants, known as 'Quaking' and 'Jimpy', have been described[14], the latter showing the more serious deficiency. The primary defect leading to these blocks in myelination is unknown. Until this is determined it cannot be concluded that all myelin components will necessarily be diminished in these animals; however, a decrease in the level of any protein presents strong supporting evidence that it is intimately involved with myelin. In all cases where proteins satisfying the two criteria discussed above have been examined in neurological mutants, lower levels have been found than in normal controls (Figure 6.3).

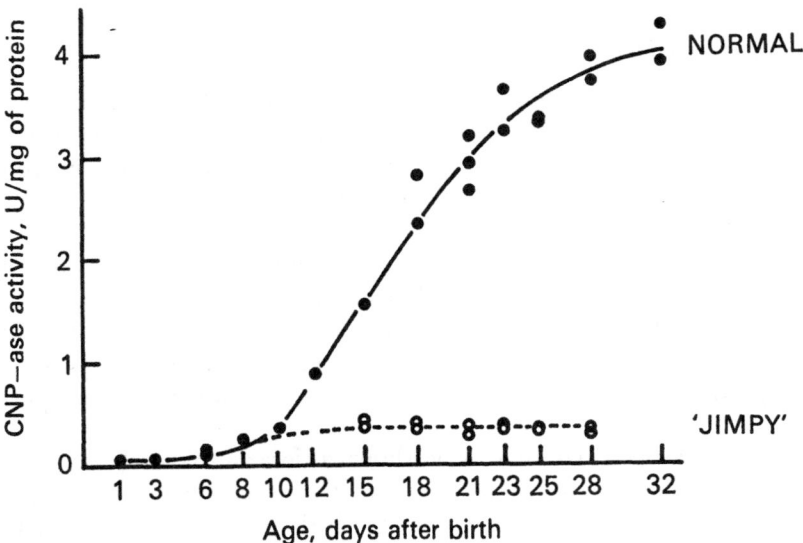

Figure 6.3 In normal mice between 10 and 20 days of age there is a period of rapid synthesis of myelin in the brain; 2′,3′-cyclic nucleotide 3′-phosphohydrolase (CNPase) activity increases rapidly in this period in normal mice but not in the 'Jimpy' mutant where there is a failure to synthetize myelin proteins and lipids (modified from Kurihara et al.[14])

In this chapter some or all of the above criteria will be discussed. As the properties of the basic protein and the proteolipid protein have frequently been reviewed only important features will be outlined. Since there is no review on the minor but possibly important proteins of myelin, these will be considered in detail. Any evidence for involvement of the proteins of myelin in multiple sclerosis will be given and speculations on their role in the pathogenesis of multiple sclerosis will be discussed.

Myelin basic protein

The basic protein is the most thoroughly studied protein from myelin. Interest in the basic protein was generated by the discovery that it could induce experimental allergic encephalomyelitis (EAE), an autoimmune disease of the brain which occurs readily in guinea-pigs (reviewed by Kies[15]). Whether or not this autoimmune disease can be taken as a model of part of the pathogenesis in multiple sclerosis is controversial.

Protein as a myelin component

The protein is well established as a myelin component and its isolation[16,17], properties[10,18] and immunological activity[15] have recently been reviewed in detail. This section will summarize its properties and emphasize recent work on enzymic modification of the basic protein and its possible involvement in multiple sclerosis.

The basic protein can readily be prepared from myelin by extraction with acid. To prepare large quantities of the basic proetin, the usual starting material is a chloroform–methanol extract of whole brain or spinal cord. The protein is a major component of the brain and accounts for 30% of the total protein of myelin and thus about 1% of the wet weight of spinal cord[16].

Several developmental studies have shown a close association between the appearance of basic protein in brain and the development of myelin[10]. Although it is generally assumed that the basic protein is synthetized by oligodendrocytes, direct evidence is lacking. It is possible that the basic protein is synthetized as a larger protein or a glycosylated protein which is modified in the process of myelin formation.

Physical properties

The physical properties of myelin basic protein are listed in Table 6.1. The isolated protein has an open conformation where the amino acid residues are readily accessible to enzymes and chemical reagents. Although there is no α helical or β pleated sheet there is some form of ordered structure which confers an ellipsoid shape with dimensions $15 \times 15\text{Å}$[19]. At present there is no information on its conformation in myelin but from studies on its interaction with lipids[20] it is likely to have a more ordered structure in a lipid environment.

Table 6.1 Physical properties of bovine myelin basic protein (adapted from Eylar et. al.[17])

Molecular weight	18 400
Intrinsic viscosity	9·3
Axial ratio a/b	10 prolate
(minimum solvation)	14 oblate
Diffusion constant $D_{20, w}$	$7·8 \times 10^{-7}$ cm^2 s^{-1}
Sedimentation constant S_{20w}	1·72S
Isoionic point	above pH 12
Absorbance 1% solution 276 nm	5·89

Amino acid sequence

The amino acid composition of myelin basic protein from a number of species is closely similar, with a high percentage of basic amino acids (17%) and a high content of glycine (15%)[10]. The protein from frog brain is unusual as it contains a cysteine residue[21].

The complete amino acid sequence has been determined for the human[22], bovine[23], and rat[24] proteins and partial sequence information is available on some other species. Errors and disputed sequences were discussed by Carnegie and Dunkley[10] and historical developments leading to the amino acid sequences of human and bovine proteins were described by Kies[15].

Some regions of the protein appear to have been more conserved than others during evolution (Figure 6.4). Rats, mice and other members of the *Myomorpha* and *Sciuromorpha* have a large and a small form of myelin basic protein[25]. The smaller form has apparently arisen from the larger as a result of an unusually long deletion of 40 amino acid residues within the molecule[24]. Bauer[26] has postulated that the myelin basic protein evolved by duplication from an ancestral gene which gave rise to histones and some other basic proteins.

Enzymic modification of myelin basic protein

Myelin basic protein is subject to a number of interesting modifications which presumably occur after synthesis. Thus myelin basic protein is actually a heterogeneous mixture of proteins with the differences being due to incomplete enzymic modification. These modifications (Table 6.2) will be described and their possible implications with regard to demyelinating disease will be discussed. Unfortunately no information is available on the extent of modification of the basic protein from multiple sclerotic brain.

```
                                                                    5                        10                       15                       20
Bovine                      Ala
Human        Ac- Ala- Ser- Gln-Lys-Arg-Pro-Ser-Gln-Arg-His-Gly-Ser- Lys-Tyr-Leu-Ala- Thr-Ala-Ser- Thr-Met-Asp-His-Ala-
Rat (small)

                    25                      30                       35                       40            45
                                                                                                                  Ser
Bovine
Human        Arg-His-Gly-Phe-Leu-Pro-Arg-His-Arg-Asp-Thr-Gly-Ile- Leu-Asp-Ser-Ile- Gly-Arg-Phe-Phe-Gly-Gly-Asp-Arg-
Rat (small)                                                                                                        Ser

                    50                55              60            65                 70
Bovine                                        Gly           Ala  Thr
Human        Gly-Ala-Pro- Lys-Arg-Gly-Lys- Asp-Ser-His- His-Pro- Ala-Arg-Thr-Ala-His-Tyr-Gly-Ser- Leu-Pro-Gln-
Rat (small)                                                  —          Thr

                        75        80                  85                    90                      95
                     Ala Gln     His    Pro          Glu Asn
                                  ↑
Bovine
Human        Lys-Ser- His-Gly-Arg-Thr-Gln-Asp-Gln-Asp-Pro-Val-Val-His- Phe-Phe-Lys-Asn-Ile- Val-Thr-Pro-Arg-Thr-Pro-
Rat (small)          Gln—                        Glu Asn

                          100      105              110                    115                     120
                                (MeArg)                                                          Lys
Bovine
Human        Pro-Pro-Ser- Gln-Gly-Lys-Gly-Arg-Gly-Leu-Ser-Leu-Ser-Arg-Phe-Ser-Trp-Gly-Ala-Glu-Gly- Gln-Arg-Pro-Gly-
Rat (small)             (Me4Arg)                          ————————————————

                          125              130                135              140     145
                                                                            Leu     His
Bovine
Human        Phe-Gly-Tyr-Gly-Gly-Arg-Ala-Ser-Asp-Tyr-Lys-Ser- Ala-His- Lys-Gly-Phe-Lys-Gly- Val-Asp-Ala-Gln-Gly-Thr-
Rat (small)  ——————————————————————————————————————————————————————————————————————————

                          150              155                160              165           170
Bovine
Human        Leu-Ser-Lys- Ile- Phe-Lys-Leu-Gly-Gly-Arg-Asp-Ser-Arg-Ser-Gly-Ser- Pro-Met-Ala-Arg-Arg
Rat (small)  ——————————————————————————————————————————————————————————————————————————
```

Figure 6.4 Amino acid sequence of myelin basic proteins. The full sequence of the human protein is shown in the centre with changes in the bovine above and the rat below. The sequences of the bovine and rat proteins are the same as those of the human protein except where substitutions, insertions (↑) or deletions (—) are shown. The residue numbers used in the text refer to the human protein (from Carnegie and

Table 6.2 Enzymic modifications of myelin basic protein

Modification	Site	Demonstrated in vitro	Demonstrated in vivo	Influence
Acetylation	Ala-1	No	Yes	Protects from digestion
Methylation	Arg-107	Yes	Yes	Increases hydrophobicity, protects against digestion
Phosphorylation	Ser-12	Yes	Yes	Increases negative charge; protects against digestion
	Thr-35	Yes	Yes?	
	Ser-56	Yes	Yes?	
	Ser-110	Yes	No?	
Glycosylation	Thr-98	Yes	No	Potential major change in antigenicity
Carboxypeptidase	Arg-170	Yes	Yes?	Lowers positive charge
(Deamidation)*	Gln-103	Yes	Yes?	Increases negative charge

* Maybe non-enzymic; for references see text

ACETYLATION

The N-terminal residue from a number of species has been shown to be blocked[10]. In the human and bovine proteins an acetyl group has been shown[22,23]. A number of other proteins also have blocked N-terminal residues and it has been suggested that the acetyl residue protects the protein from digestion by aminopeptidase. This could be important in myelin as there are claims that myelin contains aminopeptidase activity.

METHYLATION

Amino acid residue-107 in the human protein was found to be present as arginine, ω-N-monomethylarginine (MMA)or as ω-N,N'-dimethylarginine (sym-DMA)[22]. It is relatively simple to determine the ratio of the MMA to the sym-DMA form of the basic protein but because of the high content of arginine in the protein it is difficult to obtain reliable estimates of the amount of unmodified arginine at residue 107. The ratio of MMA to DMA varies with the species studied but appears to be constant for a given species[10,27]. This raises a major problem in understanding how this type of modification can remain constant and how the methylase is regulated.

The enzyme (methylase I) which methylates myelin basic protein is localized in the cytoplasmic fraction of brain[28–30]. Its concentration in neurones and glial cells remains to be determined. The enzyme is difficult to purify and may exist in several physical forms[29]. The methyl donor is S-adenosyl methionine and the enzyme is readily inhibited by the product

S-adenosyl-homocysteine[29]. Isolated bovine myelin was found to be a substrate which suggests that at least a portion of the protein is accessible to the enzyme in myelin[29]. Enzymes involved with the process of myelination show a characteristic rapid change in specific activity during the period of myelination. Although there is a slight increase in methylase activity during the period of myelination, the increase is not as dramatic as for example with enzymes involved in cerebroside synthesis[13]. In contrast to phosphorylation, methylation appears to be a relatively stable modification but the presence or absence of a 'demethylase' remains to be determined. There was no change in the ratio of MMA to DMA during the development of myelin in the rat[27].

The function of methylarginine in myelin basic protein is not known. One possibility is to protect this region of the protein from digestion by proteolytic enzymes which have similar properties to trypsin. However, the lysine residue at 105 would be expected to be digested. Thus it is less likely a possibility than the second which is to enable the arginine to move into a more hydrophobic environment. It has been suggested that methylation of arginine is necessary to complete a hydrophobic 'pocket' into which serotonin would neatly fit[31].

It is well established that deficiency of vitamin B_{12} in man and other animals leads to abnormal myelin. Although the main lesion is vacuolation of myelin, areas of demyelination have been observed in the optic nerve of B_{12}-deficient monkeys[32]. The reason for this dysmyelination is not known and the involvement of lipid methylation has been considered. However, because of the need for B_{12} in the reformation of S-adenosyl-homocysteine in the central nervous system, and because of the ready inhibition of arginine methylases by S-adenosyl-homocysteine it is possible that the dysmyelination is due to a failure to sufficiently methylate myelin basic protein during turnover.

The postulated viral agent in multiple sclerosis (Chapter 5) could influence myelination by altering the efficiency of methylation of myelin basic protein; such an effect is known for RNA[33]. The possibility of such an abnormality in multiple sclerosis has not been examined.

PHOSPHORYLATION

Because of its similarity in physical properties to histones, myelin basic protein was tried as a substrate for cyclic AMP-dependent protein kinase, and was found to be readily phosphorylated[34-36]. Several sites were phosphorylated and the main ones in the human protein were serine-12, threonine-35 and serine-110. In species where the content of dimethylarginine, at residue 107, was lower, relatively more phosphorylation of serine-110 occurred[34]. Protein kinases from rabbit skeletal muscle, bovine cardiac muscle, bovine brain and chicken kidney all phosphorylated the same sites in the basic protein. For phosphorylation to occur the intact protein was not essential and quite small peptides acted as substrates[37]. A synthetic peptide Gly-Arg-Gly-Leu-Ser-Leu-Ser-Arg was useful in ascertaining the structural requirements for phosphorylation and it appears that an arginine must be present to the N-terminal side of the serine to be phosphorylated[38].

Myelin was shown to contain a protein kinase which was not stimulated by cyclic AMP and myelin basic protein was the main substrate for this kinase[35,36,39]. It phosphorylated a different site from the cytoplasmic kinase; over 80% of the radioactivity was found to be associated with the equivalent of serine-56 in the human protein[39].

Although the basic protein as usually isolated cannot be considered to be a phosphoprotein, a small proportion has been found to contain phosphate as phosphoserine[35,40]. Radioactive phosphate, when injected, was readily incorporated into myelin basic protein in rat[36] and chicken brains[41].

The biological significance of phosphorylation of the basic protein of myelin remains to be determined. In contrast to the widely held view that myelin is metabolically inert, the in vivo turnover of phosphate on myelin basic protein suggests a much more dynamic role for the protein. One wonders if the effects of calcium on the stability of myelin are related to the binding of calcium to the basic protein. In multiple sclerosis Davis et al. have claimed that lowering the serum calcium has a beneficial effect on the patient's symptoms[42,43].

GLYCOSYLATION

Myelin basic protein can act as a substrate in vitro for N-acetyl-galactosaminyl transferases[44], the sugar residue being attached to threonine-98. There is no evidence that the basic protein is glycosylated in vivo, but a glycosylated form might not be readily extracted nor identified. The main protein of peripheral myelin appears to be a glycosylated form of a peripheral myelin basic protein and it is not readily solubilized[10].

CARBOXYPEPTIDASE AND DEAMIDATION

Microheterogeneity of myelin basic protein has been clearly demonstrated in a number of studies by Kies and colleagues. Recently they showed[41] that part of the heterogeneity was due to phosphorylation and part was due to removal of C-terminal arginine residues. It is not clear if this modification occurs in vivo or takes place during the isolation. Because of the denaturing conditions used during isolation it is more likely to be an in vivo modification.

Selective deamidation of glutamine residues has been demonstrated[24] and it is probable that this modification contributes to the heterogeneity. It is probable that this may be a spontaneous change not requiring an enzyme and it occurs during the extract with acid.

Robinson and Rudd[45] have suggested that spontaneous deamidation might be involved in degradation of proteins; removal of the amide group would increase the negative charge, change the conformation and start the degradative process. There is a need to examine the basic protein from multiple sclerotic brains with regard to these modifications.

Synthesis and degradation of myelin basic protein

Studies on the turnover of myelin basic protein have yielded confusing results as to the precise half-life of the protein in animals (reviewed by Carnegie and Dunkley[10]). Burton and Agrawal[3] have attempted to resolve the confusion by examining the turnover of myelin proteins over an extended period and have suggested that there is a precursor pool which is degraded if the proteins are not incorporated into the myelin sheath. Once laid down in the sheath the proteins apparently are stable (see Figure 6.1).

The normal in vivo procedure for the degradation of myelin basic protein is not known. In diseases such as multiple sclerosis and experimental autoimmune encephalomyelitis (EAE) where there is infiltration of lymphocytes into nervous tissue, myelin basic protein has been observed to be extensively degraded[46,47]. Because the concentration of lysomal acid proteinase is highest at the edge of the plaque in multiple sclerosis, it has been suggested that the proteolysis of the protein is a key event in the formation of the plaque[48]. Acid proteinase from brain[49] and thymocytes selectively hydrolyses myelin basic protein at the two Phe–Phe bonds thus producing three large fragments.

Localization

The precise localization and concentration of the basic protein within the lamellar structure of myelin is not known. One difficulty is that it is not clear how much reorganization and exposure of proteins has occurred during the isolation of myelin. With isolated myelin it appeared that the basic protein was associated with the period line (P in Figure 6.2) observed in the electron-microscope[50]. This would imply that it was originally present in vivo on the inner side of the oligodendrocyte membrane, if one accepts the conventional model for myelination. Attempts to establish the localization of myelin proteins in vivo with lactoperoxidase and ingeneous spinal cord preparation met with limited success but supports its localization in the period line[51].

Wherever the basic protein is located in vivo some of it at least is accessible to lymphocytes in experimental autoimmune encephalomyelitis (EAE)[52] (see Chapter 8). In this disease lymphocytes are sensitized to the basic protein by immunization in the hind footpad. The lymphocytes migrate to the brain where they produce a lesion only where they meet their target—myelin basic protein*. However, there is evidence that in native and thus undamaged myelin, most of the myelin basic protein is not accessible to antibody[53]. It is possible that a modified form of the basic protein is recognized on the surface of oligodendrocytes or at the equivalent of the nodes of Ranvier (see Figure 6.2). Wherever it is located it must be much more accessible to lymphocytes than other brain proteins, for example S-100 protein which is a good antigen but which does not induce lymphocytic infiltration into the brain nor any neurological disease.

Recently Wood et al.[54] used a non-penetrant probe for localization of membrane proteins on myelin from acute and chronic multiple sclerotics. They claimed that myelin basic protein was much more exposed in the myelin from the acute form. If confirmed this could be of major importance in understanding the breakdown of myelin.

Encephalitogenic determinants

Myelin basic protein when injected with appropriate adjuvants will produce experimental autoimmune encephalomyelitis (EAE), which is characterized by paralysis especially of the hind quarters and infiltration of lymphocytes into the central nervous system (see Chapter 8 and [15]).

One difficulty in studying this type of autoimmune disease is that different species respond preferentially to different regions of myelin basic protein. This is probably a reflection on the extent of immunological control over self-antigens rather than the exposure of different regions of the protein in the central nervous system. One would expect the protein to have a similar function in all mammals and an immune response to any part of it would disrupt its function and cause similar clinical symptoms. The sites which induce clinical EAE in various species are listed in Table 6.3. Although the

Table 6.3 Encephalitogenic regions of myelin basic protein

Region	Induces EAE	Reference
Phe-Ser-Trp-Gly-Ala-Glu-Gly-Gln-Lys or Arg	Guinea-pig	55, 56
Thr-Thr-His-Tyr-Gly-Ser-Leu-Pro-Gln-Lys-Gly	Rabbit	57
Phe-Lys-Leu-Gly-Gly-Arg-Asp-Ser-Arg-Ser-Gly-Ser-Pro-Met	Monkey	58
Between residues 45 and 86 in rat and mouse proteins	Rat and mouse	24, 59, 60, 61

* This view is by no means universally held by microscopists (see Chapter 1, page 7). Editor.

site for the monkey is known, it cannot be assumed that the human would respond to the same region of the protein. Two different assays[62,63] for cell-mediated immune response have claimed that lymphocytes from patients with multiple sclerosis respond to the tryptophan region of myelin basic protein.

In relation to multiple sclerosis

IMMUNOLOGICAL STUDIES

Because of the ability of myelin basic protein to induce experimental auto-immune disease of the central nervous system it has been widely studied as a possible antigen in multiple sclerosis. These studies provide no evidence for a humoral immune response to the basic protein; there are controversial results on the possibility of it being an antigen in cell-mediated responses. It is possible that the lack of agreement between laboratories[64] may reflect the difficulty of obtaining patients at a particular stage in the disease. It is conceivable that the differences reflect differences in the basic protein used as test antigen. Although there is considerable homology of amino acid sequence between the human protein and that from other species, the non-homologous regions could be important in assessing the response of lympho-cytes from patients. In addition another source of variation is the extent of enzymic modification of myelin basic protein. The extent of methylation of arginine varies quite markedly between species and the amount of phosphate remaining will vary with the purification procedure used. If the cell-mediated immune response were directed against a region of the human protein which is subject to modification then variation in results from laboratory to laboratory would be expected. There is a need for a preparation of human basic protein to be made available and used as a standard in work on cell-mediated immunity in multiple sclerosis.

IS MULTIPLE SCLEROSIS AN IMMUNOPHARMACOLOGICAL DISEASE?

The concept that clinical disease could result from a block of antibodies directed against cell surface receptors[65] evolved from consideration of the cause of paralysis in EAE. As was discussed above the basic protein of myelin in contrast to other brain proteins can readily induce marked neurological symptoms as a consequence of immunization. It was found that the whole protein was not required for the induction of EAE and that guinea-pigs responded to a small peptide Phe-Ser-Trp-Gly-Ala-Glu-Gly-Gln-Arg[56]. Carnegie[52] observed that this region of the protein fulfilled the requirements for a binding site for serotonin and that the clinical disease could result from antibody directed against serotonin receptors. Antibody has been implicated in the disruption of electrical activity in isolated cultures of central nervous tissue[66] but the precise site of action of the antibody, whether at the synapse, nodal region or at the oligodendrocyte has not been defined. Myelin basic protein was shown to interact with serotonin and related indoles[62] and support for the concept of a block or damage to serotonin receptors in EAE have come from neurophysiological studies[67] and determination of serotonin levels in the brain[68]. Moreover, when the level of brain serotonin was raised either by administration of tryptophan[69] or by monoamine oxidase inhibitors[70], the induction of EAE was suppressed.

Lennon and Carnegie[65] extended the concept to other diseases possibly caused by antibody to receptors. Their hypothesis has been validated by the demonstration that in myasthenia gravis there is an immune response to acetylcholine receptors, in Graves' disease there is an immune response to receptors for thyroid-stimulating hormone, and in insulin-resistant diabetes there is a response to insulin receptors.[71]

Multiple sclerosis is a likely addition to the list of immunopharmacological diseases. In multiple sclerosis abnormal levels of immunoglobulin are clearly demonstrated in cerebrospinal fluid but the antigen to which it is directed has not been identified. Serum from patients with multiple sclerosis contains antibody which will cause a block of bioelectric activity in tissue culture[66]. It is well established that multiple sclerotics have a peculiar sensitivity to small increases in temperature and the extent of their deterioration can be determined by tests of optic tract function, for example flicker fusion test. The deterioration in function induced by hyperthermia could be completely prevented by injection of the precursors of neurotransmitters tyrosine and tryptophan, but not by other compounds[72]. Moreover three groups have reported abnormalities in metabolites of serotonin in cerebrospinal fluid[73-75]. Our suggestion is that in multiple sclerosis there is a block by antibody of receptors for serotonin on oligodendrocytes (Figure 6.5) and that this type of reaction could account for the fluctuating clinical symptoms observed in the disease; demyelination would result from a prolonged immunological attack on the oligodendrocyte rendering it incapable of maintaining the myelin sheath. Receptors for serotonin must be present on oligodendrocytes as serotonin will alter their rate of pulsation[76].

Lymphocytes from patients with multiple sclerosis did not react to myelin but did react with oligodendrocytes[77]. Alvord et al.[78] found a similar lack of reactivity to myelin but obtained a response to a membrane fraction which although labelled 'synaptosomal membranes' could easily have included oligodendrocyte membranes. There is thus a need for further work on the antigen involved in the membrane and we speculate that it will be found to

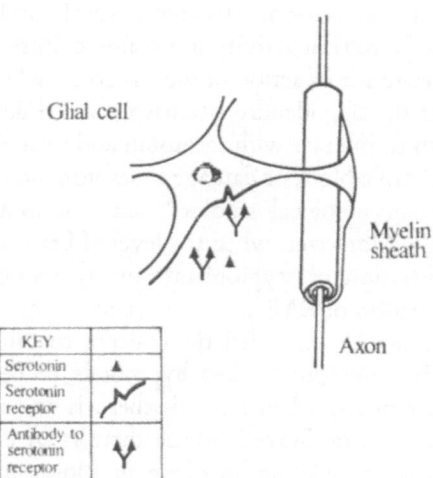

Figure 6.5 Concept of an immunopharmacological block in EAE and multiple sclerosis. Antibody to the serotonin receptor would interfere with the response of the glial cell to serotonin and disrupt its support of the myelin sheath. In myasthenia gravis it is now well established that antibody to acetylcholine receptor is involved in the pathogenesis

be an enzymically modified form of myelin basic protein acting as a serotonin receptor.

Should multiple sclerosis turn out to be an immunopharmacological disease similar to myasthenia gravis new approaches would appear with regard to treatment. To alleviate some of the symptoms, precursors of serotonin or certain monoamine oxidase inhibitors would be used to raise the level of serotonin at the receptor. In myasthenia gravis the use of anticholinesterase drugs is well established. It is of interest in this connection that monoamine oxidase inhibitors have been administered to multiple sclerotics with controversial results[52]. In the future it might be possible to specifically manipulate the immune response thus selectively restoring immunological tolerance to the receptors.

Recently Hyyppä et al.[79] found that L-tryptophan, a precursor of serotonin, had a beneficial effect on motility and bladder function in patients with multiple sclerosis. In this short-term trial there was no dramatic change in the condition of the patients. In future trials L-hydroxytryptophan should be used as it is a more direct precursor of serotonin. However more detailed trials should perhaps await experimental evidence to support the concept of an immunopharmacological block in multiple sclerosis. This may come from an investigation of the effects of serum from patients on serotonin receptors on cells cultured from the central nervous system.

OTHER STUDIES

Myelin basic protein has been implicated in studies on the proteolytic activity in the region of plaques of demyelination[80,81]. The claim[54] that the basic protein was more exposed in myelin from a patient with multiple sclerosis was discussed above.

Proteolipid protein

Protein as a myelin component

In most areas of the central nervous system the main protein of myelin is the proteolipid protein. This is a peculiarly hydrophobic protein with an unknown function. From electrophoretic studies it is clearly associated with the appearance of myelin during development. It is present in myelin through extensive purification and is not produced when myelin synthesis stops in mutant mice. Detailed references are given in recent reviews on the properties of the protein[82,83].

Isolation and properties

The protein is peculiar in that it is soluble in chloroform–methanol. A chloroform–methanol (2:1 by volume) extract of brain or myelin makes a convenient starting material for the isolation of the proteolipid protein[82]. It is readily denatured and great care must be taken to prevent aggregation during the separation of the protein from lipid. The physical properties alter during the conversion to the lipid-free protein. Even after extensive purification the protein retains a small amount of fatty acid which is covalently linked to some unidentified site[82,83]. It is possible that a glycosylated form of the protein exists in myelin but this remains to be substantiated[84].

The molecular weight (25 000 daltons) is slightly higher than that of the myelin basic protein[82]. The protein has an unusually high content of hydrophobic amino acids which presumably helps to explain its ready solubility in chloroform–methanol[82,83]. The aggregation which readily occurs during isolation probably involves crosslinking through disulphide bonds. The isolated protein is extremely resistant to digestion by proteolytic enzymes[85] and it has not so far been possible to obtain detailed information on the amino acid sequence, apart from a short segment at the N-terminal end[86]. This region from the human protein had the sequence Gly-Leu-Leu-Glu-Cys-Cys-Ala-Arg-Cys-Leu-Val-Gly-Ala-Pro-Phe-Ala-X-Leu-Val-Ala. It is noteworthy that there is a high proportion of hydrophobic amino acids in this section.

Protein in relation to multiple sclerosis

In contrast to the basic protein, proteolipid protein does not induce EAE. It does not appear to have been examined as a possible antigen in multiple sclerosis. Although very resistant to proteolytic digestion *in vitro*, when it is present in myelin proteolytic enzymes appear to be able to digest it readily[87]. In studies on plaques from multiple sclerotic brains the proteolipid protein was found to have disappeared along with other myelin components[80].

2',3'-Cyclic nucleotide-3'-phosphohydrolase

2',3'-cyclic nucleotide-3'-phosphohydrolase (CNPase) is an enzyme which catalyses hydrolysis of 2',3'-cyclic nucleotides to produce 2' derivatives.

Because of its application in studies of demyelination in multiple sclerosis and in experimental animals, it is reviewed in detail.

Although activity of this nature was first demonstrated in bovine spleen[88] and pancreas[89] it was shown in 1962 by Drummond *et al.*[90], in a more detailed study in the dog, that the specific activity in the central nervous system was at least ten times greater than in a wide range of other tissues.

CNPase as a myelin enzyme

Determination of the regional distribution of CNPase in the central nervous system of several vertebrates indicated a correlation with the distribution of myelinated fibres[91]. Unmyelinated invertebrate nerves contained no activity[92]. As cerebroside had been shown to increase simultaneously with myelination and was demonstrated to be a major myelin lipid it was considered the most characteristic myelin marker and accordingly Drummond *et al.*[90] examined the ratios of CNPase to cerebroside for different CNS regions of a number of vertebrates including dog, skate, dogfish and turtle. The ratio varied widely between different regions in a single animal and especially between comparable regions in the different species. The authors concluded that the absolute amounts of CNPase and myelin were independent although they also suggested the results could arise if cerebroside did not represent a universal myelin marker. As the species studied are widely separated on a phylogenetic scale, differences in CNPase/cerebroside ratio may only reflect different evolutionary development with respect to these components.

FRACTIONATION

Subcellular fractionation of rabbit brain showed that the enzyme was associated with particulate fractions especially with those demonstrated by electronmicroscopy primarily to contain myelin sheaths[91]. Similar results were found for a subcellular fractionation of bovine brain[93]. A more recent study[94] of CNPase activity of myelin isolated from different regions of bovine brain showed variations resembling those observed by Drummond et al.[90] for CNPase activity in dog brain.

When purified myelin from rat was further fractionated on a discontinuous sucrose gradient, CNPase activity was shown to increase from light to heavy fractions as did glycoprotein and other high molecular weight protein in contrast to basic protein[95]. The observed changes of CNPase levels both between different brain regions and within myelin may reflect localization of the enzyme in specific regions and may in turn be of functional significance for the enzyme.

DEVELOPMENT

In the developing central nervous system of chicks[96], mice[14] and rats[93] the appearance of CNPase activity closely paralleled active myelination, but was not associated with axonal development.

NEUROLOGICAL MUTANTS

Studies on two neurological mutant mice which exhibit a deficiency of myelination indicated that CNPase was decreased to 25–50% in 'Quaking' mutant[14,93] and to 10% in 'Jimpy'[92,97] when compared to controls. This is consistent with the observation that 'Jimpy' shows the more serious myelin deficiency. In normal mice CNPase specific activity increases rapidly from 10–28 days after birth. By contrast it has been demonstrated[14] that CNPase levels in 'Jimpy' brains do not increase beyond the 21st day level whilst in 'Quaking' an increase is observed to day 21 (Figure 6.3).

Whether or not there is a strictly quantitative relationship between CNPase activity and myelin content the weight of evidence indicates that CNPase is a true myelin enzyme satisfying all criteria listed in the introduction. As such, this has proven a useful 'marker' for myelin in isolation and developmental studies involving higher animals.

Properties

Myelin CNPase is conveniently measured by determining the rate of hydrolysis of 2′,3′-cyclic nucleotides to their 2′ derivatives. The adenosine cyclic nucleotide is maximally hydrolysed[90] and is the substrate used in most assay systems. Other 2′,3′-cyclic nucleotides are hydrolysed to a lesser extent whilst 3,5′-cyclic nucleotides and non-cyclic phosphate diesters do not act as substrates. Unless indicated, studies discussed below have used 2′,3′-cyclic adenosine monophosphate (cyclic AMP) as substrate.

Several-fold activation of the enzyme in myelin has been shown to occur by treatment with the detergents sodium deoxycholate[98], Triton X-100[92], Cetavlon[99] and Sulphobetaine-DLH[100]. This activation is probably a result of lipid removal allowing increased access of substrate to active sites. Some support for this idea comes from the observation that sonication results in partial activation[91]. From studies performed, it is not possible to determine whether any of the activating effect observed results from a direct action of the detergents on the enzyme.

In our work on solubilization of the enzyme using Triton X-100, we showed that solubilization required ionic strength of above 0·5 but maximal activation is obtained at greater than 2% Triton X-100 independently of the ionic strength[101].

The pH optimum of the detergent-activated enzyme from mammals is 6·2–6·5[102,103] although earlier work involving material that was not pre-activated showed a pH optimum of 7·5. The temperature optimum for rat brains was shown to be 30 °C[103]. An optimal pH of around 6·5 and a temperature optimum of 30 °C was obtained for shark brain[102-105] which had not been activated[104]. Several values of apparent K_m have been reported and whilst these vary fairly widely they fall in the range of 1·3–5 mM. This wide variation is not surprising as source and conditions of sample and assay differ drastically, but as will be discussed later, the values obtained are generally higher than would be expected for a physiological substrate.

Data on inhibition of the enzyme is confused, probably because studies have been performed using different assays on material processed in various ways. The enzyme shows no metal requirement but inhibition has been shown to occur with cupric sulphate, zinc acetate and mercuric chloride[90]. A form of the enzyme solubilized using Tween/guanidinium was shown[105] to be inhibited by high levels of sodium acetate, sodium chloride and guanidinium chloride although work in our laboratory has shown no effect of sodium chloride on a Triton X-100–salt solubilized form of the enzyme.

Early studies using a fixed time assay containing $7\frac{1}{2}$ mM 2′,3′-cyclic AMP reported no inhibition by 2' or 3' AMP at concentrations up to 10 mM[90,93]. A more recent study[105], however, using a rapid spectral assay and substrate concentration of 1 mM (cyclic AMP) reported 50% inhibition by both these compounds at 0·5 mM. Adenosine-5'-phosphate and adenosine-5'-triphosphate were shown to inhibit at slightly higher levels (0·52 and 0·96 mM respectively for 50% inhibition) and adenosine 3'-5-cyclic phosphate, orthophosphate and adenosine (4·4, 8·5 and 16·0 mM) at much higher levels. Pyridoxal phosphate was also inhibitory but the extent of its inhibition was not determined.

The physiological substrate for the enzyme has not been determined but the observed action and inhibition of the enzyme would seem to suggest that a sterically restricted phosphate group is required in the substrate. The recent observations of phosphorylation[34] in basic protein make it tempting to suggest the enzyme may perform a role in modifying the pattern of phosphorylation of the basic protein (for example as a phosphotransferase). Initial studies in this direction (unpublished) have shown that CNPase and phosphoprotein phosphatase activities are unrelated. A synthetic peptide Gly-Arg-Gly-Leu-Ser-Leu-Ser-Arg, related to myelin basic protein was phosphorylated with cyclic AMP-dependent protein kinase[39]. The phosphopeptide was readily dephosphorylated by the phosphoprotein phosphatase associated with myelin but not by a CNPase purified by ion exchange chromatography[106].

CNPase activity in other membranes

CNPase activity was originally reported in non-neural material[88,89] and a later study[90] indicated that activity was fairly widespread although always at least ten times lower than the levels in the nervous system. The peripheral nervous system was shown[90,107] to have five to ten times lower activity than the central nervous system. Detailed studies of CNPase from human erythrocyte[108] and spleen[109] showed in both cases the enzyme was associated with membrane material and for the properties examined was identical to the myelin CNPase. This would suggest that the enzyme could perform a function of general importance in membranes and not just one peculiar to myelin.

With cells from the central nervous system, marked differences were found in CNPase content. Oligodendroglial cells were found to have eight times more enzyme than astrocyte or neurones[110]. The specific activity of CNPase in the plasma membrane fraction of oligodendrocytes was half that of myelin[5]. As it is generally accepted that oligodendroglial cells are involved in myelin formation it is not surprising that these cells contain this myelin component. The higher specific activity of CNPase in myelin compared to oligodendroglial cells would suggest CNPase exists in myelin not merely through passive transfer with other oligodendroglial proteins, but that it is either produced for incorporation into myelin or selectively maintained during the myelination process.

Using different isolation procedures, two subfractions, labelled 'myelin-like'[98, 111–113] and 'membrane fraction'[114], which bear some resemblance to myelin by a number of criteria, have been isolated from young rat brains. These two fractions have similar chemical compositions and both appear as single-walled vesicles in electronmicroscopy, but differ in the detailed morphology of the vesicle wall[114]. Both subfractions are virtually devoid of cerebroside but have high activities of CNPase, and electrophoresis indicates that they contain basic protein. Labelling studies[114] suggest that there may be a precursor–product relationship between these fractions and mature myelin. The presence of CNPase in myelin-like material has recently[115] been confirmed and was also shown to be present in microsomal fractions in the early stages of postnatal development. Basic protein was also detected electrophoretically in these fractions and it has been suggested that the microsomes contain precursor membrane fragments at a stage prior to myelin formation.

CNPase in myelination, demyelination and disease

The intimate relationship between CNPase and myelin has led to the study of this enzyme in relation to a number of diseases or treatments which result in changes or loss of myelin. The extensive studies on CNPase in relation to defective myelination in mutant mice have already been described. In the human genetic disease, Down's syndrome, myelin levels are usually decreased. The protein composition of the myelin seems generally unchanged, but three cases examined for CNPase activity showed a 20–30% reduction of this enzyme[116].

The production of EAE by injection of myelin basic protein and its relationship to multiple sclerosis have been discussed in Chapter 6. Drummond *et al.*[92] examined CNPase activity in spinal cords of guinea-pigs in the terminal stages of EAE, but no significant difference in activity was found between diseased and control animals. However, another study[117] claimed a slight increase at early stages in the disease. A study of EAE in the monkey revealed that enzyme levels in the plaques of demyelination were lower than those found in apparently normal white matter from the diseased brain from animals with EAE[118]. Bornstein and Raine[119] reported that serum from animals with EAE, when added to embryonic mouse spinal cord cultures, inhibited visible myelination. Under normal conditions these cultures show an increase in sulphatide synthesis as followed by ^{35}S uptake just prior to myelination and an increase of CNPase activity during myelination, both of which mimic the situation in the whole animal. In the presence of EAE serum, CNPase activity did not increase in the cultures but on removal of the serum visible myelination and CNPase activity increased in parallel[120]. A similar response was observed when sulphatide synthesis was examined[121].

Tumour cell lines of glial origin were found to have CNPase activity[122]. Later studies[123] on series of brain tumours showed that CNPase levels in all cases were considerably less than normal brain white matter. For typical tumours CNPase activity decreased in the order oligodendroglioma> neurinoma and astrocytoma>glioblastoma>medulloblastoma>meningioma. Pfeiffer and Weschler[124] established four neoplastic clonal cell lines from a transplantable tumour of the PNS, and showed by several criteria including a relatively high CNPase activity that one of these was a Schwannoma. Konings and Pierce[109] examined a lymphosarcoma in spleen and found approximately double the activity observed in normal spleen tissue. Whether this represents a general phenomenon of these tumours has not yet been reported.

Thyroid hormones appear to exert some effect during CNS maturation. Thyroxine administration leads to precocious myelination and hypothyroidism results in a deficiency of myelin lipids. Hyperthyroidic animals exhibited an 80% increase of CNPase activity on the fifth day of life. In hypothyroidism CNPase levels followed a similar pattern of increase to normal but were retarded in actual level so that at 20 days CNPase activity was approximately equivalent to 15-day activity of a control animal[125]. Injection of triiodothyronine to hypothyroidic animals resulted in complete restoration in four days to a normal CNPase level in brain. It would appear therefore, that the rate of appearance of the enzyme is, at least partially, under the influence of thyroid hormones. Another study of this type on hypothyroid rats reported essentially the same results[126].

Chronic administration of triethyltin (TET) to rats results in a demyelination process which proceeds in the presence of severe oedema and without the intervention of macrophage activity. Several hypotheses exist as to the mechanism of TET disruption and one such theory suggests that the mode of action of several enzymes has been affected. Wassenaar and Kroon[127] studied a number of enzymes from rabbits with TET-induced oedema as well as effects of TET on these enzymes *in vitro*. CNPase levels in treated animals were not reported but TET was shown to have no effect on CNPase *in vitro*.

The compound 1,1,3-tricyano-2-amino-1-propene (TCAP) increases neuronal metabolism and production of nucleoprotein in rabbit cerebral cortex pyramidal cells and spinal cord motor neurons. When TCAP was injected into chick embryos, and the CNPase level in sciatic nerve was examined 24 hours later, an increase in activity was observed. The increase was not the result of direct activation of the enzyme by TCAP. Cerebroside production was also stimulated but to a lesser extent and CNPase in the brain and other enzymes studied from the sciatic nerve were not affected. Labelling studies indicated production of a single protein (or group of proteins) and it was suggested that TCAP selectively stimulated *de novo* synthesis of CNPase by Schwann cells[128].

In relation to multiple sclerosis

CNPase activity in multiple sclerosis patients was shown to be the same or marginally lower than controls in the white matter of the temporal region outside plaques of demyelination and to decrease towards the centre of plaques[129,130]. In nearly all cases, changes were reflected by changes in cerebroside levels[129]. Two samples from the corresponding temporal region of the patients with the virally induced demyelinating disease, subacute sclerosing panencephalomyelitis (SSPE), were also examined and showed much lower values than controls and again these were reflected by similar decreases in cerebroside levels[129].

Myelination and CNPase activity in tissue cultured from newborn mouse cerebellum was shown to increase to 20 days and then plateau off. Addition of EAE or MS serum at 20 days caused demyelination, and CNPase activity fell by 80% within a few hours. No CNPase activity was detected in the culture medium, indicating that the enzyme was blocked or destroyed before release[131]. Unfortunately this interesting observation has not been further examined.

Cell cultures derived from autopsy and biopsy material from multiple sclerosis patients showed no significant differences in their CNPase activity when compared to cultures from patients with other diseases not involving the central nervous system. All cultures showed increased CNPase specific activity with increasing cell density, or after transformation with SV40 virus[132].

These studies would seem to suggest that CNPase is not involved directly in the pathogenesis of multiple sclerosis. However, until the physiological substrate for this enzyme is determined and further studies performed this possibility cannot be completely eliminated. The ability of this enzyme to serve as a marker for myelin has been indicated in this section and because it is not altered drastically in multiple sclerosis it remains a useful marker in material isolated from patients.

Cholesteryl ester hydrolase

Several cholesteryl ester hydrolases exist in the brain. One of these, distinguishable by pH optimum, was shown to be almost exclusively localized in fractions containing purified myelin from rat brain. Levels of the enzyme are markedly decreased in grey matter, in seven-day-old (unmyelinated) rat brains and in 'Quaking' and 'Jimpy' mice[133]. This strongly suggests it is truly associated with myelin.

Properties

The enzyme is activated by taurocholate but inhibited by Triton X-100, Tween 20 and sodium deoxycholate[133]. Furthermore the enzyme in myelin has a lipid requirement being stimulated by some phospholipids, saturated fatty acids and neutral glycolipids and inhibited by unsaturated fatty acids, lysolecithin and acidic glycolipids[134]. Of the lipids examined, phosphatidyl serine produced the greatest stimulation but even this could not completely replace the taurocholate activation. Stimulation was independent of the enzyme source but dependent on the amount of substrate present, and the K_m and linearity of the enzyme response were not significantly affected.

In relation to multiple sclerosis

It has commonly been observed that cholesteryl ester is increased in demyelinating disease whether demyelination is primary to or secondary to the disease process. Furthermore, the cholesteryl esters formed usually show variation with respect to the esterified fatty acid when compared to the trace amounts of cholesteryl esters in normal myelin. There is some conjecture[135,136] as to whether the pattern of esterification varies according to the disease or is the same regardless of the demyelinative process. In multiple sclerosis it has been suggested that cholesteryl esters are altered in the apparently normal white matter as well as the plaques of demyelination, an observation which could imply a causative role for these lipids in the disease. A recent paper[137] concluded that this observation was probably due to the presence of plaques in the normal white matter which escaped detection.

The existence of a cholesteryl ester hydrolase which seems to be almost exclusively localized to myelin suggests that it may be involved, directly or indirectly, in the metabolism of cholesteryl esters. The role of the enzyme is not known although it may be involved in maintaining low cholesteryl ester levels in the myelin. In the disruption caused by demyelination the enzyme may be destroyed or become inhibited by interaction with lipids with which it is not normally in contact, hence resulting in increases in the levels of cholesteryl esters. A further possibility, which has not been investigated, is that this enzyme may be capable of catalysing the reverse reaction under the influence of certain lipids. It could then be seen to play an active role in the production of cholesteryl esters during demyelination. Whatever the involvement (if any) of this enzyme in demyelination, the observation that it is strongly inhibited by unsaturated fatty acids is intriguing in view of the controversy over the role of fatty acids in multiple sclerosis (see Chapters 8, 9).

Other proteins and enzymes of myelin

In this section a number of proteins and enzymes which have been claimed to be associated with myelin will be described. The presence of these components serves to emphasize that myelin is a much more complex membrane than previously thought.

Glycoprotein

Compared to other membrane fractions myelin has a relatively low glycoprotein content[138]. However, Quarles et al.[139] using SDS gel electrophoresis and [14C] fucose, injected into rat brain, showed that the radioactivity was incorporated into myelin primarily into a single band. Extraction with chloroform–methanol results in solubilization of less than 10% radioactivity suggesting it was neither labelled glycolipid nor part of the chloroform–methanol soluble proteins which constitute a large amount (~90%) of the myelin proteins[140]. A glycoprotein of similar electrophoretic mobility was also found in human and bovine brain[141]. From the ratio of carbohydrate to protein it was determined that in rats the glycoprotein represented only less than 2% of the total myelin protein[140]. A number of experiments were therefore necessary to confirm that this protein was truly myelin associated and not merely a contaminant from a richer source.

GLYCOPROTEIN AS A MYELIN COMPONENT

It was reasoned that if glycoprotein were a contaminant, a preparation of myelin from white matter would contain less glycoprotein than one from mainly grey matter which is rich in glycoproteins from neuronal membranes. Despite the great differences in yield of myelin from the two sources, the specific radioactivity was approximately the same suggesting that the glycoprotein was a true component of myelin[140].

When pure myelin was isolated and separated into four fractions on a discontinuous gradient the glycoprotein was shown to increase from the light to heavier fractions similarly to CNPase[95].

That the labelled glycoproteins were not introduced to the myelin from other fractions during myelin isolation was shown by examining the myelin fraction from mixtures of brains of adult and neonatal rats bearing different isotopic labels. By similarly examining brains from animals aged 10–22 days it could be shown there was a good correlation between the amount of radioactive glycoprotein in the myelin and the amount of myelin in the brain[140]. A fraction isolated from 'Jimpy' mice using the procedure for immature myelin was shown to contain virtually none of the characteristic myelin markers nor the major glycoprotein[142]. Myelin isolated from fucose-labelled 'Quaking' mice brains contained less radioactive fucose than controls and was incorporated into a protein of apparently larger molecular weight[143]. It has been suggested that the smaller glycoprotein may be required for normal maturation of myelin and hence it was proposed that the absence of this form may be the defect responsible for impaired myelination of 'Quaking' mice.

The plant lectin, concanavalin A, binds to isolated myelin providing further evidence for the existence of glycoprotein. Lectins specific for fucose and N-acetylhexosamine residues did not bind but it was suggested this may be due to these residues being sterically inaccessible in the myelin[144].

GLYCOPROTEIN IN MYELINATION

A detailed study[145] of myelin isolated from brains of rats aged 14–60 days and examined by electrophoresis showed an insignificant variation in the amount of glycoprotein relative to total protein. Injection of labelled glucose and fucose into 13-day-old animals showed increasing total radioactivity in myelin for several weeks in contrast to total brain which decreased in radioactivity over the same time. The authors suggested these results are best explained by the existence of a precursor material for myelin which has different density characteristics to myelin and is not isolated with it. Radioactivity would incorporate rapidly into this precursor and would appear more slowly in the myelin as it was formed by modification of the precursor.

Electrophoretic studies of the glycoprotein from rats indicated a molecular weight of approximately 110 000 daltons although mobility of glycoproteins in SDS is partially dependent on the carbohydrate groups present. When myelin fractions isolated from 14-day and 22-day-old rats, injected with different isotopes, were run on a single gel, the major glycoprotein from the older animals had a slightly greater mobility[146]. This effect was also observed[147] in hamsters, gerbils and other strains of rats but could not be shown for strains of mice or for prairie deer mice. The glycoprotein in the latter two groups had a mobility corresponding to the faster glycoprotein of the former species. As this faster glycoprotein is present in all species, it has been suggested that it is necessary for normal myelin maturation. The small change in mobility was proposed to be a result of changes in carbohydrate composition of the protein, or alternatively could have resulted from a decrease in the molecular weight of 15000–200000 daltons[148].

As glycoproteins are believed to be involved in cell–cell interactions it has been suggested[148] that myelin glycoprotein could function in the recognition of axonal sites for myelination or in promoting the formation of compact myelin from loose layers as a result of alteration or removal of the glycoprotein.

GLYCOPROTEIN IN RELATION TO MULTIPLE SCLEROSIS

No studies have been reported on the myelin glycoprotein in multiple sclerosis. However, there is a report that a brain-specific glycoprotein, obtained from human white matter, will stimulate lymphocytes from patients with multiple sclerosis. It is unlikely that this component of white matter is the same as the myelin glycoprotein as the former is readily soluble in EDTA-saline[149].

DM20

A protein observed on SDS gel electrophoresis to run between basic protein and proteolipid protein and which seems to be unique to central nervous system myelin has been reported and named DM20[150]. It has been shown that DM20 is enriched in parallel with proteolipid and basic proteins during myelin isolation and is present in myelin prepared from a number of species suggesting that it is a general component of this membrane. It remains in the acid insoluble fraction and a band of similar mobility has been observed in SDS gels of chloroform–methanol extracts suggesting it might be a component of proteolipid protein; however, further clarification of the nature of the protein and its relationship to proteolipid is required. Studies on DM20 in relation to multiple sclerosis have not been performed.

Non-specific esterase

NON-SPECIFIC ESTERASE AS A MYELIN COMPONENT

Whilst the presence of non-specific esterase activity in the brain is beyond doubt[151], the association of some of this activity with myelin remains controversial. Early histochemical studies[152,153] indicated that myelin was not a major site of esterase activity, but precise location of activity using such techniques is difficult. Direct assay of myelin obtained by subcellular fractionation from rat[153], human[154], bovine[155,156] and guinea-pig[155] brains indicated the presence of some non-specific esterase. It has also been shown[157,158], however, that levels of non-specific esterase activity as well as the activities of several 'marker' enzymes usually regarded as characteristic of non-myelin subfractions, vary markedly with myelin according to the media used for its isolation. It has been suggested that redistribution of some enzymes occurs during fractionation by release into solution from their native site and subsequent reabsorption by other components, and this may be responsible for the observed variation in enzyme levels. Nonetheless myelin has been produced which retains low esterase activity in the absence of significant activity from the 'marker' enzymes[158-160] and no cases have been reported of isolated myelin which completely lacks esterase activity. Whilst this would seem to suggest the existence of esterase activity in normal myelin, it is far from definitive. Determinations of levels of esterase activity during active myelination and in the neurological mutant mice 'Quaking' and 'Jimpy' would help to clarify the problem.

PROPERTIES

The enzyme remaining in purified myelin shows a marked preference for esters of short-chain fatty acids as substrates although activity is still detectable with longer-chain substrates[154,157,160]. It has been suggested[159] that two enzymes may be responsible for the observed activity—a lipase attacking longer-chain esters and an esterase for short-chain substrates. Whilst this has not been examined in detail, investigation of the variation in specific activity in developing guinea-pig (15 days to one year) gave different results depending on whether short or long-chain esters were used as substrates. The physiological substrate of the enzyme is not known.

The enzyme remaining in purified myelin is partially released into the soluble fraction by the action of non-ionic detergents but is not released by aqueous buffers and salt solutions of various ionic strengths and pH[160,161]. This adds further evidence of its intimate association with myelin.

IN RELATION TO MULTIPLE SCLEROSIS

No work has been reported on the levels of non-specific esterase in myelin isolated from multiple sclerosis patients. Early work involving examination of esterase activity in white matter using zymogram techniques revealed major changes with short-chain esterase activity between multiple sclerosis and control samples, although these were not always reflected by changes for homogenates when assayed directly[162,163].

Aminopeptidase and arylamidase

A problem arises in interpreting the data on the localization of amino-peptidase activity as early studies used L-leucyl-β-naphthylamide as substrate as it was thought this reflected a leucine aminopeptidase-type activity. It has now been shown[164] that hydrolysis of this may result from action of enzymes unrelated to leucine aminopeptidase which have been termed arylamidases (or aminopeptidase N). Only in recent studies has the distribution of sub-strates hydrolysed by true aminopeptidases have been examined.

As with non-specific esterase there has been difficulty in determining if any arylamidase or aminopeptidase activity, which is apparently associated with myelin, is present merely as an artifact of myelin preparation or not. As-sociation of arylamidase activity with myelin was first suggested by Adams et al.[152] from assay of subfraction activity although histochemical staining failed to support this. Early reports[152,165] claimed that activities in myelin represented between 15 and 20% of the total brain activity but more rigorous purification of myelin results in only 2–4% being retained[166]. It was further demonstrated[167] that arylamidase activity in isolated myelin decreased if gradient centrifugations of the myelin were repeated but reached a plateau after several such centrifugations. Enzymatic markers for other membranes were generally reduced to negligible levels by such isolation procedures. D'Monte et al.[168] also showed a marked decrease in arylamidase activity accompanied by decreased specific activity during rigorous myelin purifica-tion but reported that the specific activity of an aminopeptidase (using Leu-Gly-Gly as substrate) was increased.

Only marginal changes were found in arylamidase during myelination in the rat[111] or chicken[169]. It was found however, that arylamidase was present, along with CNPase, in 'early' myelin from the rat[111], a fraction for which a possible precursor role to myelin may exist.

A slight increase in the specific activity of the tripeptide aminopeptidase in chicken brain during myelination (13 days prenatal to 7 days postnatal) was observed[169]. This did represent a doubling of activity expressed relative to wet weight of brain but was far from the dramatic change observed for CNPase.

These results seem to suggest that arylamidase activity is absent, or present only at very low levels in myelin. The possibility of myelin-associated amino-peptidase activity has not been completely ruled out.

No studies on these enzymes in relation to multiple sclerosis have been reported although it has been shown that arylamidase activity was not greatly affected in experimental autoimmune encephalomyelitis (EAE)[165].

UDP-galactose:ceramide galactosyltransferase

UDP-galactose:ceramide galactosyltransferase catalyses the last step of synthesis of galactosyl ceramide which is a major lipid of the myelin sheath. Recently it was claimed, from studies on its subcellular distribution, that it is a component of myelin[170].

Protein kinase and phosphoprotein phosphatase

Protein kinases are enzymes which phosphorylate selected serine or threonine residues in proteins. Brain contains, in the cytoplasmic fraction, protein kinase which is activated by adenosine 3',5'-cyclic monophosphate (cyclic AMP). *In vitro* this enzyme was found to utilize myelin basic protein as a substrate. Among the enzymes of myelin are a protein kinase[35,36,39], not regulated by cyclic AMP, and a phosphoprotein phosphatase[39,171]. Both use myelin basic protein as substrate but as they were only recently discovered little information is available on their properties and role in myelin. Because of the presence in myelin of both a kinase and a phosphatase only a small proportion of the basic protein would be expected to be phosphorylated at any one time and the extent of phosphorylation would depend upon a difference in rate between the kinase and phosphatase.

Phosphorylation of myelin basic protein has been demonstrated *in vivo* in rats[35,36] and chickens[172]. Several sites are phosphorylated in chicken myelin basic protein and both the cyclic AMP-dependent protein kinase and the myelin kinase appear to be responsible for phosphorylation of basic protein. In addition small amounts of phosphoserine have been located in bovine basic protein[35,40]. There is a need to investigate the role of these enzymes in demyelinating disease.

Conclusion

Basic protein of myelin has long been examined as the prime candidate for playing a direct role in the aetiology and/or pathogenesis of multiple sclerosis. In this chapter the other proteins of myelin have also been examined in some detail and whilst there is no strong evidence to suggest any of these may play primary roles in the disease process, the paucity of information on most of these proteins, especially in relation to multiple sclerosis, would suggest there is a real need for further study. As indicated there are a number of enzymes responsible for modification of basic protein and these could all be candidates for primary or secondary involvement in multiple sclerosis. Until the importance of these modifications *in vivo* is determined there is little basis for speculation.

Evidence seems to be increasing for involvement of oligodendroglial cells in multiple sclerosis. One hypothesis in which basic protein is proposed to be a receptor in oligodendroglial cells has been outlined. Again it is obvious that further work on the oligodendroglial cell and its relationship to myelin is required before any hypothesis can be critically examined.

One problem faced in framing any hypothesis for the aetiology of multiple sclerosis is that whilst, statistically, differences between multiple sclerosis, patients and controls, and correlations between a number of factors and geographic distribution of multiple sclerosis can be demonstrated, none of these has been shown to be true for all, or even nearly all, multiple sclerosis patients. It could perhaps be argued that this is merely a reflection of the fact that the true causative agent for multiple sclerosis has not been 'discovered', but it is also possible that a number of different primary insults to the central nervous system result in the clinical condition labelled multiple sclerosis.

References

1. Giorgi, P. P., Karlsson, J. O., Sjostrand J. and Field, E. J. (1973). Axonal flow and myelin protein in the optic pathway. *Nature (London)*, **244**, 121
2. Prensky, A. L., Fujimoto, K. and Agrawal, H. C. (1975). Are myelin proteins synthesized in retinal ganglion cells? *J. Neurochem.*, **25**, 883
3. Burton, R. M. and Agrawal, H. C. (1975). The turnover of protein and lipid components of myelin membranes. In R. M. Burton and L. Packer (eds.). *Biomembranes, Lipids, Proteins and Receptors*, pp. 27–50 (Webster Groves, Missouri: B.I. Science publications division)
4. Adams, D. H. and Osborne, J. (1973). A developmental study of the relationship between the protein components of rat CNS myelin. *Neurobiology*, **3**, 91
5. Poduslo, S. (1975). The isolation and characterization of a plasma membrane and a myelin fraction derived from oligodendroglia of calf brain. *J. Neurochem.*, **24**, 647
6. Morell, P., Bornstein, M. B. and Norton, W. T. (1972). Diseases of myelin. In R. W. Albers, G. J. Siegel, R. Katzman, B. W. Agranoff (eds.). *Basic Neurochemistry*, pp. 497–515 (Boston: Little, Brown and Co.)
7. Smith, M. E. (1973). Studies of the mechanism of demyelination: Triethyltin induced demyelination. *J. Neurochem.*, **21**, 357
8. Lumsden, C. E. (1972). The clinical immunology of multiple sclerosis. In D. McAlpine, C. E. Lumsden, and E. D. Acheson (eds.). *Multiple Sclerosis: A Reappraisal*, pp. 512–621 (London: Churchill, Livingstone)
9. Raine, C. S., Hummelgard, A., Swanson, E. and Bornstein, M. B. (1973). Multiple sclerosis: serum-induced demyelination *in vitro*, a light and electron microscope study. *J. Neurol. Sci.*, **20**, 127

10. Carnegie, P. R. and Dunkley, P. R. (1975). Basic proteins of central and peripheral nervous system myelin. *Adv. Neurochem.*, **1**, 95

11. Norton, W. T. (1972). Myelin. In R. W. Albers, G. J. Siegel, R. Katzman, B. W. Agranoff (eds.). *Basic Neurochemistry*, pp. 365–386 (Boston: Little, Brown and Co.)

12. Zimmerman, A. W., Quarles, R. H., Webster, H. de F., Matthieu, J.-M. and Brady, R. O. (1975). Characterization and protein analysis of myelin subfractions in rat brain, developmental and regional comparisons. *J. Neurochem.*, **25**, 749

13. Davison, A. N. (1970). The biochemistry of the myelin sheath. In A. N. Davison and A. Peters (eds.). *Myelination*, pp. 80–161 (Illinois: Charles C. Thomas)

14. Kurihara, T., Nussbaum, J. L. and Mandel, P. (1970). $2',3'$-cyclic nucleotide $3'$-phosphohydrolase in brains of mutant mice with deficient myelination. *J. Neurochem.*, **17**, 993

15. Kies, M. W. (1973). Experimental allergic encephalomyelitis. In G. E. Gaul (ed.). *Biology of Brain Dysfunction*, Vol. 2, pp. 185–224 (New York: Plenum Press)

16. Dunkley, P. R. and Carnegie, P. R. (1974). Isolation of myelin basic proteins. In N. Marks and R. Rodnight (eds.). *Research Methods in Neurochemistry*, Vol. 2, pp. 219–245 (New York: Plenum Press)

17. Eylar, E. H., Kniskern, P. S. and Jackson, J. J. (1974). Myelin basic proteins. *Methods Enzymol.*, **32**, 323

18. Eylar, E. H. (1973). Myelin-specific proteins. In D. J. Schneider, R. H. Angeleti, R. A. Bradshaw, A. Grasso and B. W. Moore (eds.). *Proteins of the Nervous System*, pp. 27–44 (New York: Raven Press)

19. Epand, R. M., Moscarello, M. A., Zierenberg, B. and Vail, W. J. (1974). The folded conformation of the encephalitogenic protein of human brain. *Biochemistry*, **13**, 1264

20. London, Y. and Vossenberg, F. G. A. (1973). Specific interaction of central nervous system myelin basic protein with lipids: Specific regions of the protein sequence protected from proteolytic action of trypsin. *Biochim. Biophys. Acta*, **307**, 478

21. Martenson, R. E., Deibler G. E., and Kramer, A. J. (1975). The presence of cysteine in frog myelin basic protein. *J. Neurochem.*, **24**, 959

22. Carnegie, P. R. (1971). Amino acid sequence of the encephalitogenic basic protein of human myelin. *Biochem. J.*, **123**, 57

23. Brostoff, S. W., Reuter, W., Hichens, M. and Eylar, E. H. (1974). Specific cleavage of the A^1 protein from myelin with cathepsin D. *J. Biol. Chem.*, **249**, 559

24. Dunkley, P. R. and Carnegie, P. R. (1974). Sequence of a rat myelin basic protein. *Biochem. J.*, **141**, 243

25. Martenson, R. E., Deibler, G. E. and Kies, M. W. (1971). The occurrence of two myelin basic proteins in the central nervous system of rodents in the suborders *Myomorpha* and *Sciuromorpha*. *J. Neurochem.*, **18**, 2427

26. Bauer K. (1972). Evidence for the homology of the main determinant of the human encephalitogenic protein and an ancestral histone IV sequence. *Biochem. J.*, **126**, 1245

27. Kakimoto, Y., Matsuoka, Y., Miyake, M. L. and Konishi, H. (1975). Methylated amino acid residues of proteins of brain and other organs. *J. Neurochem.*, **24**, 893

28. Baldwin, G. S. and Carnegie, P. R. (1971). Specific enzymic methylation of an arginine in the experimental allergic encephalomyelitis protein from human myelin. *Science*, **171**, 579

29. Jones, G. and Carnegie, P. R. (1974). Methylation of myelin basic protein by enzymes from rat brain. *J. Neurochem.*, **23**, 1231

30. Miyake, M. (1975). Methylases of myelin basic protein and histone in rat brain. *J. Neurochem.*, **24**, 909

31. Smythies, J. R., Benington, F. and Morin, R. D. (1972). Encephalitogenic protein: a β-pleated sheet conformation (102–120) yields a possible molecular form of a serotonin receptor. *Experientia*, **28**, 23

32. Hind, V. M. D. (1972). The histology of vitamin B_{12} deficiency optic neuropathy in monkeys. In J. S. Cant (ed.). *The Optic Nerve*, pp. 257–269 (London: Henry Kimpton).

33. Cantoni, G. L. (1975). Biological methylation: selected aspects. *Ann. Rev. Biochem.*, **44**, 435

34. Carnegie, P. R., Kemp, B. E., Dunkley, P. R. and Murray, A. W. (1973). Phosphorylation of myelin basic protein by a cyclic AMP-dependent protein kinase. *Biochem. J.*, **135**, 589

35. Miyamoto, E. and Kakiuchi, S. (1974). *In vitro* and *in vivo* phosphorylation of myelin basic protein by exogenous and endogenous adenosine 3',5'-monophosphate-dependent protein kinases from brain. *J. Biol. Chem.*, **249**, 2769

36. Steck, A. J. and Appel, S. H. (1974). Phosphorylation of myelin basic protein. *J. Biol. Chem.*, **249**, 5416

37. Daile, P. and Carnegie, P. R. (1974). Peptides from myelin basic protein as substrates for 3',5'-cyclic monophosphate-dependent protein kinases. *Biochem. Biophys. Res. Comm.*, **61**, 852

38. Daile, P., Carnegie, P. R. and Young, J. D. (1975). Synthetic substrate for cyclic AMP-dependent protein kinase. *Nature (London)*, **257**, 416

39. Carnegie, P. R., Dunkley, P. R., Kemp, B. E. and Murray, A. W. (1974). Phosphorylation of selected serine and threonine residues in myelin basic protein by endogenous and exogenous protein kinases. *Nature (London)*, **249**, 147

40. Deibler, G. E., Martenson, R. E., Kramer, A. J., Kies, M. W. and Miyamoto, E. (1975). The contribution of phosphorylation and loss of COOH-terminal arginine to the microheterogeneity of myelin basic protein. *J. Biol. Chem.*, **250**, 7931

41. Dunkley, P. R., Jones, G. M. and Mudie, D. (1975). Phosphorylation of CNS myelin protein. *Abstracts 5th Meeting, Internat. Soc. Neurochem.*, p. 402

42. Davis, F. A., Becker, F. O., Michael, J. A. and Sorensen, E. (1970). Effect of intravenous sodium bicarbonate, disodium edetate (Na_2 EDTA) and hyperventilation on visual and oculomotor signs in multiple sclerosis. *J. Neurol., Neurosurg. Psychiatry*, **33**, 723

43. Schauf, C. L. and Davis, F. A. (1974). Impulse conduction in multiple sclerosis: a theoretical basis for modification by temperature and pharmacological agents. *J. Neurol., Neurosurg. Psychiatry*, **37**, 152

44. Hagopian, A., Westall, F. C., Whitehead, J. S. and Eylar, E. H. (1971). Glycosylation of the A_1 protein from myelin by a polypeptide N-acetylgalactosaminyl transferase: Identification of the receptor sequence. *J. Biol. Chem.*, **246**, 2519

45. Robinson, A. B. and Rudd, C. J. (1974). Deamidation of glutaminyl and asparaginyl residues in peptides and proteins. *Curr. Top. Cell. Regul.*, **8**, 247

46. Rauch, H. C., Einstein, E. R. and Csejtey, J. (1973). Enzymatic degradation of myelin basic protein in central nervous system lesions of monkeys with experimental allergic encephalomyelitis. *Neurobiology*, **3**, 195

47. Riekkinen, P. J., Clausen, J., Frey, H. J., Fog, T. and Rinne, U. K. (1970). Acid proteinase activity of white matter and plaques in multiple sclerosis. *Acta Neurol. Scand.*, **46**, 349

48. Einstein, E. R., Csejtey, J., Dalal, K. B., Adams, C. W. M., Bayliss, O. B. and Hallpike, J. F. L. (1972). Proteolytic activity and basic protein loss in and around multiple sclerosis plaques: combined biochemical and histochemical observations. *J. Neurochem.*, **19**, 653

49. Marks, N., Benuck, M. and Hashim, G. (1974). Hydrolysis of myelin basic protein with brain acid proteinase. *Biochem. Biophys. Res. Comm.*, **56**, 68

50. Herndon, R. M., Rauch, H. C. and Einstein, E. R. (1973). Immunoelectron microscopic localization of the encephalitogenic basic protein in myelin. *Immunol. Comm.*, **2**, 163

51. Poduslo, J. F. and Braun, P. E. (1975). Topographical arrangement of membrane proteins in the intact myelin sheath. Lactoperoxidase incorporation of iodine into myelin surface proteins. *J. Biol. Chem.*, **250**, 1099

52. Carnegie, P. R. (1971). Properties, structure and possible neuroreceptor role of the encephalitogenic protein of human brain. *Nature (London)*, **229**, 25

53. Cohen, S. R., McKhann, G. M. and Guarnieri, M. (1975). A radioimmunoassay for myelin basic protein and its use for quantitative measurements. *J. Neurochem.*, **24**, 371

54. Wood, D. D., Vail, W. J. and Moscarello, M. A. (1975) The localization of the basic protein and N-2 in diseased myelin. *Brain Res.*, **93**, 463

55. Westall, F. C., Robinson, A. B., Caccam, J., Jackson, J. and Eylar, E. H. (1971). Essential chemical requirements for induction of allergic encephalomyelitis. *Nature (London)*, **229**, 22

56. Lennon, V. A., Wilks, A. V. and Carnegie, P. R. (1970). Immunologic properties of the main encephalitogenic peptide from the basic protein of human myelin. *J. Immunol.*, **105**, 1223

57. Shapira, R., Chou, F. C.-H., McKneally, S. S., Urban, E. and Kibler, R. F. (1971). Biological activity and synthesis of an encephalitogenic determinant. *Science*, **173**, 736

58. Karkhanis, Y. D., Carlo, D. J., Brostoff, S. W. and Eylar, E. H. (1975). Allergic encephalomyelitis, isolation of an encephalitogenic peptide active in the monkey. *J. Biol. Chem.*, **250**, 1718

59. McFarlin, D. E., Blank, S. E., Kibler, R. F., McKneally, S. and Shapira, R. (1973). Experimental allergic encephalomyelitis in the rat: Response to encephalitogenic proteins and peptides. *Science*, **179**, 478

60. Dunkley, P. R., Coates, A. S. and Carnegie, P. R. (1973). Encephalitogenic activity of peptides from the smaller basic protein of rat brain myelin. *J. Immunol.*, **110**, 1699

61. Bernard, C. C. A. and Carnegie, P. R. (1975). Experimental autoimmune encephalomyelitis in mice: immunologic response to mouse spinal cord and myelin basic proteins. *J. Immunol.*, **114**, 1537

62. Carnegie, P. R., Smythies, J. R., Caspary, E. A. and Field, E. J. (1972). Interaction of hallucinogenic drugs with encephalitogenic protein of myelin. *Nature (London)*, **240**, 561

63. Berg, O., Bergstrand, H., Kallen, B. and Nilsson, O. (1975). Effect of encephalitogenic protein on the migration in agarose of leucocytes from patients with multiple sclerosis. *Acta Neurol. Scand.*, **52**, 303

64. Mackay, I. R., Carnegie, P. R. and Coates, A. S. (1973). Immunopathological comparisons between experimental autoimmune encephalomyelitis and multiple sclerosis: A review. *Clin. Exp. Immunol.*, **15**, 471

65. Lennon, V. A. and Carnegie, P. R. (1971). Immunopharmacological disease: a break in tolerance to receptor sites. *Lancet*, **i**, 630

66. Bornstein, M. B. and Crain, S. M. (1965). Functional studies of cultured brain tissue as related to demyelinative disorders. *Science*, **148**, 1242

67. Lyck, E. and Roos, B. E. (1973). Brain monoamines in guinea-pigs with experimental allergic encephalomyelitis. *Int. Arch. Allergy*, **45**, 341

68. White, S. R., White, F. P., Barnes, C. D. and Albright, J. F. Increased shock sensitivity in rats with experimental allergic encephalomyelitis and reversal by 5-hydroxy tryptophan. *Brain Res.*, **58**, 251

69. Lennon, V. A. (1972). Cellular and humoral immune responses in experimental autoimmune encephalomyelitis. *Ph.D. Thesis, Melbourne University*

70. Saragea, M. and Vladutiu, A. (1965). L'influence de la nialamide sur l'encéphalomyelite allergique expérimentale. *Naturwissenchaften*, **52**, 564

71. Carnegie, P. R. and Mackay, I. R. (1975). Vulnerability of cell-surface receptors to autoimmune reactions. *Lancet*, **ii**, 684

72. Harrer, G. and Fishback, R. (1973). Über die wirkung bestimmter aminosäuren auf das ergebnis des überwärmungstests bei multiplesklerose-kranken. *J. Neural Transm.*, **34**, 205

73. Sonninen, V., Riekkinen, R. and Rinne, U. K. (1973). Acid monoamine metabolites in cerebrospinal fluid in multiple sclerosis. *Neurology*, **23**, 760

74. Johansson, B. and Roos, B. E. (1974). 5-hydroxysindoleacetic acid and homovanillic acid in cerebrospinal fluid of patients with neurological diseases. *Eur. Neurol.*, **11**, 37

75. Claveria, K. E., Curzon, G., Harrison, M. J. G. and Kantamaneni, B. D. (1974). Amine metabolites in the cerebrospinal fluid of patients with disseminated sclerosis. *J. Neurol., Neurosurg. Psychiatry*, **37**, 715

76. Murray, M. R. (1958). Responses of oligodendrocytes to serotonin. In W. F. Windle (ed.). *Biology of Neuroglia*, pp. 176–190 (Springfield, Ill.: Charles C. Thomas)

77. Myers, L. W., Ellison, G. W., Fewster, M. E. and Wolfgram, F. (1975). Cell-

mediated immunity to isolated human oligodendroglia in multiple sclerosis. *Arch. Neurol.*, **32,** 354

78. Alvord, E. C., Hsu, P. C. and Thron, R. (1974). Leucocyte sensitivity to brain fractions in neurological diseases. *Arch. Neurol.*, **30,** 296

79. Hyyppä, M. T., Jolma, T., Riekkinen, P. and Rinne, U. K. (1975). Effects of L-tryptophan treatment on central indoleamine metabolism and short-lasting neurological disturbances in multiple sclerosis. *J. Neural Transm.*, **37,** 297

80. Einstein, E. R. (1972). Basic protein of myelin and its role in experimental allergic encephalomyelitis and multiple sclerosis. In A. Lajtha (ed.). *Handbook of Neurochemistry*, Vol. 7, pp. 107–129 (London: Plenum Press)

81. Hallpike, J. F. and Adams, C. W. M. (1969). Proteolysis and myelin breakdown. A review of recent histochemical and biochemical studies. *Histochem. J.*, **1,** 559

82. Folch-Pi, J. and Stoffyn, P. J. (1972). Proteolipids from membrane systems. *Ann. N.Y. Acad. Sci.*, **195,** 86

83. Folch-Pi, J. (1973). Proteolipids. In D. J. Schneider (ed.). *Proteins of the Nervous System*, pp. 45–66 (New York: Raven Press)

84. Agrawal, H. C., Fujimoto, K. and Burton, R. M. (1975). Incorporation of ^{3}H-5, 6 fucose into CNS myelin PLP. *Abstracts 5th International Meeting of the International Society for Neurochemistry*, p. 400

85. Lees, M. B. and Chan, D. S. (1975). Proteolytic digestion of bovine brain white matter proteolipid. *J. Neurochem.*, **25,** 595

86. Nussbaum, J. L., Romayrene, J. F., Jolles, J., Jolles, P. and Mandel, P. (1974). Amino acid analysis and N-terminal sequence determination of P7 proteolipid apoprotein from human myelin. *FEBS Lett.*, **45,** 295

87. Royatta, M., Frey, H., Riekkinen, P. J., Laaksonen, H. and Rinne, U. K. (1974). Myelin breakdown and basic protein. *Exp. Neurol.*, **45,** 174

88. Whitfield, P. R., Heppel, L. A. and Markham, R. (1955). The enzymic hydrolysis of ribonucleoside-2′,3′ phosphates. *Biochem. J.*, **60,** 15

89. Davis, F. F. and Allen, F. W. (1956). A specific phosphodiesterase from beef pancreas. *Biochim. Biophys. Acta*, **21,** 14

90. Drummond, G. I., Iyer, N. T. and Keith, J. (1962). Hydrolysis of ribonucleoside 2′,3′–cyclic phosphates by a diesterase from brain. *J. Biol. Chem.*, **237,** 3535

91. Kurihara, T. and Tsukada, Y. (1967). The regional and subcellular distribution of 2′,3′–cyclic nucleotide 3′–phosphohydrolase in the central nervous system. *J. Neurochem.*, **14,** 1167

92. Drummond, G. I., Eng, D. Y. and McIntosh, C. A. (1971). Ribonucleoside 2′,3′–cyclic phosphate diesterase activity and cerebroside levels in vertebrate and invertebrate nerve. *Brain Res.*, **28,** 153

93. Olafson, R. W., Drummond, G. I. and Lee, J. F. (1969). Studies on 2′3′–cyclic nucleotide 3′–phosphohydrolase from brain. *Can. J. Biochem.* **47,** 961

94. Lees, M. B., and Paxman, S. A. (1974). Myelin proteins from different regions of the central nervous system. *J. Neurochem.*, **23,** 825

95. Matthieu, J. M., Quarles, R. H., Brady, R. O., and Webster, H. de F. (1973). Variation of proteins, enzyme markers and gangliosides in myelin subfractions. *Biochim. Biophys. Acta*, **329,** 305

96. Kurihara, T. and Tsukada, Y. (1968). 2′,3′-cyclic nucleotide 3′-phosphohydrolase in the developing chick brain and spinal cord. *J. Neurochem.*, **15**, 827

97. Kurihara, T., Nussbaum, J. L. and Mandel, P. (1969). 2′,3′-cyclic nucleotide 3′-phosphohydrolase in the brain of the 'Jimpy' mouse, a mutant with deficient myelination. *Brain Res.*, **12**, 401

98. Agrawal, H. C., Banik, N. L., Bone, A. H., Davison, A. N., Mitchell, R. F. and Spohn, M. (1970). The identity of a myelin-like fraction isolated from developing brain. *Biochem. J.*, **120**, 635

99. Lees, M. B., Sandler, S. W. and Eichberg, J. (1974). Effect of detergents on 2′,3′-cyclic nucleotide 3′-phosphohydrolase activity in myelin and erythrocyte ghosts. *Neurobiology*, **4**, 407

100. Sims, N. R. and Carnegie, P. R. Unpublished observation.

101. Sims, N. R. and Carnegie, P. R. (1975). Release of 2′,3′-cyclic nucleotide 3′-phosphohydrolase from myelin. *Proc. Aust. Biochem. Soc.*, **8**, 75

102. Kurihara, T. and Takahashi, Y. (1973). Potentiometric and colorimetric methods for the assay of 2′,3′-cyclic nucleotide 3′-phosphohydrolase. *J. Neurochem.*, **20**, 719

103. Prohaska, J. R., Clark, D. A. and Wells, W. W. (1973). Improved rapidity and precision in the determination of brain 2′,3′-cyclic nucleotide 3′-phosphohydrolase. *Anal. Biochem.*, **56**, 275

104. Trams, E. G. and Brown, E. A. B.(1974). The activity of 2′,3′-cyclic adenosine monophosphate 3′-phosphoesterhydrolase in Elasmobranch and teleost brain. *Comp. Biochem. Physiol. (B)*, **48**, 185

105. Hugli, T. E., Bustin, M. and Moore, S. (1973). Spectrophometric assay of 2′,3′-cyclic nucleotide 3′-phosphohydrolase: Application to the enzyme in bovine brain. *Brain Res.*, **58**, 191

106. Guha, A. and Moore, S. (1975). Solubilization of 2′,3′-cyclic nucleotide 3′-phosphohydrolase from bovine brain without detergents. *Brain Res.*, **89**, 279

107. Uyemura, K., Tobari, C., Hirano, S. and Tsukada, Y. (1972). Comparative studies on the myelin proteins of bovine peripheral nerve and spinal cord. *J. Neurochem.*, **19**, 2607

108. Sudo, T., Kikuno, M. and Kurihara, T. (1972). 2′,3′-cyclic nucleotide 3′-phosphohydrolase in human erythrocyte membranes. *Biochim. Biophys. Acta*, **255**, 640

109. Konings, A. W. T. and Pierce, D. A. (1974). Hydrolysis of 2′,3′-cyclic adenosine monophosphate and 3′,5-cyclic adenosine monophosphate in subcellular fractions of normal and neoplastic mouse spleen. *Life Sci.*, **15**, 491

110. Poduslo, S. E. and Norton, W. T. (1972). Isolation and some chemical properties of oligodendroglia from calf brain. *J. Neurochem.*, **19**, 727

111. Banik, N. L. and Davison, A. N. (1969). Enzyme activity and composition of myelin and subcellular fractions in the developing rat brain. *Biochem. J.*, **115**, 1051

112. Wachneldt, T. V. (1975). Ontogenetic study of a myelin-derived fraction with 2′,3′-cyclic nucleotide 3′-phosphohydrolase activity higher than that of myelin. *Biochem. J.*, **151**, 435

113. Agrawal, H. C., Trotter, J. L., Mitchell, R. F. and Burton, R. M. (1973).

Criteria for identifying a myelin-like fraction from developing brain. *Biochem. J.*, **136**, 1117

114. Agrawal, H. C., Trotter, J. L., Burton, R. M. and Mitchell, R. F. (1974). Metabolic studies on myelin. Evidence for a precursor role of a myelin subfraction. *Biochem. J.*, **140**, 99

115. Sabri, M. I., Tremblay, C., Banik, N. L., Scott, T., Gohil, K. and Davison, A. N. (1975). Biochemical and morphological changes in the subcellular fractions during myelination of rat brain. *Biochem. Soc. Trans.*, **3**, 275

116. Banik, N. L., Davison, A. N., Palo, J. and Savlovainen H. (1975). Biochemical studies on myelin isolated from the brains of patients with Down's syndrome. *Brain*, **98**, 213

117. Pechan, I. and Simekova, J. (1972). 2',3'-cyclic nucleotide 3'-phosphohydrolase activity of the central nervous tissue in experimental allergic encephalomyelitis. *J. Neurochem.*, **19**, 557

118. Govindarajan, K. R., Rauch, H. C., Clausen, J. and Einstein, E. R. (1974). Changes in cathepsins B-1 and D, neutral proteinase and 2',3'-cyclic nucleotide 3'-phosphohydrolase activities in monkey brain with experimental allergic encephalomyelitis. *J. Neurol. Sci.*, **23**, 295

119. Bornstein, M. B. and Raine, C. S. (1970). Experimental allergic encephalomyelitis. Antiserum inhibition of myelination *in vitro*. *Lab. Invest.*, **23**, 536

120. Fry, J. M., Lehrer, G. M. and Bornstein, M. B. (1973). Experimental inhibition of myelination in spinal cord tissue cultures: enzyme assays. *J. Neurobiol.*, **4**, 453

121. Fry, J. M., Lehrer, G. M. and Bornstein, M. B. (1972). Sulfatide synthesis: Inhibition by experimental allergic encephalomyelitis serum. *Science*, **175**, 192

122. Zannetta, J. P., Benda, P., Gombos, G. and Morgan, I. G. (1972). The presence of 2',3'-cyclic AMP 3'-phosphohydrolase in glial cells in tissue culture. *J. Neurochem.*, **19**, 881

123. Kawakami, S., Kurihara, T., Ueki, K. and Takahashi, Y. (1974). 2',3'-cyclic nucleotide 3'-phosphohydrolase activity in human brain tumours. *J. Neurochem.*, **22**, 1143

124. Pfeiffer, S. E. and Wechsler, W. (1972). Biochemically differentiated neoplastic clone of Schwann cells. *Proc. Nat. Acad. Sci. USA*, **69**, 2885

125. Wysocki, S. J. and Segal, W. (1972). Influence of thyroid hormones on enzyme activities of myelinating rat central nervous tissues. *Eur. J. Biochem.*, **28**, 183

126. Einstein, E. R. (1974). Protein and enzyme changes with brain development. In A. Vernadakis and N. Weiner (eds.). *Drugs and the Developing Brain*, pp. 375–391 (New York: Plenum Press)

127. Wassenaar, J. S. and Kroon, A. M. (1973). Effects of triethyltin on different ATPases, 5'-nucleotidase and phosphodiesterases in grey and white matter of rabbit brain and their relation with brain edema. *Eur. Neurol.* **10**, 349

128. Dreiling, C. E. and Newburgh, R. W. (1972). Effect of 1,1,3-tricyano-2-amino-1-propene on 2',3'-cyclic AMP 3'-phosphohydrolase in the sciatic nerve of the chick embryo. *Biochim. Biophys. Acta*, **264**, 300

129. Riekkinen, P. J., Rinne, U. K., Arstila, A. U., Kurihara, T. and Pelliniemi, T. T. (1972). Studies on the pathogenesis of multiple sclerosis. 2',3'-cyclic nucleotide

3'-phosphohydrolase as marker of demyelination and correlation of findings with lysomal changes. *J. Neurol. Sci.*, **15**, 113

130. Braun, P. E. and Barchi, R. L. (1972). 2',3'-cyclic nucleotide 3'-phosphodiesterase in the nervous system. Electrophoretic properties and developmental studies. *Brain Res.*, **40**, 437

131. Tsukada, Y., Shibuya, M. and Ogawa Y. (1973). Changes in 2',3'-cyclic nucleotide 3'-phosphohydrolase on myelinating heural tissue grown in culture. In *Abstracts 4th International Meeting of the International Society for Neurochemistry (Tokyo, Japan)*, p. 299

132. Duch, D., Mandel, P. and Koprowski, H. (1975). Demonstration of enzymes related to myelinogenesis in established human brain cell cultures. *J. Neurol. Sci.*, **26**, 99

133. Eto, Y, and Suzuki, K. (1973). Cholesterol ester metabolism in rat brain. A cholesterol ester hydrolase specifically localized in the myelin sheath. *J. Biol. Chem.*, **248**, 1986

134. Igarashi, M. and Suzuki K. (1976). Effect of exogenous lipids on activities of the rat brain cholesterol ester hydrolase localised in the myelin sheath. *J. Neurochem.*, **27**, 859

135. Eto, Y. and Suzuki, K. (1971). Fatty acid composition of cholesterol esters in brains of patients with Schilder's disease, Gm1-gangliosidosis and Tay-Sachs disease, and its possible relationship to the β-position fatty acids of lecithin. *J. Neurochem.*, **18**, 1007

136. Wender, M., Filipek-Wender, H. and Stanislawska, J. (1974). Cholesteryl esters of the brain in demyelinating diseases. *Clin. Chim. Acta*, **54**, 269

137. Wender, M., Filipek-Wender, H. and Stanislawska, B. (1973). Cholesteryl esters in apparently normal white matter in multiple sclerosis. *Eur. Neurol.*, **10**, 340

138. Brunngraber, E. G. (1970). Glycoproteins in neural tissue. In A. Lajtha (ed.), *Protein Metabolism of the Nervous System*, pp. 383–407. (New York: Plenum Press)

139. Quarles, R. H., Everly, J. L. and Brady, R. O. (1972). Demonstration of a glycoprotein which is associated with a purified myelin fraction from rat brain. *Biochem. Biophys. Res. Commun.*, **47**, 491

140. Quarles, R. H., Everly, J. L. and Brady, R. O. (1973). Evidence for the close association of a glycoprotein with myelin in rat brain. *J. Neurochem.*, **21**, 1177

141. Quarles, R. H. and Everly, J. L. (1973). Evidence for the close association of a glycoprotein with myelin. *Fed. Proc.*, **32**, 486

142. Matthieu, J.-M., Quarles, R. H., Webster, H. de F., Hogan, E. L., and Brady R. O. (1974). Characterization of the fraction obtained from the CNS of 'Jimpy' mice by a procedure for myelin isolation. *J. Neurochem.*, **23**, 517

143. Matthieu, J.-M., Brady, R. O. and Quarles, R. H. (1974). Anomalies of myelin-associated glycoproteins in 'Quaking' mice. *J. Neurochem.*, **22**, 291

144. Matthieu, J.-M., Daniel, A., Quarles, R. H. and Brady, R. O. (1974). Interactions of conconavalin A and other lectins with CNS myelin. *Brain Res.*, **81**, 348

145. Druse, M. J., Brady, R. O. and Quarles, R. H. (1974). Metabolism of a myelin-associated glycoprotein in developing rat brain. *Brain Res.*, **76**, 423

146. Quarles, R. H., Everly, J. L. and Brady, R. O. (1973). Myelin-associated glyco-protein: a developmental change. *Brain Res.*, **58**, 506

147. Matthieu, J.-M., Brady, R. O. and Quarles, R. H. (1974). Developmental change in a myelin-associated glycoprotein: a comparative study in rodents. *Dev. Biol.*, **37**, 146

148. Brady, R. O. and Quarles, R. H. (1973). The enzymology of myelination. *Mol. Cell Biochem.*, **2**, 23

149. Brunngraber, E. G., Susz, J. P., Javaid, J., Aro, J. and Warecka, K. (1975). Binding of conconavalin A to the brain-specific proteins obtained from human white matter by affinity chromatography. *J. Neurochem.*, **24**, 805

150. Agrawal, H. C., Burton, R. M., Fishman, M. A., Mitchell, R. F. and Prensky, A. L. (1972). Partial characterization of a new myelin protein component. *J. Neurochem.*, **19**, 2083

151. Seiler, N. (1969). In A. Lajtha (ed.). Enzymes. In *Handbook of Neurochemistry*, Chemical architectuie of the nervous system, pp. 325-468 (New York: Plenum Press)

152. Adams, C. W. M., Davison, A. N. and Gregson, N. A. (1963). Enzyme inactivity of myelin: histochemical and biochemical evidence. *J. Neurochem.*, **10**, 383

153. Bernsohn, J., Barron, K. D., Doolin, P. F., Hess, A. R. and Hedrick, M. T. (1966). Subcellular localization of rat brain esterases. *J. Histochem. Cytochem.*, **14**, 455

154. Barron, K. D., Bernsohn, J. and Mitzen, E. (1972). Non-specific esterases of human peripheral nerve and centrum ovale. A comparison and observation on esteratic activity of myelin fractions. *J. Neuropathol. Exp. Neurol.*, **31**, 562

155. Rumsby, M. G., Riekkinen, P. J. and Arstila, A. V. (1970). A critical evaluation of myelin purification. Non-specific esterase activity associated with central nerve myelin preparations. *Brain Res.*, **24**, 495

156. Riekkinen, P. J. and Rumsby, M. G. (1969). Esterase activity in purified myelin preparations from beef brain. *Brain Res.*, **14**, 772

157. Frey, H. J., Arstila, A. U., Rinne, U. K. and Riekkinen, P. J. (1971). Esterases in developing CNS myelin. *Brain Res.*, **30**, 159

158. Koeppen, A. H., Barron, K. D. and Bernsohn, J. (1969). Redistribution of rat brain esterases during subcellular fractionation. *Biochim. Biophys. Acta*, **183**, 253

159. Mitzen, E. J., Barron, K. D., Koeppen, A. H. and Harris, H. W. (1974). Enzyme activity of human central nervous system myelin. *Brain Res.*, **68**, 123

160. Rumsby, M. G., Getliffe, H. M. and Riekkinen, P. J. (1973). On the association of non-specific esterase activity with central nerve myelin preparations. *J. Neurochem.*, **21**, 959

161. Torrie, S. and Rumsby, M. G. (1975). Purification of non-specific esterase activity from isolated central nerve myelin preparations. In *Abstracts 5th International Meeting of the International Society for Neurochemistry (Barcelona, Spain)*, p. 415

162. Barron, K. D., Bernsohn, J. and Hess, A. R. (1963). Abnormalities in brain esterases in multiple sclerosis. *Proc. Soc. Exp. Biol. Med.*, **113**, 521

163. Barron, K. D. and Bernsohn, J. (1965). Brain esterases and phosphatases in multiple sclerosis. *Ann. N.Y. Acad. Sci.* **122**, 369

164. Patterson, E. K., Hsiao, S. H. and Keppel, A. (1963). Studies on dipeptidases and aminopeptidases. Distinction between leucine aminopeptidase and enzymes that hydrolyze L-leucyl-b-naphthylamide. *J. Biol. Chem.*, **238**, 3611

165. Beck, C. S., Hasionoff, C. W. and Smith, M. E. (1968). L-analyl-β-naphthylamidase in rat spinal cord myelin. *J. Neurochem.*, **15**, 1297

166. Riekkinen, P. J. and Clausen, J. (1970). Peptidase activity of purified myelin *Acta Neurol. Scand.*, **46**, 93

167. Riekkinen, P. J. and Rumsby, M. G. (1972). Aminopeptidase and neutral proteinase activity associated with central nerve myelin preparations during purification. *Brain Res.*, **41**, 512

168. D'Monte, B., Mela, P. and Marks, N. (1971). Metabolic instability of myelin protein and proteolipid fractions. *Eur. J. Biochem.*, **23**, 355

169. Mezei, C. and Palmer, F. B. St. C. (1974). Hydrolytic enzyme activities in the developing chick central and peripheral nervous system. *J. Neurochem.*, **23**, 1087

170. Constantino-Ceccarini, E. and Suzuki, K. (1975). Evidence for presence of UDP-galactose: ceramide galactosyltransferase in rat myelin. *Brain Res.*, **93**, 358

171. Miyamoto, E. and Kakiuchi, S. (1975). Phosphoprotein phosphatases for myelin basic protein in myelin and cytosol fractions of brain. *Biochim. Biophys. Acta*, **384**, 458

172. Carnegie, P. R., Dunkley, P. R. and Mudie, D. L. (1977). Phosphorylation of chicken myelin basic protein *in vivo*. (In preparation)

7

The problem of cerebrospinal fluid

A. Lowenthal

Introduction

The examination of the cerebrospinal fluid (CSF) in multiple sclerosis (MS) is an essential step to arrive at a diagnosis and to study the physiopathology of the disease.

It is known that serum of MS slows conduction in the spinal cord of the frog[1] and demyelinizes nerve fibres in culture[2]. However, no other biological blood anomaly is known. It is clear that one finds important organic anomalies in the central nervous system (CNS), both morphological and biochemical. The examination of this material is practically impossible during the patient's lifetime. The contribution to our understanding of MS has not been greatly enhanced after biopsies during stereotaxic operations or examination of post-mortem material.

To confirm biologically the diagnosis of MS, one has thus to rely on the CSF. This means that first and foremost one has to discard the preconceived idea that a CSF examination (that is to say, a lumbar puncture) is dangerous for patients suffering from MS. Our experience, based on hundreds of lumbar punctures carried out on such patients, completely negates this hypothesis. Moreover, the danger of effecting a wrong diagnosis, through failure to examine CSF, is a real one. We have, on numerous occasions, seen the clinical diagnosis of MS being altered, sometimes after many years, by the discovery of a significant increase in total CSF proteins, caused by a medullary compression or the development of a tumour of the posterior fossa. Therefore it seems to us indispensable that before the diagnosis of MS is established, a lumbar puncture should always be made. Certainly, from a scientific point of view, no case of MS can be accepted as such unless a lumbar puncture has been made and also, as we will show later, an electrophoretic examination of the CSF proteins, either in agar gel, agarose gel or on cellulose acetate.

It is therefore most important to discuss the different methods used to examine CSF, on the one hand, and on the other to try to assess the significance of the results of the different examinations, both for diagnostic and for physiopathological ends.

Techniques and results

We will discard straight away the examination of the CSF pressure: in MS, it is normal. Queckenstedt's procedure gives no indication. To the naked eye the appearance of CSF is normal.

On the other hand the morphological and chemical examinations can give valuable indications.

Morphological examinations

Morphological examination cannot be confined to cell count though this may often give important information. Pleiocytosis[3] is common, some workers putting its occurrence at more than 50% of cases[4]. We ourselves do not, however, think it so frequent. The number of cells does not usually exceed 25 to 30 per mm^3, though much higher figures have been reported. The cells are usually mononuclear leukocytes[5], lymphocytes or plasmacytes. However, morphological appearance of the cells in a counting chamber is not adequate for their assessment. For significant results, a proper cytological examination of the cells should be carried out. In general it gives informative results, not only in cases of tumour, but also where there are inflammatory lesions, and it is amongst this last group that MS is to be classified. Cytological examination, in our opinion, is too neglected in Western Europe and North America. This morphological study shows the presence of leukocytes and plasmacytes in CSF of patients suffering from MS and it immediately poses the question of the part such cells, which may be immunoactive, play in the immunological manifestations of the disease. This will be discussed later.

Chemical examinations

In the abundant literature that we have been able to gather, dealing with CSF of patients suffering from MS, numerous and varied chemical examinations[6] have been suggested. Some have been carried out (for example, colloidal precipitation) with techniques which today are no longer accepted.

We must mention that, in spite of some abnormal values, such as for the ionic concentration of sodium, potassium, chloride, and phosphate[7,8] on the one hand, and the amino acid concentrations[9] on the other, no constant or characteristic anomaly has been found. The techniques used are often open to criticism: it has been said, for example, that the level of glutamine is decreased in CSF[10] and this is after paper chromatography.

Notwithstanding the many papers dealing with the level of trace metals, in particular copper[11], and iron[7], we are convinced that clear and consistent anomalies of copper and iron levels do not occur. We underline this point, because a relationship is sometimes thought to exist between copper metabolism and some demyelinating diseases. This assumption rests on observations made on swayback lambs. We would emphasize, however, that swayback can, neither clinically, nor morphologically, nor immunologically, be compared to MS[12].

Some authors have paid particular attention to more complex factors in spinal fluid, such as blood coagulation factors[13,14] and enzymes[6,15]. A few results have suggested anomalies associated with the disease, but these have not been confirmed nor has the increased level of real cholinesterase[8,11]. We must admit that, up till now, these researches, which may ultimately turn out to be of interest, have led nowhere. The same applied to hexoses or the substrates involved in the metabolism of hexoses, such as pyruvate, ketoglutarate, or citrate[16]. Here again, relatively large series have been examined but no significant conclusions can be drawn. Even the mesoinositol[17] concentration does not supply any information.

Above all, since MS is considered a 'demyelinating disease' the intensive study of lipids was indicated. It may not be one of the least important paradoxes in the biochemical study of MS that the study of CSF lipids[18] has been unrewarding and, although we do not discuss it here, this probably also applies to the central nervous system. In the central nervous system, apart from some results concerning fatty acids[19], more or less long-chained and unsaturated, not much has emerged and the same is true for the CSF. Increases in sphingomyelin[20], cerebrosides[21], cholesterol esters and cholesterol[22,23], mainly of cholesterol esters, and hexosamine[24,25] have been observed. We are willing to accept the existence of such anomalies, although they do not seem specific. They are probably a consequence of a non-specific secondary demyelinating process. In our opinion the lipid anomalies, observed in MS, are secondary ones, not only in the central nervous system but also in CSF. However we have to make some reservations. We mentioned previously the fatty acid anomalies and the decrease of relatively unsaturated fatty acids in the central nervous system. These are comparable to the anomalies found in the serum[26]. We think that to date these results have not yet been confirmed in CSF.

In fact, in the biochemical field, the most interesting study in MS CSF is that of the proteins. The changes observed are not only quantitative but significantly qualitative too. Apart from a few instances, the total protein level in the fluid of patients suffering from MS is normal. Numerous authors [3,27] including ourselves have seen examples in which the total protein level is increased to a considerable extent. Although we have not seen an increase as great as that recorded by Dowzenko *et al.*[28], levels up to 100 mg % are found, and are commonly between 40 and 50 mg %. We do not believe, as some authors claim, that those levels exist in 50 % of MS spinal fluids and we maintain that in 80 % the total protein level is not above 40 and is usually lower, closer to 20 mg %.

Qualitative modifications have been observed in early phases of the disease. These qualitative modifications have been demonstrated by techniques of which the physicochemical characteristics are not fully understood—colloidal precipitations, for example. Though many of these techniques have been, and are still, in use, we shall not discuss them here for two reasons:

(1) These techniques are never very rigorously adhered to and the methods indeed often differ from one laboratory to another so that results cannot easily be compared.

(2) All such techniques must be replaced by electrophoresis, which has rightly supplanted them since it permits more precise standardization and interpretation.

Right from the outset electrophoretic studies of CSF proteins in MS revealed anomalies, such as an increase of γ-globulins[29]. This increase was first observed through free electrophoresis, by the method of Tiselius, and later shown by paper electrophoresis[30-33]. At once this increase posed the important question as to whether the increase in γ-globulins in MS was similar to that observed in a great number of other diseases, such as meningeal and inflammatory diseases, syphilis, cerebral trypanosomiasis or diseases with modification of haematoencephalic barrier (such as Guillain–Barré's syndrome); or yet diseases producing compression, for example, due to cerebral or medullary tumours. In addition, anomalies observable in myeloma patients also lead to γ-globulin increases. Analysis of the phenomenon of γ-globulin increase becomes essential. We did try, like many others, to analyse these proteins and classify them according to their composition, as lipoproteins[31] and glucoproteins[5]. Lipidograms and glucidograms of CSF from patients affected with MS showed that the γ-globulins in this disease appeared richer in glucoproteins than were normal γ-globulins.

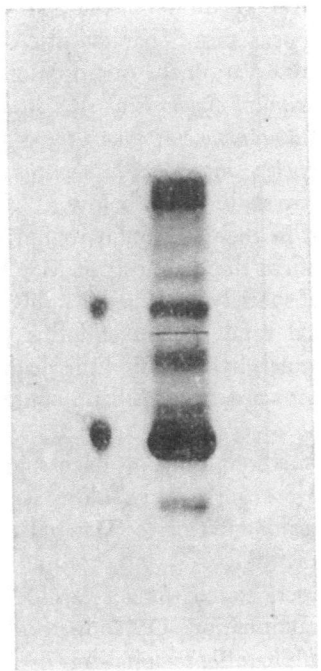

Figure 7.1 Agar gel electrophoresis of CSF proteins in a case of multiple sclerosis. The γ-globulins are increased and fractionated

An important advance was made, when we were able to show that the γ-globulins in MS do not show up in agar gel electrophoresis as do the γ-globulins in other illnesses; that the main characteristic of these globulins was not only their increase (which one does not always find), but a qualitative modification in the sense that the γ-globulins appear as separate fractions[29,34,35]. These fractions are only separated after agar gel, agarose gel[36] or cellulose acetate electrophoresis. By analogy with myeloma protein one refers to them as M-components. These fractions are also considered as oligoclonal, which would imply that they are formed as the myeloma paraprotein, by one cell clone. The more precise term, which has no physiopathological implication, is γ-globulins with restricted heterogeneity[37]. Normally the γ-globulins in CSF spread over a region being made up of numerous different immunoglobulins and are thus heterogeneous. In MS a number of homogeneous γ-globulins appear in this region which are typical of the disease and the heterogeneity of the entire γ-globulin fraction is thus restricted. This has, since then, been confirmed by many authors and can be accepted as a fact admitted by all[38].

Tourtelotte's column fractionation[39] of the CSF γ-globulins in MS yields some fractions which appear more characteristic of MS than others. This corroborates our own observation. In our opinion the *most important biochemical fact to confirm a clinical diagnosis of MS is this fractionation of the γ-globulins, the formation of M-components among the γ-globulins, these γ-globulins being of restricted heterogeneity, oligoclonal or sometimes monoclonal γ-globulins.* The significance of this we shall discuss below.

It is this modification in the γ-globulin region of the CSF pherogram which enables us to confirm the diagnosis of MS. We must add that these modifications are not absolutely confined to this disease, but where the spinal fluid has a normal total protein and this γ-globulin fractionation appears, one must very much bear in mind the diagnosis of MS especially if the clinical examination is suggestive. Gilland confirms this hypothesis in a very thorough study[38].

Whilst several other methods may produce suggestive results, they are usually inadequate. Agarose gel[40] or cellulose acetate electrophoresis, although generally technically inferior to agar gel electrophoresis, give the same results.

Electrophoresis on paper, starch, or acrylamide[6,29], does not show up clearly the γ-globulin fractionation. Other methods of γ-globulin estimation, for example zinc sulphate[41] precipitation, or IgG determinations[42-44], by electroimmunodiffusion[45] or any other method of immunoglobulin estimation, do not show the γ-globulin fractionation. Radial immunodiffusion and several other techniques used for quantitative assessment of IgG all fail to reveal the restricted heterogeneity of the γ-globulins. We shall refer to it again later.

The γ-globulin fractionation implies an important and significant qualitative and quantitative modification of the CSF immunoglobulins. Several methods have been used to establish the chemical composition of these γ-globulins. The first method used was immunoelectrophoresis[46], which in fact showed some morphological anomalies in the precipitation lines but little more. On the other hand methods of quantitation of immunoglobulins[43,47] have undoubtedly added to our knowledge of these γ-globulins and proved that the increase is essentially by IgG (Immunoglobulin G). This leads us to the conclusion that *in MS, the level of CSF IgG is increased and also, but to a lesser degree IgA (Immunoglobulin A), but not IgM (Immunoglobulin M). In addition the IgGs are shown to be of restricted heterogeneity.*

Whilst we may set aside most methods, apart from agar gel, agarose gel or cellulose acetate electrophoresis, we must refer to two recent technical advances.

(1) Agar gel, agarose gel and cellulose acetate electrophoresis call for concentration of the spinal fluid, which can itself introduce errors or artifacts. In attempting to avoid this, Kerenyi and Gallegas[48] have suggested staining the pherograms by a silver method, based on histological methods. We studied this method with Kerenyi and Verheecken[49] and believe that it is not yet available for routine work. However the method will probably enable examination of non-concentrated CSF, as soon as the technique has been further developed and perfected.

(2) Delmotte[50], on the other hand, has studied the CSF proteins by thin layer isoelectric focusing in acrylamide gel. He was able to show that the γ-globulin fractionation could be achieved by a different method from electrophoresis in agar gel, agarose gel or cellulose acetate. The fractionation obtained by Delmotte is much more efficient than that achieved so far. This method, therefore, would appear to have possibilities for expansion.

To indicate the fractionation of the IgGs is a very important fact, but the aim should be to identify the different bands which can thus be separated. The *qualitative study* of the γ-globulin fractions is most important.

This qualitative study has already been started in various laboratories in two different ways. Some authors have tried to define the CSF γ-globulin activity as antibodies. The search for nervous tissue antibodies[51], or autoantibodies has failed. On the other hand, by analogy with the findings in other diseases, such as subacute sclerosing panencephalitis (SSPE), and nonneurological diseases, measles antibodies have been sought[52-55]. All authors agree that there is definitely an increase of measles antibodies in the serum and in CSF of patients affected with MS. They also agree that this activity is less constant and quantitatively much less important than in SSPE. Nevertheless one should bear in mind that some at least of the antibodies found in CSF of patients suffering from MS are measles antibodies.

Attempts have also been made to obtain more data on CSF antibodies by studying their structure. Whilst some studies failed to elicit anything specific to MS[56], Link[40] was able to demonstrate a modification of the κ/λ ratio and a predominance of κ chains. On the other hand Ishiwata *et al.*[57] found (by immunodiffusion) a double ring formation for the κ chains. This double ring formation is certainly not specific for MS. Ishiwata himself points out that it is also present in SSPE spinal fluid.

We checked these results. In our studies[58] this ring was not observed for the λ chains. Free κ and γ chains were present besides those bound in IgG

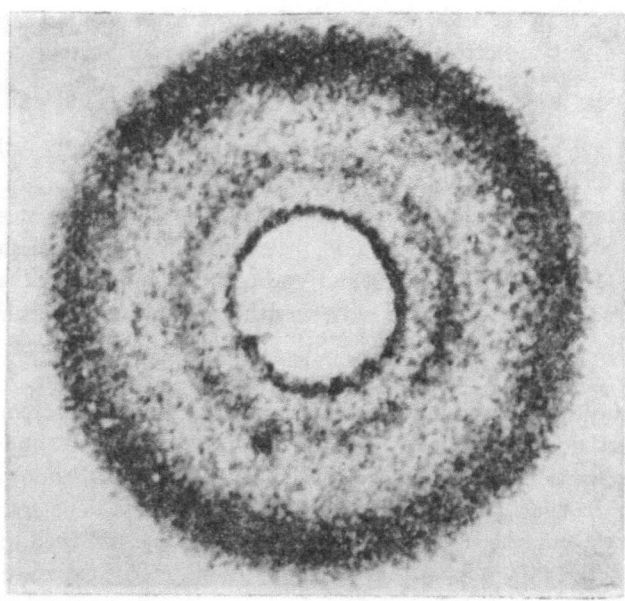

Figure 7.2 Double ring formation after immunodiffusion with rabbit serum antihuman chains against SSPE CSF proteins

molecules so that the problem appears very complex. The double ring formation apparently indicates only the presence of oligoclonal γ-globulins. Predominance of κ chains has been found in CSF and serum of MS patients. This predominance of κ chains might be specific since it does not appear in SSPE.

We tend to have here the first indications of a qualitative modification, or more precisely, of a specific characteristic of the MS IgG molecule.

A problem we have not yet tackled is the relation between the quantitative and qualitative modifications of IgG and the clinical condition of the patient though several authors[47,59,60] have dealt with this subject. It seems certain that at the onset of the disease, especially if it starts with an optic neuritis[45,61], there is no qualitative or quantitative modification of the immunoglobulins, these only appearing after several months, and becoming more pronounced after years. Do they progress much during the course of the disease? Are they more pronounced at some stage of the disease? That is difficult to assess. In the cases we examined, we have often been surprised to note, in periods of remission with relatively few neurological clinical symptoms, high levels of CSF oligoclonal γ-globulins. However we can state that in optic neuritis, modifications of CSF immunoglobulins are uncommon. It is difficult to draw a definite conclusion. Perhaps research based on newer and more precise biochemical methods may yield more rewarding results.

Certain authors have also analysed other substances occurring in the immunological reactions, among them the complement[51,62,63], but no firm conclusion has resulted.

Discussion

Whilst we have outlined many aspects of the CSF problem in MS and the biochemical phenomena mentioned related to them as well as the morphological aspects of pleicytosis, we shall, however, focus our attention on one particular problem only, as those concerned with spinal fluid in MS do generally. This is the problem of proteins, and various questions may be considered:

(1) Is the study of the CSF proteins of diagnostic and therapeutic value?

(2) Are the modifications of the CSF proteins related to the permeability of the haematoencephalic barrier?

(3) What is this immune reaction seen in CSF?

(4) Can one find similar immune reactions in other diseases, such as experimental allergic encephalomyelitis or slow viral diseases?

(5) What is the relationship between the immune reaction observed and the cell reaction described?

Of what value is the study of CSF proteins?

For diagnosis, let us repeat that the IgG anomalies are found in approximately 75% of all cases, from the time the clinical diagnosis is made. This percentage increase and approaches 100% in advanced stages of the disease. Whilst exact figures vary, we think that approximately three out of four cases show clearly IgG anomalies. We will repeat that, for the time being, until the introduction of Kerenyi's silver staining method is routine or Delmotte's isoelectrofocusing available, electrophoresis in agar gel, agarose gel or in cellulose acetate remains the best method for CSF protein examination.

Do these examinations help prognosis and therapy control? This is not proven. During treatment with ACTH, a reduction of these IgG levels has been observed, but this does not warrant any conclusion as to the efficacy of the therapy.

Modifications of the CSF proteins

The appearance of these IgG in CSF has been explained by a permeability change of the haematoencephalic barrier. Authors, such as Tourtelotte[64] and Roboz-Einstein et al.[65], have in fact shown that modifications of the haematoencephalic barrier exist in patients suffering from MS, so that the CSF IgGs might be derived from blood and possibly originate in other haematopoietic structures. We agree that a modification of the haemato-encephalic barrier could exist and the problem is to ascertain where the CSF IgG originates in the central nervous system or in other organs. This will now be discussed.

The immune reaction in CSF

Indeed the question is: what is the significance of the putative immune reaction observed in CSF, and where does the IgG originate? Many authors claim that it originates in the central nervous system since IgG of this character is not found in the serum. Frick and Schneid-Seidel[66] and Cutler et al.[69] have shown that, in cases of MS and SSPE, some of the IgG is synthetized in the central nervous system. In the nervous tissue hydrosoluble extracts of MS we were the first[29] to show, as Tourtelotte did later[68], increases of IgG and that these IgG have an oligoclonal distribution as in CSF.

We do not, however, consider this as conclusive evidence that these IgGs are synthesized in the central nervous system. Indeed one would have to define the central nervous system; can we accept that these IgG are synthetized in the neurones, in the glial cells or in the perivascular spaces? Indeed the IgG can pass from these various cells into CSF, but one cannot yet accept the very attractive hypothesis that cells of neuroectodermal or even meningeal origin are responsible for IgG synthesis. Simply because a substance is found in a relatively higher concentration in CSF than in blood or any other biological media, it does not necessarily follow that it is a synthetized in the central nervous system.

Another hypothesis has been suggested: that these proteins are synthetized by cells in the spinal fluid. Thus, in one case of MS, which had an unusually large number of cells in the CSF, Cohen and Bannister[69] succeeded in culturing them and showed that they were able to produce IgG and to a lesser degree IgA. Tourtelotte[70] made precise, if somewhat complicated, calculations to prove that such cells could not produce all the IgG found in CSF.

At present, one cannot be sure of the origin of these IgGs. Some may originate from the peripheral blood, but need not be specific to the disease, some may be synthetized in one or other group of cells in the central nervous system as we have already mentioned, whilst yet others may be synthetized by cells of the CSF. For the time being we must admit these three alternatives to explain the presence of IgG in CSF.

Another question of paramount importance is the nature of these IgGs and their role as antibody.

Their antibody activity implies that their production is triggered by the stimulation of an antigen. Is it a single antigen or are these IgG directed against several antigens? If only one is involved, is it an exogenous factor? May it be a virus or other agent causing the disease, or on the contrary is it an endogenous protein and more specifically one derived from the central nervous system itself? Whilst antibody activity directed against an exogenous antigen has been observed, and authors like ter Meulen et al.[71] have isolated a virus from the central nervous system of patients suffering from MS, it has not been proved that those antibodies combine with one of the central nervous system proteins or one of the body proteins to produce an autoimmune reaction. It is evident that CSF, from patients suffering from MS, can bring about demyelinization of nerve fibres in tissue culture. This still does not mean an immune reaction with the myelin proteins.

Some authors have tried to combine both hypotheses, accepting that the CSF IgGs are antibodies, against an exogenous factor such as a virus, and against a nervous tissue protein. This attractive hypothesis has to be confirmed. So far, the evidence put forward by Schuller et al.[72] is only indirect, and should be distinguished from facts. The oligoclonal reaction in CSF is very similar to the one observed in the serum of hyperimmunized animals[37]. We consider the oligoclonal reaction in MS as a hyperimmunization phenomenon, which can only be explained by the fact that the organism remains subjected to the action of one or more antigens during the whole illness. The antigen could thus perhaps be a persistent agent. So why is there an oligoclonal reaction, which is also observed in experimental animals? We still do not know. We have been able to prove that the oligoclonal phenomena in SSPE serum consists of homogenous IgG[37], but this has still to be established for CSF. The difficulty of establishing such proof is chiefly technical owing to insufficient quantities of protein being available. The hypothesis that we deal with a similar phenomenon as in experimental hyperimmunization is not conducive to the action of several antigens. In animals the repeated administration of one antigen produces the fractionated serum γ-globulin with two main and as many as five secondary fractions similar to the ones seen in CSF of MS patients, so that the fractionation of the CSF IgGs in MS might also result from a single antigen.

The relation of immunological reaction in MS to those in other diseases

This naturally brings us to the fourth point: the relation of this immunological reaction to that observed in other neurological diseases, for clearly this must help to classify MS. The problem has been discussed elsewhere at length[73]. The oligoclonal reaction observed in CSF of patients affected with MS is not seen in the serum but is comparable to the oligoclonal reaction seen in the serum of viral diseases with slow evolution, such as sheep visna[74], SSPE distemper in the dog or mink Aleutian disease[73], although the elevation of total protein and γ-globulin in spinal fluid of monkeys during the acute phases of EAE has long been known[75]. However, so far as we know the oligoclonal reaction is not observed in experimental allergic encephalomyelitis, although more study is needed especially of CSF proteins by electrophoresis in agar gel, agarose gel or cellulose acetate. The relatively few studies

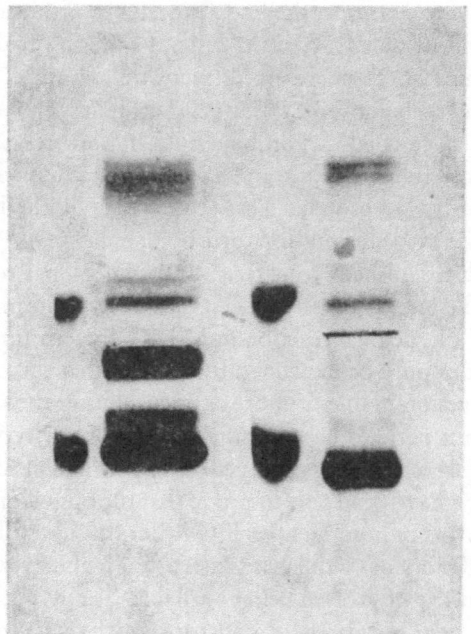

Figure 7.3 CSF proteins left and agar gel electrophoresis right in the case of subacute sclerosing panencephalitis (SSPE). The γ-globulins are clearly fractioned

published do not indicate an oligoclonal reaction. It may be noted that diseases considered to be 'slow' viral infections, such as kuru, and Creutzfeldt–Jakob in man, scrapie or rida in sheep[73] do not show any immunological reaction and certainly not the oligoclonal CSF immunoglobulins observed in MS. The oligoclonal reaction observed in MS CSF is the real basis for considering MS as belonging to the group of slow viral diseases, with persistent antigen. Nevertheless, the antigen has not been identified and anomalies are not

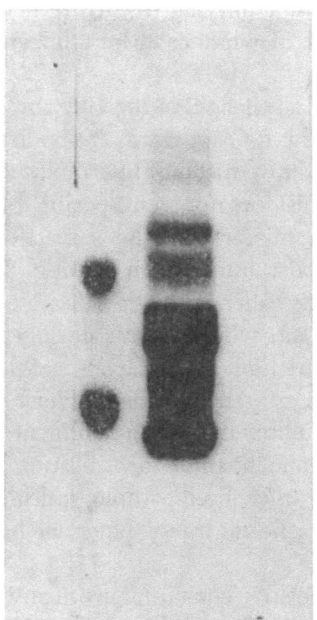

Figure 7.4 Agar gel electrophoresis of serum proteins in a case of mink Aleutian disease. The γ-globulins are clearly fractionated

present in serum. They are, however, seen in hydrosoluble extracts of the central nervous system.

The relationship between immune reaction and cell reaction in CSF

This has already been discussed; CSF cells could play a part in the production of IgG in CSF though quantitatively they cannot account for it all. The presence of these and their morphology prove that MS is an inflammatory disease.

MS must definitely not be classified as a degenerative disease. Nor can it be considered as an entirely autoimmunological phenomenon, such as the Guillain–Barré syndrome or experimental allergic encephalomyelitis[42]. The evidence suggests that it is probably a slow viral disease with an immune reaction similar to that seen in experimental hyperimmunization.

Conclusions

From a survey of the study of the CSF of patients affected with MS we may draw two clear and positive conclusions:

(1) In the CSF of patients suffering from MS there are cell modifications and primarily an increase of white cells, lymphocytes and even more often plasmacytes.

(2) There are biochemical changes in the CSF and especially an increase of the IgG concentration. This IgG appears as antibodies with restricted heterogeneity. There is a larger proportion of IgG molecules with bound κ chains than with λ chains but this does not seem specific for MS. Free κ chains are also detected in CSF. A similar oligoclonal reaction is seen in slow viral diseases, such as sheep visna, distemper in the dog, SSPE, etc. and this leads us to believe that patients suffering from MS are undergoing exposure to at least one antigenic agent, which persists during the entire course of the disease. We should bear in mind that at the onset of the disease, the triggering factor may initially be an exogenous antigen which may last many years, to be superseded later by another endogenous antigenic agent, though this still has to be proved. Immunochemical identification of IgG in CSF might confirm this. Apart from the physiopathological interest the modifications of the IgG have a real diagnostic value, which we have mentioned and emphasized many times.

We cannot draw any positive conclusion from any other analyses made on CSF. However they indicate that lipid anomalies and amino acid changes as well as abnormal metal concentrations and enzyme level variations may occur. More precise research methods are needed for such further studies.

References

1. Cerf, J. A. and Carels, G. (1966). Multiple sclerosis serum factor producing reversible alterations in bioelectric responses. *Science*, **152**, 1066

2. Bornstein, M. B. (1973). The immunopathology of demyelinative disorders examined in organotypic cultures of mammalian central nerve tissues. *Prog. Neuropathol.*, **II**, 69

3. De Crousaz, G. (1966). Le liquide céphalo-rachidien dans la sclérose en plaques. *Rev. Med. Suisse Romande*, **11**, 737

4. Koufen, H. and Consbruck, U. (1967). Untersuchungen zur Bedeutung der Liquorelektrophorese für Diagnose und Differentialdiagnose der multiplen Sklerose. *Arch. Psychol. Z. Ges. Neurol.*, **209**, 148

5. Sayk, J. and Schmidt, R. M. (1956). Zur Liquordiagnostik bei der multiplen Sklerose. *Ärztlich. Wochenschr.*, **36**, 788

6. Lowenthal, A. (1972). Chemical physiopathology of the cerebrospinal fluid. *Handb. Neurochem.*, **7**, 429

7. Plum, C. M. (1961). Biochemical studies of the composition of cerebrospinal fluid in multiple sclerosis. *Int. J. Neurol.*, **2**, 121

8. Plum, C. M. and Fog, T. (1959), Studies in multiple sclerosis. *Acta Psychol. Neurol. Scand.*, **34**, suppl. 128, 54

9. Van Sande, M., Mardens, Y., Adriaenssens, K. and Lowenthal, A. (1970). The free amino acids in human cerebrospinal fluid. *J. Neurochem.*, **17**, 125

10. Diessner, H. and Schmidt, R. M. (1967). Das Aminosäurespektrum des Liquor cerebrospinalis bei entzündlichen Erkrankungen des Zentralnervensystems. *Arch. Psychol. Z. Ges. Neurol.*, **209**, 395

11. Plum, C. M. and Hansen, S. E. (1960). Studies on variations in serum copper and serum copper oxidase activity, together with studies on the copper content of the cerebrospinal fluid, with particular reference to the variations in multiple sclerosis. *Acta Psychol. Neurol. Scand.* **35**, suppl. 148, 41

12. Karcher, D. (1962). Approche biochimique d'une carence spontanée en cuivre chez l'agneau. *Bull. Soc. R. Zool. (Anvers)*, **24**, 1

13. Feldman, S., Izak, G. and Nelken, D. (1957). Blood coagulation studies and serotonin determinations in serum and cerebrospinal fluid in multiple sclerosis. *Acta Psychol. Neurol. Scand.*, **32**, 37

14. Konyves-Kolonics, L. and Huszak, I. (1949). Der Normal-Haemolysingehalt des Liquors bei multiplen Sklerose und verschiedenen anderen Erkrankungen des Nervensystems. *Wien Z. Nervenheilkd.*, *Deren Grenzgeb.*, **2**, 296

15. Lowenthal, A. (1968). Enzymes du liquide céphalo-rachidien in 'Der Liquor Cerebrospinalis' (Berlin: VEB Verlag Volk und Gesundheit)

16. Haerer, A. F. (1972). Pyruvate, citrate, alphaketo glutarate and glucose in the cerebrospinal fluid and blood of neurologic patients. *Acta Neurol. Scand.*, **48**, 306

17. Baumgarten, F. and Saar, M. (1960). Der Gehalt des Liquor cerebrospinalis an Meso-inosit bei Meningitis und anderen Erkrankungen des ZNS. *Dtsch. Z. Nervenheilkd.* **180**, 125

18. Clausen, J. and Fog, T. (1969). Polar lipids and proteins in the cerebrospinal fluid. *Int. Arch. Allergy, Appl. Immunol.*, **36** suppl., 649

19. Seidel, D. and Lindlar, F. (1970). Über die Fettsäuren der Liquorlipide bei demyelinisierenden Erkrankungen. *Z. Neurol.*, **198**, 223

20. Tourtelotte, W. and Haerer, A. F. (1964). A study of lipids in the cerebrospinal fluid. XI. In multiple sclerosis. *Neurology*, **14**, 256

21. Christensen Lou, H. O. and Matzke, J. (1965). Cerebrosides and other polar lipids of the cerebrospinal fluid in neurological diseases. *Acta Neurol. Scand.*, **41**, 445

22. Green, J. B., Papadopoulos, N., Cevallos, W., Forster, F. M. and Hess, W. C. (1959). The cholesterol and cholesterol ester content of cerebrospinal fluid in patients with multiple sclerosis and other neurological diseases. *J. Neurol. Neurosurg. Psychiatry*, **22**, 117

23. Tichy, J. (1966). Cholesterol in the cerebrospinal fluid. An analysis of 447 neurological patients. *Rev. Czech. Med.*, **12**, 265

24. Dyrbye, M. and Fog, T. (1962). The hexosamine concentration in the spinal fluid in patients with disseminated sclerosis. *Acta Neurol. Scand.*, **38**, 1

25. Worm-Petersen, J. (1960). Determination of hexosamine on lipid-free brain tissue. Studies in multiple sclerosis. *Acta Psychol. Neurol. Scand.*, **35**, suppl. 148,

28

26. Mertin, J., Shenton, B. K. and Field, E. J. (1973). Unsaturated fatty acids in multiple sclerosis. *Br. Med. J.*

27. Bizouard, P., Guisard, S., André, J. M. and Arnould, G. (1970). La formule protéique du liquide céphalorachidien dans les affections du système nerveux central et de la sclérose en plaques en particulier. *Sem. Hôp. Paris*, **46**, 2151

28. Dowzenko, A., Wender, M. and Patelski, J. (1958). Beitrag zu ungewöhnlich grossen Liquorveränderungen bei der multiplen Sklerose. **81**, 144

29. Lowenthal, A. (1964). *Agar electrophoresis in neurology* (Elsevier: Amsterdam)

30. Shinko, H. and Tschabitscher, H. (1958). Der γ-quotient als differentialdiagnostisches Kriterium zwischen multipler Sklerose und degenerativen Erkrankungen des Nervensystems unter besonderer Berücksichtigung der Krankheitsdauer. **24**, 417

31. Steger, J. (1955). Blut- und Liquorveränderungen bei der Multiplen Sklerose mit kritischen Bemerkungen zur Eiweiss- und Lipoid-Elektrophorese. *Verh. Dtsch. Ges. Inn. Med.*, **61**, Kongress, 377

32. Van Sande, M., Karcher, D. and Lowenthal, A. (1957). Examens électrophorétiques des protéines du sérum et du liquide céphalo-rachidien chez des patients atteints de sclérose en plaques. *Acta Neurol. Psychol. Belg.*, **57**, 407

33. Weber, E. L. (1972). Electrophoretic analysis of cerebrospinal fluid proteins in patients with central nervous system mass lesions. *J. Neurosurg.*, **36**, 679

34. Fadiloglu, M. (1967). Les γ-globulines du sérum et du liquide céphalo-rachidien dans la leucoencéphalite sclérosante subaigüe et la sclérose en plaques. *Acta Med. Belg.*, **67**, 763

35. Laterre, E. C. (1966). Les γ-globulines du liquide céphalo-rachidien dans la sclérose en plaques. *Acta Neurol. Psychol. Belg.*, **66**, 305

36. Link, H. (1973). Comparison of electrophoresis on agar gel and agarose gel in the evaluation of γ-globulin abnormalities in cerebrospinal fluid and serum in multiple sclerosis. *Clin. Chim. Acta*, **46**, 383

37. Strosberg, A. D., Karcher, D. and Lowenthal, A. (1975). Structural homogeneity of human subacute sclerosing panencephalitis antibodies. *J. Immunol.*, pp. 115–157

38. Gilland, O. (1967). Cerebrospinal fluid. *Prog. Neurol. Psychol.*, **34**, 338

39. Tourtelotte, W., Parker, J. A. and Haerer, A. F. (1962). Subfractionation of multiple sclerosis γ-globulin. *Z. Immun. und Allerg.*, **126**, 85

40. Link, H. (1972). Oligoclonal immunoglobulin G in multiple sclerosis brains. *J. Neurol. Sci.*, **16**, 103

41. Hanok, A. (1961). A micromodification of a method for the measurement of globulin in cerebrospinal fluid and its application in diagnosis of multiple sclerosis. *J. Lab. Clin. Med.*, **57**, 42

42. Paterson, P. Y. (1973). Multiple sclerosis: an immunologic reassessment. *J. Chron. Dis.*, **26**, 119

43. Schmidt, R. M. (1963). Immunoelektrophorese des Liquor cerebrospinalis. *Psychol. Neurol. Med. Psychol.*, **11**, 429

44. Skrabanek, P., Staunton, H., Holland, P. D. J. and Lawlor, L. (1973). Immunoglobulins in cerebrospinal fluid in multiple sclerosis and other neurological diseases. *J. Irish Med. Ass.*, **66**, 692

45. Schneck, S. A. and Claman, H. N. (1969). Cerebrospinal fluid immunoglobulins in multiple sclerosis and other neurologic diseases. *Arch. Neurol.*, **20**, 132

46. Schmidt, R. M. (1963). Beitrag zur Agarelektrophorese des Liquor cerebrospinalis. *Psychol. Neurol. Med. Psychol.*, **10**, 393

47. Vymazal, J. and Polacek, L. (1966). γ-globulinwerte im Liquor und ihre Beziehung zum klinischen Bild und Verlauf der multiplen Sklerose. *Psychol. Neurol. Med. Psychol.*, **4**, 136

48. Kerenyi, L. and Gallegas, F. (1972). A highly sensitive method for demonstrating proteins in electrophoretic, immunoelectrophoretic and immunodiffusion preparations. *Clin. Chim. Acta*, **38**, 465

49. Verheecke, P. (1974). Agar gel electrophoresis of unconcentrated cerebrospinal fluid: the degenerative type. *Acta Neurol. Belg.*, **74**, 376

50. Delmotte, P. (1972). Comparative results of agar electrophoresis and isolectric focusing examination of the γ-globulins of the cerebrospinal fluid. *Acta Neurol. Belg.*, **72**, 226

51. Laurell, A. B. and Link, H. (1972). Complement-fixing antibrain antibodies in multiple sclerosis. *Acta Neurol. Scand.*, **48**, 461

52. Brown, P., Cathala, F., Gadjusek, C. D. and Gibbs, C. J. (1971). Measles antibodies in the cerebrospinal fluid of patients with multiple sclerosis. *Proc. Soc. Exp. Biol. Med.*, **137**, 956

53. Ebinger, G. and Matthyssens, G. (1971). Cerebrospinal measles antibody titer and γ-globulins, in subacute sclerosing panencephalitis. *Z. Neurol.*, **200**, 1

54. Norrby, E., Link, H. and Olsson, J. E. (1974). Measles virus antibodies in multiple sclerosis. *Arch. Neurol.*, **30**, 285

55. Novalez, E., Link, H. and Olsson, J. E. (1974). Measles virus antibodies in multiple sclerosis. *Arch. Neurol.*, **30**, 285

56. Grimm, R. R., Alter, M. and Williams, R. C. Jr. (1966). Gm and Inv. antigenic character of serum, cerebrospinal fluid IgG in multiple sclerosis. *Proc. Soc. Exp. Biol. Med.*, **122**, 554

57. Ishiwata, H., Grundwald, F. and Bauer, H. (1974). Double ring formation in single radial immunodiffusion for kappa chains in multiple sclerosis cerebrospinal fluid. *J. Neurol.*, **207**, 45

58. Bollengier, F., Lowenthal, A. and Henrotin, W. (1975). Bound and free light chains in subacute sclerosing panencephalitis and multiple sclerosis serum and cerebrospinal fluid. *Z. Klin. Chem. Klin. Biochem.*, **13**, 305

59. Goldstein, N. P., McKenzie, B. F. and McGuckin, W. F. (1962). Changes in cerebrospinal fluid of patients with multiple sclerosis after treatment with intrathecal methylprednisolone ace: a preliminary report. *Proc. Mayo Clin.*, **37**, 657

60. Olsson, J. E. and Link, H. (1973). Immunoglobulin abnormalities in multiple sclerosis. Relation to clinical parameters: exacerbations and remissions. *Arch. Neurol.*, **28**, 391

61. Sandberg, M. and Bynke, H. (1973). Cerebrospinal fluid in 25 cases of optic neuritis. *Acta Neurol. Scand.*, **49**, 443

62. Dube, V. E., McDuffie, F. C., Burton, R. C. and Ilstrup, D. (1973). Cerebrospinal fluid complement in multiple sclerosis. *J. Lab. Clin. Med.*, **81**, 530

63. Link, H. (1972). Complement factors in multiple sclerosis. *Acta Neurol. Scand.*, **48**, 521

64. Tourtelotte, W. (1963). Multiple sclerosis and cerebrospinal fluid. *Med. Clin. N. Am.*, **47**, 1619

65. Roboz, E., Hess, W. C., Forster, F. M. and Temple, D. M. (1954). Paper electrophoretic studies in multiple sclerosis. *Neurology*, **4**, 811

66. Frick, E. and Scheid-Seidel, L. (1957). Immunologische Untersuchungen an Liquoreiweisskörpern. *Z. Ges. Exp. Med.*, **129**, 221

67. Cutler, R. W., Merla, E. and Hammerstal, S. P. (1968). Production of antibody by the central nervous system in subacute sclerosing panencephalitis. *Neurology*, **18**, 129

68. Tourtelotte, W. (1974). Data to support the immunogenesis of the multiple sclerosis plaque. The international symposium on multiple sclerosis. *Acta Neurol. Scand.*, **50**, suppl. 58, 60

69. Cohen, S. and Bannister, R. (1967). Immunoglobulin synthesis within the central nervous system in disseminated sclerosis. *Lancet*, **i**, 366

70. Tourtelotte, W. (1970). On cerebrospinal fluid immunoglobulin G (IgG) quotients in multiple sclerosis and other diseases. *J. Neurol. Sci.*, **10**, 279

71. ter Meulen, V., Moller, D., Kackell, Y. and Katz, M. (1972). Isolation of infectious measles virus in measles encephalitis. *Lancet*, **ii**, 1172

72. Schuller, E., Delasnerie, N., Deloche, G. and Loridan, M. (1973). Multiple sclerosis: a two-phase disease. *Acta Neurol. Scand.*, **49**, 453

73. Lowenthal, A. (1973). La sclérose en plaques dans le cadre des maladies virales lentes. *Acta Neurol. Belg.*, **73**, 165

74. Sigurdsson, B., Karcher, D., Van Sande, M. and Lowenthal, A. (1960). Electrophoresis of serum and cerebrospinal proteins in sheep neurological diseases. The protides of the biological fluids. *7th Colloquium Bruges.* 110–111. (Amsterdam: Elsevier)

75. Kabat, E. A., Wolf, A., Bezer, A. E., and Murray, J. P. (1951). Studies on acute disseminated encephalomyelitis produced experimentally in rhesus monkeys. VI. Changes in cerebrospinal fluid proteins. *J. Exper. Med.*, **93**, 615

8

Lipids and multiple sclerosis

A. D. Smith and R. H. S. Thompson

Introduction

The outstanding problem in multiple sclerosis remains the aetiology and pathogenesis of the disease, and theories which have been advanced concerning its origin embrace viral, immunological, nutritional and metabolic considerations, alone or in various combinations. The paramount role of lipids lies in their contribution to the functions of cell membranes of all kinds. Whichever of the above theories one favours, it is more than likely that cellular membranes will enter into the argument at some stage. For example, the lymphocyte plasma membrane will be involved in immune processes; viruses of the paramyxovirus group, thought possibly to be of the type which could play a part in the disease, utilize the host plasma membrane during one stage of their replication, and nutritional or metabolic approaches often advance the suggestion that there may be some degree of abnormal instability in the myelin sheath, or in the oligodendroglial membrane from which it is derived.

Thus it can be seen that scope exists for the involvement of membrane lipids in any of the major hypotheses concerning the aetiopathogenesis of the disease. Evidence for such involvement is, however, as yet fragmentary. This may be due partly to inability in the past to investigate lipids at an adequate level of detail. It could also be due to our former lack of awareness of the importance to membrane function of different types of lipid, and of their arrangements within the membrane, not to mention the lack of techniques with which to investigate these matters. This is now being rectified by the rapid and far-reaching advances which have recently been made in factual knowledge, technical capacity and theoretical concepts in the membrane field. These basic achievements are now ripe for application to problems of lipid pathology.

The possible impact of these innovations on multiple sclerosis research is an exciting prospect, and we therefore propose to outline very briefly some of the more salient features of the area (referring the reader to reviews for more detailed study) before proceeding to describe known lipid abnormalities in this disease. We believe that by introducing these concepts at the outset, we may enable existing findings, which tend to emphasize the state of lipids in isolation from their natural environment, to be set in their proper context, and may stimulate thought concerning future investigations.

Biological membranes

Much diverse evidence was resolved by Singer and Nicolson[1] in their fluid mosaic model of membrane structure, the success of which has been ensured by its usefulness in the interpretation of a wide range of membrane experiments. Recent reviews which discuss these ideas in greater detail are those of Lee[2] and of Marsh[3].

The essential features of this now familiar model, illustrated in Figure 8.1,

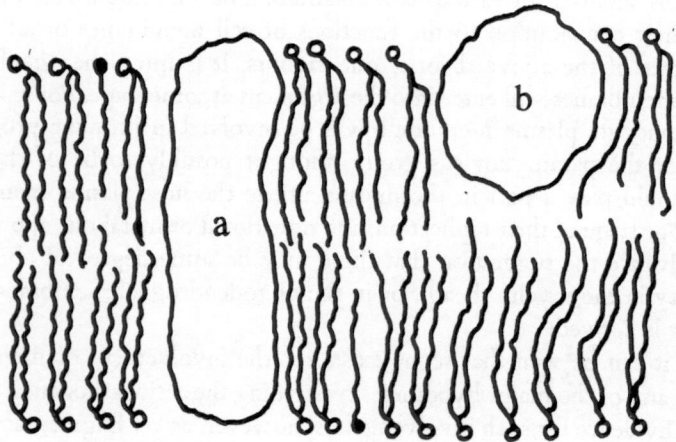

Figure 8.1 Diagrammatic representation of a bilayer membrane. Open circles represent the polar head groups of phospholipids with their fatty acids oriented towards the interior of the bilayer. Closed circles represent cholesterol. Protein marked 'a' penetrates the whole span of the bilayer; protein marked 'b' less deeply embedded.

are that the membrane consists of a two-dimensional sheet of lipid, within which are suspended a variety of membrane proteins. The lipid is mainly phospholipid, arranged as a bilayer, with the fatty acid chains oriented towards the interior and the polar head groups facing out from the membrane interior. Proteins may penetrate the entire depth of the bilayer or be more loosely attached at one of the surfaces. The proteins are free to diffuse laterally at quite rapid rates[4]. Many membrane-bound enzymes are inactivated when freed of lipid, and reactivated when lipid is added back, and it is thought that the properties of the bilayer lipid can influence the function of membrane proteins.

The study of these proteins, which encompass not only all those enzymes known to be membrane-bound, including transport enzymes, but antigens and other non-enzymic proteins also, is less advanced than is the study of the lipid bilayer, although it must be stressed that these latter studies have for the most part been carried out with more simple mixtures of lipid than are found in the cell.

In considering the influence of the bilayer lipids on membrane protein function a property of the bilayer known as fluidity is of special interest. This concept derives from studies using physical methods and is covered by the reviews cited above. Essentially, there is a temperature, known as the transition temperature and characteristic for each phospholipid or mixture, above which the lipid exhibits markedly different physical properties from those that are found below that temperature. These changes in physical properties are interpreted as being due to a change from a relatively rigid gel-like structure in the phospholipid array, to a more mobile or fluid state, resulting, it is suggested, from a greater degree of mobility in the fatty acid chains. In particular, the microviscosity decreases, facilitating lateral movement within the bilayer not only of the lipids but also of any proteins associated with them. Changes in fluidity affect the kinetic properties of a number of membrane enzymes[5].

The importance of the fatty acids in influencing fluidity is shown by the fact that if a phospholipid contains saturated acids its transition temperature is higher than that of a corresponding phospholipid containing unsaturated fatty acids. The transition temperatures of mixtures of lipids extracted from cell membranes are usually less sharp than those of pure lipids and usually span the physiological temperature of 37 °C. In this region, therefore, it is possible that the phospholipids, in whole or in part, may be in an intermediate phase between the two physical states which exist on either side of the transition. It may be, therefore, that comparatively small changes in the degree of unsaturation of the acids in a biological membrane could exert local effects within the membrane bilayer which could considerably alter a specific function of the membranes by, say, affecting the function of a membrane protein.

Polyunsaturated fatty acids

Apart from oleic and palmitoleic acids, the unsaturated acids in biological membranes are of the polyunsaturated series deriving from either linoleic acid (the $n6$ group) or linolenic acid (the $n3$ group) as shown in the footnote below*. The work on lipid bilayers is throwing new light on the function of these groups of acids. In the past, however, a great deal of work has been carried out on their metabolism in the investigation of essential fatty acid deficiency[6].

Interest in these acids in multiple sclerosis research was aroused by the early suggestions by Swank[7], Sinclair[8] and Allison[9] that a relative dietary deficiency of these acids could contribute to the onset of multiple sclerosis.

The essential fatty acids (EFA) are generally defined as those which support the growth of animals maintained on an otherwise fat-free diet, and for practical purposes may be listed as linoleate, arachidonate, and to some extent linolenate. These acids have double bonds all of which are in the *cis* configuration and separated by one methylene ($-CH_2-$) group. It is important to distinguish the difference between these acids, and those included under the

---

$*CH_3CH_2CH_2CH_2CH_2CH=CHCH_2CH=CHCH_2CH_2CH_2CH_2CH_2CH_2COOH$
Linoleate

$CH_3CH_2CH=CHCH_2CH=CHCH_2CH=CHCH_2CH_2CH_2CH_2CH_2CH_2COOH$
Linolenate

Acids are often designated by a convention which gives first (before a colon) the total number of carbons and then (after the colon) the number of double bonds; thus $18:2=$ linoleate, $18:3=$ linolenate. The position of the double bonds can be indicated by numbering either from the carboxy carbon, in which case the prefix Δ is used (thus linoleate would be $\Delta 9,12$) or from the methyl carbon, in which case the prefix n is used (in older literature ω is used instead of n). Linoleate would thus be $n6,9$. The n system of numbering has the advantage of emphasizing the metabolic origin of the acids as indicated below, and is the accepted IUPAC–IUB system. *Biochem. J.*, **105**, 897 (1967).

The $n6$ group

Linoleate (18:2) metabolically converted to arachidonate (20:4):

Δ 9, 12	Δ 5, 8, 11, 14
n 6, 9	n 6, 9, 12, 15

The $n3$ group

Linolenate (18:3) metabolically converted to docosahexaenoate (22:6):

Δ 9, 12, 15	Δ 4, 7, 10, 13, 16, 19
n 3, 6, 9	n 3, 6, 9, 12, 15, 18

more general term polyunsaturated fatty acid, which embraces a number of other long-chain fatty acids with several double bonds, which do not fulfil the requirements for definition as essential fatty acids, especially when the double bonds are in the *trans* configuration. Polyunsaturated fatty acids of the more general type are found widely distributed in plant and marine materials, and sometimes but not always they may have similar biochemical properties to the essential fatty acids. Thus, in discussing the aetiology of multiple sclerosis, in which for example comment is often made of the relative immunity of fish-eating populations, it should be borne in mind that fish oils contain little linoleate, arachidonate or linolenate, but do contain appreciable quantities of other longer-chain acids, mainly of the linolenate series, which can be regarded for some purposes as being in the class of essential fatty acids.

EFA deficiency

If animals are maintained for a sufficiently long period on a fat-free diet the essential fatty acid deficiency syndrome occurs. It is important to emphasize the difference between this extreme condition, in which essential fatty acid concentrations in the tissues are at the very lowest levels, and other conditions in which the levels of essential fatty acids are varied within what might be considered a normal range. Often, in experimental situations, the extreme condition of EFA deficiency is used to reveal abnormalities arising from the lack of essential fatty acids. EFA deficiency, however, is a pathological condition, in which the animal is responding to severe stress, and results obtained with such animals need to be interpreted accordingly. The extreme condition is seldom found in humans, although the appearance of 5,8,11-eicosatrienoic acid (a sign that deficiency of essential fatty acids is reaching severe levels) is known[10]; it has never been reported, however, in MS patients.

With these reservations, work with EFA-deficient animals may nevertheless yield results which can subsequently be tested in less extreme conditions, and may point to abnormalities which might otherwise remain undetected, for example, in MS patients. As indicated in the previous section, it has recently been realized that variation of essential fatty acid levels within more normal ranges may have considerable effects on membrane enzymes[5], and this is the type of effect which may be operative in multiple sclerosis.

Lipids and the CNS

Among the hypotheses that lipids may be concerned in the aetiology of MS are those which involve the concept that the myelin sheath may be chemically altered during development, principally due to a relative deficiency of unsaturated acids in the diet; others suggest that the fatty acid changes observed in the diseased brains reflect some difference in enzymic behaviour leading to altered myelin either during initial synthesis or normal maintenance. The enzymology of myelination has recently been reviewed[11, 12] (see also Chapter 6). Whether a myelin sheath which has suffered damage can be repaired in the CNS has been unclear in the past, but recent evidence suggests that under some circumstances it is possible[13].

The limitations to our understanding of the enzymic machinery responsible for these functions ensures that any hypothesis in this area concerning MS is outlined in somewhat vague terms. Evidence has however been accumulating over the past 10 to 15 years from a number of different laboratories that patients with MS may show abnormalities in the relative amounts of fatty acids present in the brain.

The starting point of this work dates back to the 1950s when the view was put forward that the high prevalence of MS in certain parts of the world might be related to the consumption of relatively large quantities of animal fats, i.e. fats containing predominantly the saturated and monounsaturated fatty acids[7]. This view was based initially on some admittedly limited studies carried out on the geographical distribution of MS in Norway, but since that time, further epidemiological observations[9, 14] have supported the view that there may be an association between high consumption of animal fat and MS.

In 1956 Sinclair pointed out[8] that in addition to containing an excess of animal fat these diets would be expected to be relatively deficient in the polyunsaturated fatty acids, and suggested that this latter deficiency may be the important factor.

It is known from animal studies that it is possible to alter the fatty acid composition of the brain lipids by varying the levels of the polyunsaturated fatty acids in the diet[15, 16], and with this background in mind a number of groups of workers have studied the fatty acid pattern of lipid fractions obtained from areas of white matter, which appeared normal on visual inspection, dissected from multiple sclerosis brains. The results obtained by these different workers have not been entirely consistent, but in a number of cases it has been reported that the amounts of various mono- or polyunsaturated fatty acids are low in the fractions isolated from the MS brains, as compared with comparable fractions derived from normal brain tissue. Unfortunately in most cases the numbers of brains that have been examined are small so that caution is needed in interpreting the findings. Thus, in 1961, Gerstl et al.[17] reported a lowering in the proportion of trienes extracted from apparently normal white matter in two MS brains. Baker et al.[18] comparing nine MS brains with six controls, found a reduction in the proportions of palmitoleic (16:1), oleic (18:1) and arachidonic (20:4) acids in the lecithin fraction of white matter. Cumings et al.[19], also using the lecithin fraction (four control brains, five MS), confirmed the finding of low levels of 18:1, while Clausen and Hansen[20], in a study of the lecithin fraction derived from myelin preparations obtained from 12 control and 17 MS brains, also found a substantial lowering of 20:4. Gerstl et al.[21] reported that the absolute amount of total polyunsaturated acids was decreased in white matter obtained from seven different areas in MS brains.

On the other hand, Arnetoli et al.[22] found no difference in the lecithin fraction (four controls, five MS), although they described a substantial lowering of both 18:1 and 20:1 in the ethanolamine phospholipid fraction. Gerstl et al.[23] also reported low levels of 18:1 and 20:1 in the ethanolamine phospholipids, and Clausen and Hansen[20] described a reduction of 18:1 in this fraction. Alling et al.[24], in a study of six MS brains and 24 controls, concluded that 'the fatty acid patterns of the MS brains were strikingly similar to those of normal brains. Nevertheless, the concentrations of some of the fatty acids characteristic of the white matter were slightly lower in the MS brains.'

The changes in brain composition that have been found are only slight, but this does not necessarily mean that they may not be of importance, since it is known from other fields of work that very small and limited changes in chemical composition may have strikingly important effects; when we turn to the field of protein biochemistry, for example, we know that the substitution of even a single amino acid by another may be of clinical significance, and the substitution of one fatty acid for another in cell membranes might also have significant effects. It remains to be determined whether, in the bilayer phospholipids, there may not be some fatty acid replacements which are forbidden, and which thus exert an effect disproportionately large compared with their quantitative importance.

One difficulty in the interpretation of work of this type with MS brain is, however, that although the areas examined were apparently normal on visual inspection it is always possible that they contained small or early demyelinating lesions not yet visible to the naked eye, and that the findings are merely reflecting early changes in the demyelinating process rather than any pre-existing abnormality of the brain tissue in which the demyelinating changes were subsequently developing.

Plasma and the blood cell fatty acids in MS

Because of these difficulties in work of this type with MS brain tissue, and since the findings prompted the question as to whether these changes in brain fatty acid composition might be associated with changes in the relative amounts of saturated and unsaturated fatty acids reaching the brain, Baker *et al.*[25] next turned their attention to the fatty acids which are present in the plasma both in the esterified (as components of cholesteryl esters and phospholipids) and non-esterified form. Blood specimens, obtained after an overnight fast, were taken from 47 patients with MS and from 38 controls (both healthy persons and patients with non-demyelinating neurological disorders). Estimation of the various fatty acids derived from the total lipid extract obtained from the serum showed that there was a small but highly significant ($P < 0.001$) lowering of the percentage of linoleate (18:2) in the MS group (see Table 8.1).

Further, when the patients were divided into groups according to the clinical severity and activity of the disease (group 1 showing no evidence of clinical deterioration over the preceding month, and groups 2, 3 and 4 showing increasing evidence of recent deterioration) it will be seen (Table 8.1) that the degree of reduction in the linoleate level appears to correlate with the activity of the disease process. The levels of fatty acids in the blood are of course influenced by dietary intake, but the general nutritional status of all these patients was good, and there was no history in any case of vomiting, difficulty in eating or of avoidance of food.

Subsequent studies on further series of patients both at Guy's Hospital and at the Courtauld Institute[26-30] have consistently confirmed this finding of a small but significant fall in the percentage of linoleate in the total lipid extract, and also the conclusion that the most marked falls are found in patients who are showing active and rapid deterioration.

These findings have since been independently confirmed by Tichy *et al.*[31], Love *et al.*[32], Crawford and Hassam[33], Paty *et al.*[34] and Kalofoutis and Jullien[35]. On the other hand, a number of conflicting reports have also been published in which no significant changes in the linoleate levels were found. In several of these studies, however, the number of patients used was small, and as minimal clinical details have been given as to the state or extent of the disease it is hard to evaluate the results[19,36].

But in a study of 30 MS patients and 33 controls, Wolfgram *et al.*[37] found no significant difference in linoleate levels, even when the patients were subdivided on the basis of severity, duration of the disease or degree of disability; they have concluded therefore that a disturbance of linoleate metabolism is not invariably associated with this disease.

The discrepancies between these various findings in the levels of serum linoleate suggest indeed that the changes that have been found may be concerned more with determining the progression of the disease rather than with its initiation.

One further point which may be highly relevant in this connection appears to emerge from these blood fatty acid studies: Love *et al.*[32], Paty *et al.*[34]

Table 8.1 Percentage composition of total fatty acids in serum lipids

Group	No. in group		14:0	16:0	16:1	18:0	18:1	18:2	20:3	20:4	Others
								Fatty acids				
Healthy controls	20	Mean	1.2	23.7	3.8	5.2	27.5	26.8	1.4	5.4	5.0
		(SEM)	(0.2)	(0.6)	(0.2)	(0.4)	(0.6)	(0.6)	(0.1)	(0.3)	—
Neurological controls	18	Mean	1.0	23.8	4.2	4.8	30.5	24.3	1.5	5.5	4.4
		(SEM)	(0.04)	(0.7)	(0.3)	(0.7)	(0.9)	(0.8)	(0.2)	(0.4)	—
All controls	38	Mean	1.1	23.8	4.2	5.0	28.9	25.6	1.4	5.5	4.7
		(SEM)	(0.1)	(0.5)	(0.2)	(0.4)	(0.6)	(0.5)	(0.1)	(0.2)	—
All multiple sclerosis patients	47	Mean	1.2	24.6	4.4	4.8	30.4	22.3	1.7	5.4	5.2
		(SEM)	(0.1)	(0.5)	(0.2)	(0.3)	(0.4)	(0.5)	(0.1)	(0.1)	—
Group 1	10	Mean	1.1	23.8	3.8	4.7	28.3	25.8	1.7	5.2	5.6
		(SEM)	(0.1)	(0.5)	(0.4)	(0.8)	(0.8)	(0.9)	(0.2)	(0.2)	—
Group 2	11	Mean	1.3	23.2	4.0	5.6	30.1	23.6	1.6	5.3	5.3
		(SEM)	(0.1)	(0.3)	(0.1)	(0.2)	(0.6)	(0.6)	(0.1)	(0.1)	—
Group 3	16	Mean	1.2	23.9	4.5	4.5	32.1	21.6	1.6	5.5	5.1
		(SEM)	(0.1)	(0.8)	(0.2)	(0.4)	(0.5)	(0.6)	(0.2)	(0.3)	—
Group 4	10	Mean	1.2	27.6	5.5	4.6	30.2	18.6	2.2	5.4	4.7
		(SEM)	(0.1)	(0.9)	(0.7)	(0.5)	(1.0)	(0.4)	(0.2)	(0.3)	—

Significance of differences between means for percentages of linoleic acid (18:2)

All controls (38) versus all multiple sclerosis patients (47): $P < 0.001$
Neurological controls (18) versus all multiple sclerosis patients (47): $P < 0.05, > 0.02$

Table 8.2 Percentage content of linoleate (18:2) in serum lipids of controls and of MS patients before, during, and after five-day period of supplementation of normal diets with sunflower seed oil emulsion

	Pre-oil (mean)	During supplementation with oil					Post-oil	
		1	2	3	4	5	1	2
Control (% ± SEM)	33·7 ±1·0 (14)	40·0 ±1·8 (5)	41·4 ±1·1 (7)	42·5 ±1·3 (10)	42·5 ±1·4 (10)	42·5 ±1·9 (7)	39·5 ±1·3 (10)	38·1 ±1·4 (13)
MS (% ± SEM)	29·7 ±0·8 (14)	36·0 ±1·3 (4)	37·7 ±1·5 (4)	39·9 ±0·9 (13)	41·1 ±0·9 (12)	41·2 ±1·2 (14)	36·7 ±0·8 (11)	34·1 ±0·9 (14)

Numbers of subjects in parentheses

Controls versus MS in pre-oil period $P < 0.01$
Controls versus MS two days after end of supplementation $P < 0.05$

and Kalofoutis and Jullien[35] have each found low levels of linoleate in patients with certain other diseases of the nervous system.

As already mentioned, it has been suggested that the prevalence of MS in certain parts of the world may be related to a dietary deficiency of unsaturated fatty acids. In addition to purely dietary considerations it is important to know whether there is any defect in the intestinal absorption of unsaturated fatty acids in patients with MS. It is of course well known that diets rich in linoleate normally cause an increase of linoleate in the serum lipids. In the main these changes have been studied over relatively long-term intervals, but Farquhar and Ahrens[38] found an increase in 18:2 in the β-lipoproteins within a few hours after a single dose of corn oil, an effect which has since been studied in greater detail in rats[39]. Belin et al.[29] have studied the fatty acid pattern in the serum lipids in fasting blood samples taken before, during and after supplementation of the normal diet with sunflower seed oil (the supplements providing 28 g linoleate/day), but found no evidence in the MS patients of deficient absorption, the rise in the 18:2 level in the serum lipids during the supplementation period being as great as in the controls (Table 8.2).

The work referred to so far has described changes in the fatty acid composition of the *total* lipid extract, i.e. the sum of the esterified and non-esterified fatty acid, but in recent studies in our laboratory[30,40], the levels of the separated 'free' (non-esterified) fatty acids have also been measured; this has

Table 8.3 Per cent linoleate in serum total lipids, serum free fatty acids, and lymphocytes, in humans

	Controls	MS	P
Total lipids	35.0 ± 1.0 (14)	28.8 ± 0.77 (19)	0.001
Non-esterified fatty acids	17.0 ± 1.1 (14)	12.1 ± 0.50 (18)	0.001
Lymphocytes	10.6 ± 0.64 (12)	8.3 ± 0.33 (19)	0.005

shown (Table 8.3) that the level of the unesterified linoleate is also significantly reduced in MS patients, and also that supplementation of the normal diet with sunflower seed oil causes a very substantial rise not only in the esterified linoleate present in the plasma lipoproteins, but also in the free linoleate. These findings may well be relevant to current observations on the effect of 18:2 and other fatty acids on lymphocyte–antigen interactions, referred to in a later section[41,42]. (See also Chapter 9.)

Blood cells

There have been many reports that the blood platelets of patients with MS are abnormally sticky, and it has been shown that in MS there is a highly significant ($P < 0.001$) inverse correlation between platelet stickiness and the serum cholesteryl linoleate level[28]. Changes have also been reported in the red blood cells of patients with MS, both increased mean red cell diameter and increased osmotic fragility having been described. A study of the fatty acid composition of the phospholipids of platelets and erythrocytes from a series of patients with MS has shown that the percentage of 18:2 is significantly lower in the MS patients as compared with healthy controls[43].

Table 8.4 Fatty acid composition of platelet and red cell phospholipids

	Platelet phospholipid fatty acids Per cent total fatty acids* ($\pm SEM$)		Red blood cell phospholipid fatty acids Per cent total fatty acids* ($\pm SEM$)	
	Control	MS	Control	MS
Cases (no.)	14	20	11	10
16:0	19·2 ±0·37	18·8 ±0·31	26·1 ±0·48	26·9 ±0·36
18:0	24·5 ±0·37	24·4 ±0·31	22·3 ±0·27	21·8 ±0·28
18:1	21·0 ±0·27	21·4 ±0·27	20·1 ±0·27	21·4 ±0·32
18:2	6·3 ±0·27	4·9 ±0·12·	14·0 ±0·42	11·0 ±0·44
20:4	29·1 ±0·62	30·5 ±0·62	17·4 ±0·60	18·8 ±0·44

* Only the five fatty acids listed were totalled. Controls and patients were reasonably matched for age. No sex differences were apparent but control and patient values are composed of similar numbers of each sex.

Per cent platelet linoleate controls versus MS $P < 0.001$
Per cent red blood cell linoleate controls versus MS $P < 0.001$

The linoleate levels in lymphocytes obtained from patients with MS have also been found to be significantly below the normal level[30], a good correlation being shown between the linoleate level of the plasma non-esterified fatty acids and that in the lymphocytes (Table 8.3 and Figure 8.2).

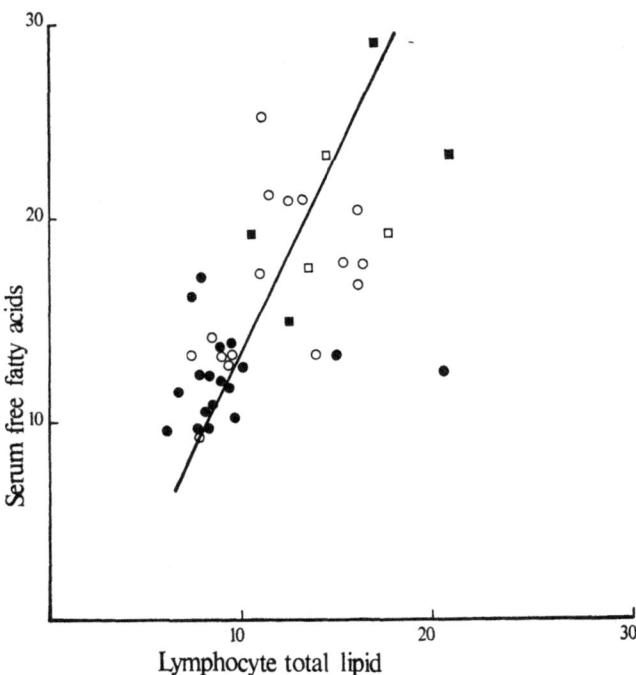

Figure 8.2 Per cent linoleate in serum-free fatty acids and in lymphocyte total lipids. O = Controls; □ = controls on oil; ● = MS; ■ = MS on oil. Correlation co-efficient = 0·62.

It remains to be determined to what extent these various findings are the result of the disease process, or whether they are playing a part in the progression of this chronic disease. They do seem to indicate however, that, as in the brain, the bilayer characteristics of these other cell membranes may be affected in MS. Again, the changes are small, and not such as would make any noticeable difference to membrane fluidity. However, it has yet to be determined whether small but specific deleterious changes, affecting a particular phospholipid species, may not have disproportionate effects on a particular membrane activity.

Lipids and the immune response

A more recent development in the connection between lipids and multiple sclerosis has been the suggestion by Mertin et al.[41] that the apparently favourable results of the sunflower seed oil trial[44] (to which we shall refer again later) might be due to an effect of the polyunsaturated acids on the immune response. There had been earlier indications of an interaction between lipids and the immune system in the work of Di Luzio[45].

A long-standing hypothesis regarding the aetiology of MS has been that some kind of autoimmune process is responsible for an attack by lymphocytes on the CNS, and this has given rise to much work on the animal model, experimental allergic encephalomyelitis (EAE). The demonstration in 1967 by Clausen and Møller[46] that the normally relatively resistant Wistar strain of rat could be rendered susceptible to EAE by EFA deficiency, and recent confirmation of this result in the Sprague–Dawley strain[47] have indicated that an autoimmune process can be affected by the lipid status of the animal.

Mertin[48] has argued that polyunsaturated fatty acids act *in vivo* to inhibit the activity of cells of the immune system, and that when the levels of polyunsaturated acids are reduced, as in EFA-deficient animals, there is a greater activity of the immune system[49]. The work cited above, demonstrating a greater susceptibility to EAE by EFA-deficient animals, might be adduced in support of this hypothesis, particularly as Selivonchick and Johnston[47] found that, in their animals, injections of linoleic acid restored resistance to the basic protein to a considerable extent. Furthermore, Mertin[48] has shown that in mice subcutaneous injections of polyunsaturated fatty acids prolong the survival of skin allografts, and correspondingly that in animals fed an EFA-deficient diet the skin grafts are rejected more rapidly than in animals fed a normal diet[49]. Not all workers, however, are in agreement with the view that linoleate prolongs the survival of skin grafts and the results have been summarized by Hughes et al.[50].

Mertin, et al.[41] had earlier advanced a similar general hypothesis as a result of *in vitro* experiments, which showed linoleic acid to inhibit the production by lymphocytes of macrophage inhibitory factor. Mertin and Hughes[42] also showed that polyunsaturated acids inhibit the blast transformation of lymphocytes, a result which was confirmed by Offner and Clausen[51] and by Paty et al.[34]. In these earlier experiments, the acids were added to the incubation mixture dissolved in ethanol. Results in our laboratory have shown that even when bound to albumin, the unsaturated acids inhibit blast transformation, but that saturated acids also inhibit[52]. However we have found that combinations of saturated and unsaturated acids inhibit very little, so before it can be said that these *in vitro* experiments support the hypothesis that polyunsaturated acids have an immunoregulatory function *in vivo*, further experiments are needed using *in vitro* conditions which more closely approach the *in vivo* situation, in particular using mixtures of fatty acids, bound to albumin, in ratios comparable with those found *in vivo* under various dietary conditions. These experiments arouse a number of interesting speculations concerning the influence of membrane fluidity on the lymphocyte response to mitogen.

The essential fatty acids act as precursors of prostaglandins, and the possibility exists that prostaglandin synthesis may be lowered in EFA deficiency, thereby causing some of the effects of the condition. The possible relevance of this situation to MS has recently been highlighted by a report[53] that incorporation of [^{14}C]acetate into prostaglandins in thrombocytes was markedly lower in MS patients than in controls (See addendum to Chapter 9.)

Therapeutic trial

As a result of the suggestions of an association between lowered linoleate intake, low blood levels of linoleate and multiple sclerosis, a double-blind trial[44] was mounted at two centres, London and Belfast. In this trial the diet of an experimental group of MS patients was supplemented with doses of a sunflower seed oil emulsion, and the diet of a control group of MS patients was supplemented with an olive oil emulsion. Each patient was studied over a two-year period and his condition assessed at the start, during, and at the end of the trial by an accepted scoring system. The outcome of this trial was that, although comparison of the overall status showed no advantage to the experimental group over this period, statistical analysis revealed that both the duration and severity of relapses were less in the patients taking sunflower seed oil. There would appear to be some incompatibility in these conclusions, in that one would expect that a decrease in the severity of relapses would ameliorate the course of the disease, but it must be concluded that over a period as short as two years, this would not emerge in the scoring system used.

This trial is currently being repeated in London, Ontario[34], and any assessment of the value of treatment with sunflower seed oil must await the outcome of this further trial.

Conclusion

This survey reveals that there is only suggestive evidence at the present time in favour of any theory associating the onset and course of multiple sclerosis with abnormal lipid chemistry or metabolism. In fairness it can be said that the same lack of hard evidence is apparent in the arguments advanced in support of the viral, immunological or any other theory. Furthermore, the circumstantial evidence in favour of lipid involvement has in recent years increased rather than diminished. Again, the growing awareness of the importance of the nature of the fatty acid chains in membrane phenomena, manifested in the influence of fatty acids on membrane fluidity, has opened up new avenues of investigation which remain to be exploited in multiple sclerosis research.

Many questions still pose themselves. Could the small differences in linoleate levels found by a number of groups have a significant effect on membrane function? Can evidence be found that abnormal fatty acid replacements specific to individual phospholipids, although making little change in overall fatty acid composition, might exert a major influence on some membrane activity?

The answers to these questions might be provided by an examination of the membrane phospholipids at a deeper level of detail, both in the MS patient and in the lymphocyte membrane modified by incubation with fatty acids. A more precise understanding of the role of individual phospholipid species in the activities of various membrane proteins will help, and more information is needed as to whether the phospholipid bilayer should be regarded as a single entity, or whether localization, possibly induced by proteins, may occur in given regions of the membrane. There are suggestions of regional variation in the fluidity state in the recent concept of 'lateral phase separation'[3]. Evidence also exists of specific interactions between membrane proteins and localized areas of lipid[3,54]. The techniques used for probing the physical properties of the membrane bilayer should be applied to accessible membranes from multiple sclerosis patients to ensure that no abnormalities at this level can be observed.

How do fatty acid replacements in membrane phospholipids affect immunological responses of lymphocytes? Why are EFA-deficient rats more susceptible to EAE? Investigation of these phenomena could be of great relevance to the problem of MS. The reservations which we expressed in the introductory remarks must be borne in mind when considering the work with EFA-deficient animals, and in whole animal experiments the wide variety of systems which may be involved must be taken into account. For example, deprivation of essential fatty acids might adversely affect the blood brain barrier which may well be involved in EAE, and it is known that injections of lipid cause large changes in the reticuloendothelial system. Nevertheless, one is tempted again to revert to the concept of membrane fluidity in speculating on these results. Indeed, current understanding of the role of unsaturated fatty acids would suggest that, apart from acting as precursors of prostaglandins, the main function of the polyunsaturated acids is concerned with fluidity phenomena.

The challenge for lipid research in MS will be to provide answers to these questions, in one direction or the other. The indications are that this will be an undertaking not lacking in intellectual stimulation.

References

1. Singer, S. J. and Nicolson, G. L. (1972). The fluid mosaic model of the structure of cell membranes. *Science*, **175,** 720
2. Lee, A. G. (1975). Functional properties of biological membranes: a physical–chemical approach. *Prog. Biophys. Mol. Biol.*, **29,** 3
3. Marsh, D. (1975). Spectroscopic studies of membrane structure. *Ess. Biochem.*, **11,** 139
4. Cherry, R. J. (1975). Protein mobility in membranes. *FEBS Lett.*, **55,** 1
5. Farias, R. N., Bloj, B., Morero, R. D., Sineriz, F. and Trucco, R. E. (1975). Regulation of allosteric membrane-bound enzymes through changes in membrane lipid composition. *Biochem. Biophys. Acta*, **415,** 231
6. Guarnieri, M. and Johnson, R. M. (1970). The essential fatty acids. *Adv. Lip. Res.*, **8,** 115
7. Swank, R. L. (1950). Multiple sclerosis: a correlation of its incidence with dietary fat. *Am. J. Med. Sci.*, **220,** 421
8. Sinclair, H. M. (1956). Deficiency of essential fatty acids and atherosclerosis, etc. *Lancet*, **i,** 381
9. Allison, R. S. (1963). Some neurological aspects of medical geography. *Proc. R. Soc. Med.*, **56,** 71
10. Shimoyama, T., Kikuchi, H., Press, M. and Thompson, G. R. (1973). Fatty acid composition of plasma lipoproteins in control subjects and in patients with malabsorption. *Gut*, **14,** 716
11. Davison, A. N. (1972). Biosynthesis of the myelin sheath. In K. Elliott and J. Knight (eds.). *Lipids, Malnutrition and the Developing Brain*, pp. 73 (Amsterdam: Elsevier)
12. Brady, R. O. (1973). The enzymology of myelination. *Mol. Cell. Biochem.*, **2,** 23
13. McDonald, W. I. (1974). Remyelination in relation to clinical lesions of the central nervous system. *Br. Med. Bull.*, **30,** 186
14. Alter, M., Yamoor, M. and Harshe, M. (1974). Multiple sclerosis and nutrition. *Arch. Neurol.*, **31,** 267
15. Mohrhauer, H. and Holman, R. T. (1963). Alteration of the fatty acid composition of brain lipids by varying levels of dietary essential fatty acids. *J. Neurochem.*, **10,** 525
16. White, H. B. Jr., Galli, C. and Paoletti, R. (1971). Brain recovery from essential fatty acid deficiency in developing rats. *J. Neurochem.*, **18,** 869

17. Gerstl, B., Kahnke, M. J., Smith, J. K., Tavaststjerna, M. G. and Hayman, R. B. (1961). *Brain*, **84,** 310

18. Baker, R. W. R., Thompson, R. H. S. and Zilkha, K. J. (1963). Fatty acid composition of brain lecithins in multiple sclerosis. *Lancet* **i,** 26

19. Cumings, J. N., Shortman, R. C. and Skrbic, T. (1965). Lipid studies in the blood and brain in multiple sclerosis and motor neurone disease. *J. Clin. Pathol.*, **18,** 641

20. Clausen, J. and Hansen, I. B. (1970). Myelin constituents of human central nervous system. *Acta Neurol. Scand.*, **46,** 1

21. Gerstl, B., Tavaststjerna, M. G., Hayman, R. B., Eng, L. F. and Smith, J. K. (1965). Alterations of myelin fatty acids and plasmalogens in multiple sclerosis. *Ann. N.Y. Acad. Sci.*, **122,** 405

22. Arnetoli, G., Pazzagli, A. and Amaducci, L. (1969). Fatty acid and aldehyde changes in choline- and ethanolamine-containing phospholipids in the white matter of multiple sclerosis brains. *J. Neurochem.*, **16,** 461

23. Gerstl, B., Eng, L. F., Tavaststjerna, M. G., Smith, J. K. and Kruse, S. L. (1970). Lipids and proteins in multiple sclerosis white matter. *J. Neurochem.*, **17,** 677

24. Alling, C., Vanier, M. T. and Svennerholm, L. (1971). Lipid alterations in apparently normal white matter in multiple sclerosis. *Brain Res.*, **35,** 325

25. Baker, R. W. R., Thompson, R. H. S. and Zilkha, K. J. (1964). Serum fatty acids in multiple sclerosis. *J. Neurol. Neurosurg. Psychiatry*, **27,** 408

26. Baker, R. W. R., Sanders, H., Thompson, R. H. S. and Zilkha, K. J. (1965). Serum cholesterol linoleate levels in multiple sclerosis. *J. Neurol. Neurosurg. Psychiatry*, **28,** 212

27. Baker, R. W. R., Thompson, R. H. S., Wright, H. P. and Zilkha, K. J. (1966). Changes in the amounts of linoleic acid in the serum of patients with multiple sclerosis. *J. Neurol. Neurosurg. Psychiatry*, **29,** 95

28. Sanders, H., Thompson, R. H. S., Wright, H. P. and Zilkha, K. J. (1968). Further studies on platelet adhesiveness and serum cholesteryl linoleate levels in multiple sclerosis. *J. Neurol. Neurosurg. Psychiatry*, **31,** 321

29. Belin, J., Pettet, N., Smith, A. D., Thompson, R. H. S. and Zilkha, K. J. (1971). Linoleate metabolism in multiple sclerosis. *J. Neurol. Neurosurg. Psychiatry*, **34,** 25

30. Tsang, W. M., Belin, J., Monro, J., Smith, A. D., Thompson, R. H. S. and Zilkha, K. J. (1976). Relationship between plasma and lymphocyte linoleate in multiple sclerosis. *J. Neurol. Neurosurg. Psychiatry*, **39,** 767

31. Tichy, J., Vymazal, J. and Michalec, C. (1969). Serum lipoproteins, cholesterol esters and phospholipids in multiple sclerosis. *Acta Neurol. Scand.*, **45,** 32

32. Love, W. C., Cashel, A., Reynolds, M. and Callaghan, N. (1974). Linoleate and fatty acid patterns of serum lipids in multiple sclerosis and other diseases. *Br. Med. J.*, **3,** 18

33. Crawford, M. A. and Hassam, A. G. (1975). Diagnostic test for multiple sclerosis. *Br. Med. J.*, **i,** 150

34. Paty, D. W., Cousin, H. K. and McDonald, K. E. (1975). Linoleic acid in multiple sclerosis. *Lancet*, **i,** 1197

35. Kalofoutis, A. and Jullien, G. (1974). A study of serum fatty acids in neurological diseases. *Biochimie*, **56**, 623

36. Karlsson, I., Alling, C. and Svennerholm, L. (1971). Major plasma lipids and their fatty acid composition in multiple sclerosis and other neurological diseases. *Acta Neurol. Scand.*, **47**, 403

37. Wolfgram, F., Myers, L., Ellison, G. and Knipprath, W. (1975). Serum linoleic acid in multiple sclerosis. *Neurology*, **25**, 786

38. Farquhar, J. W. and Ahrens, E. H., Jr. (1963). Effects of dietary fats on human erythrocyte fatty acid patterns. *J. Clin. Invest.*, **42**, 675

39. Dunn, G. D., Wilcox, H. G. and Heimberg, M. (1975). Effects of dietary triglyceride on the properties and lipid composition of plasma lipoproteins. *Lipids*, **10**, 773

40. Belin, J., Smith, A. D. and Thompson, R. H. S. (1975). Effects of short-term oral administration of sunflower seed oil on the pattern of non-esterified fatty acids in human plasma. *Clin. Chim. Acta*, **61**, 95

41. Mertin, J., Shenton, B. K. and Field, E. J. (1974). Unsaturated fatty acids in multiple sclerosis. *Br. Med. J.*, **3**, 777

42. Mertin, J. and Hughes, D. (1975). Specific inhibitory action of polyunsaturated fatty acids on lymphocyte transformation induced by PHA and PPD. *Int. Arch. Allergy Appl. Immunol.*, **48**, 203

43. Gul, S., Smith, A. D., Thompson, R. H. S., Payling-Wright, H. and Zilkha, K. J. (1970). Fatty acid composition of phospholipids from platelets and erythrocytes in multiple sclerosis. *J. Neurol. Neurosurg. Psychiatry*, **33**, 506

44. Millar, J. H. D., Zilkha, K. J., Langman, M. J. S., Payling-Wright, H., Smith, A. D., Belin, J. and Thompson, R. H. S. (1973). Double-blind trial of linoleate supplementation of the diet in multiple sclerosis. *Br. Med. J.*, **1**, 765

45. Di Luzio, N. R. (1972). Employment of lipids in the measurement and modification of cellular, humoral and immune responses. *Adv. Lip. Res.*, **10**, 43

46. Clausen, J. and Møller, J. (1967). Allergic encephalomyelitis induced by brain antigen after deficiency in polyunsaturated fatty acids during demyelination. Is multiple sclerosis a nutritive disorder? *Acta Neurol. Scand.*, **43**, 375

47. Selivonchick, D. P. and Johnston, P. B. (1975). Fat deficiency in rats during development of the central nervous system and susceptibility to experimental allergic encephalomyelitis. *J. Nutr.*, **105**, 288

48. Mertin, J. (1976). Effect of polyunsaturated fatty acids on skin allograft survival and primary and secondary cytotoxic response in mice. *Transplantation*, **21**, 1

49. Mertin, J. and Hunt, R. (1976). Influence of polyunsaturated fatty acids on survival of skin allografts and tumour incidence in mice. *Proc. Nat. Acad. Sci.*, **73**, 928

50. Hughes, D., Caspary, E. A. and Wisniewski, H. M. (1975). Immunosuppression by linoleic acid. *Lancet*, **ii**, 501

51. Offner, H. and Clausen, J. (1974). Inhibition of lymphocyte response to stimulants induced by unsaturated fatty acids and prostaglandins. *Lancet*, **ii**, 400

52. Weyman, C., Belin, J., Smith, A. D. and Thompson, R. H. S. (1975). Linoleic acid as an immunosuppressive agent. *Lancet*, **ii**, 33

53. Shivastava, K. C., Fog, T. and Clausen, J. (1975). The synthesis of prostaglandins in platelets from patients with multiple sclerosis. *Acta Neurol. Scand.*, **51**, 193

54. Warren, G. B., Houslay, M. D., Metcalfe, J. C. and Birdsall, N. J. M. (1975). Cholesterol is excluded from the phospholipid annulus surrounding an active calcium transport protein. *Nature (London)*, **255**, 684

9

Laboratory tests for multiple sclerosis: MEM–LAD and E–UFA tests; outlook for the future

E. J. Field

In the 100 years which have gone by since Charcot clearly characterized MS the only long-term treatment of the disease which has withstood a properly controlled double blind trial and found to be of some value is that published by Millar et al.[1] Not only may this work come to be regarded as a most important milestone in the treatment of MS but also a point of departure for a much deeper understanding of what goes on in the pathogenesis. It has, incidentally, led to laboratory diagnostic test(s) for MS—the lack of which was pointed out as a serious handicap in Chapter 1. At the same time, the manner in which these researches unfolded throws interesting light on the way in which new approaches develop and the limited usefulness of much of what passes for research 'planning'.

About 10 years ago, largely unremarked at the time, reports began to appear[2-8] that the composition of MS brain differed from normal in that unsaturated fatty acids (UFA) were diminished. A decreased blood level of linoleate was also reported to be present in MS[9], though this has recently been denied[10,11]. More recently reduction in UFA has also been reported in blood platelets[12] and leukocytes[13]. Attention had, of course, long been directed to dietary fatty acids in MS[14-16] largely from a deficiency or saturated/unsaturated imbalance point of view. Thompson[6], however, suggested that the deficiency might represent some inborn error in handling of UFA and in such subjects MS is prone to develop.

Intending, presumably, to effect a replacement therapy (though they do not explicitly say so) Millar et al.[1] embarked upon the diet supplementation study referred to above, adding linoleic acid in the form of sunflower seed oil. They found that 'relapses tended to be less frequent and were significantly less severe and of shorter duration in the linoleate supplemented group than in those receiving the oleate (control) mixture, but clear evidence that treatment affected the overall rate of clinical deterioration was not obtained'. This very important conclusion, marking the first occasion in the 100 years the disease has been known that any properly tested treatment has been found to be of benefit, is clearly in urgent need of independent substantiation, preferably in different countries. Moreover, the optimal dosage and conditions of absorption of UFA might be laid down as a preliminary. Thus, Shenton and Field[17] have noted the improved absorption of UFA if saturated fat has not been taken.

Apart from the stimulus which Millar et al.'s work has given to therapeutic trials in MS, it has led indirectly to a laboratory test for the disease. The test depends upon the observation that when lymphocytes are brought into contact with antigen to which they are specifically sensitized a 'lymphokine' is produced with the property of causing normal guinea-pig macrophages to travel more slowly in an electric field. Normal guinea-pig macrophages may thus be used as an indicator system for antigen–lymphocyte interaction, just as their active migratory capacity is used in the macrophage migration inhibition (MMI) test[18]. In the latter, the lymphokine produced[19] is termed macrophage inhibitory factor (MIF). In the MEM test it has been termed macrophage slowing factor (MSF), though it may well be the same as MIF.

Full technical details of the method have been described by Field and Caspary[20] and Caspary and Field[21]—the latter giving an experimental protocol in extenso—and Shenton et al.[22]. Healthy non-sensitized guinea-pigs are essential for this work[23–29], though attempts are still made to use animals from colonies in which 'a few' are sick[30]. The precautions necessary (which fall far short of SPF conditions) have been described by Shenton[27]. There is an absolute need for glass-ware thoroughly cleaned without the use of any form of detergent whatsoever. Full technical details have been set out by Shenton and Field[31], and Field and Shenton[29].

If t_c = migration time of the normal guinea-pig macrophages in the presence of the lymphocytes to be tested and t_e = migration time when antigen also present, then $t_e > t_c$ and $\dfrac{t_e - t_c}{t_c} \times 100$ is a measure of the slowing produced, and so of MSF produced by lymphocyte–antigen interaction. It would, in fact, be more accurate to take $\dfrac{t_e - t_c}{t_e} \times 100$ as the measure of slowing of speed, but with the degree of slowing observed this makes very little difference.

With the MEM method, sensitization of blood lymphocytes to human encephalitogenic factor (EF) has been found in *all* organic diseases of the nervous system and appears to be secondary to parenchymatous destruction from any cause[32]. The test may thus be used to distinguish between organic and 'functional' disease of the nervous system. It has also been possible to show that the number of cells per mm³ of blood sensitized to EF is greater in neurosyphilis (GPI) than in MS[33], so that there is nothing to suggest any specificity to the latter. It is quite clear that the demonstration of lymphocyte sensitization to brain products can have no pathogenetic bearing on the evolution of MS.

The finding by Millar *et al.*[1] that administration of linoleic acid (LA) reduced the number and severity of MS attacks raised the possibility that LA might act by depressing lymphocyte ability to take part in an antigen reaction with EF (or other antigen) believed, by those who subscribe to an immunological mechanism at work in MS, to underlie the acute attack. This would be in accord with the suggestion by Turnell *et al.*[34] that the cytolytic action of corticosteroids on normal and malignant lymphocytes may be mediated by free fatty acids in the serum. Direct study of the effect of LA (C.18:2) and arachidonic acid (C.20:4) showed that both did indeed (*in vitro*), as measured by the MEM test, dampen down normal lymphocyte–antigen interaction. This occurred whether EF, PPD (of tubercle) or F_1 (thyroglobulin fraction) of thyroid (to which everyone appears to be sensitized[35]) was used as antigen. When lymphocytes derived from MS subjects were tested with LA, they were found to be much more sensitive to it than were normal lymphocytes. The latter showed about 57% reduction in the response to thyroid antigen when 0·08 mg/ml LA (roughly twice the 'normal' level in serum) was incorporated in the *in vitro* test; MS lymphocytes showed 90% + reduction; and other neurological diseases (OND) gave about 46% reduction. There was good consistency within the groups[36], so that the effect of LA was proposed as a laboratory test for MS. The effect of arachidonic and other acids has now also been reported. Whilst arachidonic acid has a greater effect than LA, gamma linolenate has a still greater suppressive activity[37].

The original findings have been independently confirmed by Jenssen *et al.*[38,39], though Mertin *et al.*[40] were unable to do so. The reasons for this have been discussed in some detail[27,41,42]. It was found some years ago[43] that normal guinea-pigs exposed to banal viruses (such as influenza), whilst remaining clinically normal, became sensitized to EF. Under these conditions, peritoneal macrophages derived from them behave in a random manner in the MEM test, not only when lymphocytes are tested with EF, but also with PPD (which shares antigenic determinant(s) with EF[44]). This is probably due to the guinea-pig's own lymphocytes (which 10–20% of the peritoneal macrophage exudate) forming variable amounts of MSF when brought into contact with EF or PPD. In 'repeating' the work of Field et al., Mertin et al.[40] abolished the precautions detailed for keeping animals from becoming sensitized to EF and used PPD (instead of thyroid) as test antigen—hence the haphazard results. Direct experiment[45] has shown that macrophages from guinea-pigs which are inadvertently sensitized to EF may be used with thyroid as antigen but not with EF, CaBP or PPD (which share antigenic determinants to which the animals are sensitized). Mertin et al. elected to use PPD.

Apart from inadvertent sensitization of the guinea-pigs from which indicator macrophages are drawn, actual infection of the animals leads to bizarre results[29].

Recently a simplified test for MS has been developed[45,47], eliminating altogether the use of guinea-pigs. It depends simply upon the measurement of the absolute mobility of erythrocytes (μm/cm/V/cm). In the case of RBC from patients with MS, linoleic acid (LA) and arachidonic acid (AA) (at a concentration of 0·08 mg/ml) both cause a marked slowing of the cells ($p < 0·001$ in almost every individual case) whilst red cells from normal subjects and OND (other (destructive) neurological diseases) travel faster in the presence of these acids (p again $< 0·001$ in the great majority of cases).

Subjects have also been examined from families where the 'anomalous' (77% type) of result had been found with the MEM–LAD test. In such cases LA is found to slow the migration speed of RBC, whereas arachidonic acid increases it. The effects are very rapid, occurring almost as soon as the acids are added, and must be due to some 'pellicle' effect around the cells. The action is so fast (it is apparent immediately the UFA is added) that we cannot be dealing with true incorporation, but almost certainly with an adsorption effect; nor could there be time for the flip-flop phenomenon described by Bretscher[48], Renooij et al.[49] and others, to occur. Actual incorporation studies with ^{14}C marked acids are in progress in this laboratory. The small number of experiments so far completed suggest that incorporation is greater into MS RBC membranes than into those of normals (Dr M. Glover).

A full description of the E–UFA (Erythrocyte–UFA) test has been given elsewhere. Several families who have been studied by the MEM–LAD test[36] have given congruent pictures by the simplified E–UFA test. The test has the advantage that guinea-pigs are not necessary for carrying it out, but considerable attention to detail must (as before) be paid to preparation of glassware, double-distilled water, etc. and to the accurate determination of specific resistance of the medium in which the measurements are made. In our experiments we have used Medium 199 (Hanks based: Gibco Bio-Cult) and conductivity measured for every specimen used. An unexpected finding with the E–UFA test has been that the effects of LA and AA are inverted when small amounts are used (0·02 mg/ml) instead of the standard 0·08 mg/ml (Figures 9.1 and 9.2). A relative who gives the intermediate type of result (slow with 0·08 mg/ml LA; fast with 0·08 mg/ml AA) shows only partial conversion. With LA at 0·02 mg/ml such RBC still travel slowly, but with AA they travel more slowly. There must be some subtle biophysical explanation at present beyond our reach.

In some subjects the level of LA or AA may have to be lowered to 0·01

M.S. AND NORMAL
ARACHIDONIC ACID

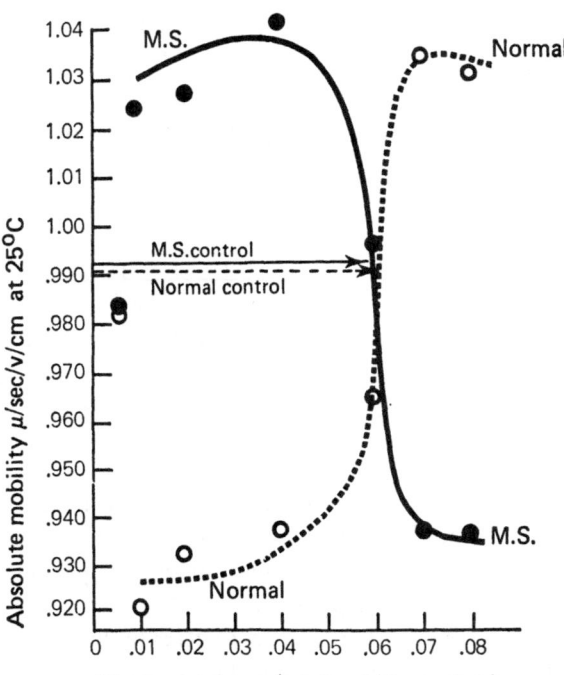

Figure 9.1 Comparison of result in an MS and normal subject as the concentration of arachidonic acid is reduced from the usual testing level of 0·08 mg/ml to 0·01 mg/ml. Below this level it becomes ineffective. Note that the MS, slowed at the higher concentration, is speeded up at the low concentration, and the reverse is true for the normal subject.

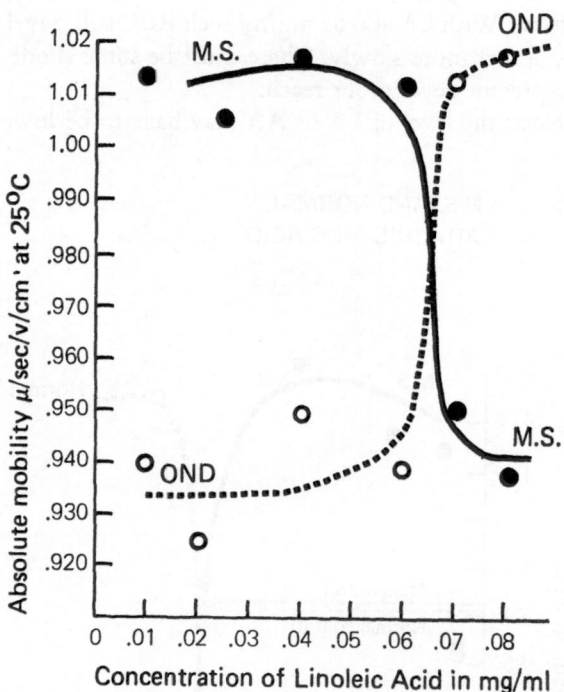

Figure 9.2 Comparison of result between a multiple sclerotic and an OND subject. Note again the reversal in effect of linoleic acid as the concentration is reduced from 0·08 mg/ml to 0·01 mg/ml.

mg/ml in order for conversion of mobility change to occur. Recently we have shown (in collaboration with Dr A. F. Rogers) that PGE_2 is active in altering the mobility of RBC and it may indeed be possible to use this material in simplifying the E–UFA method.

The erythrocyte phenomenon is perhaps of great importance, as the simple membrane of the cell may be a good model for cell membranes in general in MS. Years ago Plum and Fog[50] confirmed by Prineas[51], observed that mean erythrocyte diameter is increased in MS. The osmotic fragility of MS erythrocytes is also increased[52,53] and it is tempting to suppose both phenomena stem from unusual biochemical–biophysical make-up of the limiting red cell membrane[12] depending upon the inborn mishandling of UFA postulated by Thompson[6]. The unusual reactivity of the lymphocyte surface to UFAs which forms the basis of the MEM–LAD test described above may be but one manifestation of involvement of all membranes, the RBC phenomenon being another. If this is so, then the membrane of the oligodendroglial cell may also be abnormally constituted and this would lead to abnormal myelin make-up. Several possibilities exist. It might be that the abnormally constituted myelin is unable to stand up to the wear and tear of the normal life span and undergoes patchy perivascular 'abiotrophy'; or it may be more susceptible to an allergic process (cf. Clausen and Moller[54]); or it might form a more favourable nidus for the establishment of 'slow' virus infections, either as a sequel to attack by a banal agent (such as measles) or *ab initio*.

Both the original MEM–LAD test and the newer E–UFA test offer a means of studying MS families and scanning children born into such families as near (blood) relatives. If the test picks out young children with full MS result, then it would seem reasonable to load them with linoleic acid (or gamma linolenate) in an attempt to make up for the inborn genetic mishandling they bear[55].

Three cases of acute disseminated encephalitis following common infectious fevers have shown a negative MS result by the E–UFA test—i.e. their erythrocytes have been speeded up by LA and AA in the manner of normal subjects (or those with other neurological diseases). No special predisposition would thus appear to the development of post-exanthematous encephalomyelitis, dependent upon abnormal myelin constitution.

Devic's disease (regarded by many as a variant of MS) gives a negative result, both by the MEM–LAD and E–UFA tests. As with the former[56], the E–UFA test can be applied to the problem of optic neuritis.

Clearly MS research would appear to have entered into a new and active phase during the last 10 years with an experimentally based *leitmotif*. The E–UFA test throws a deeper light on the aetiopathogenesis of the disease than does the interpretation offered for the MEM–LAD test results in MS. There it was simply supposed that the suppression of acute MS reported by Millar *et al.*[1] could be explained simply by a depressive effect of LA on the ability of lymphocytes to react with antigen. Some disquiet was caused by the finding that exhibition of gamma linolenate (Naudicelle capsules) for some weeks led to a more normal lymphocyte reaction, i.e. they now reacted better than before to antigen[57] (see Chapter 28). The newer suggestion that LA and gamma linolenate act by altering membrane constitution (and so that of newly built up myelin) in the direction of normal means that the effect of unsaturated fatty acid therapy is on an altogether different basis. From recent determinations we now know that the slowing of RBC by both LA and AA characteristic of MS only begins to change after 4–8 months, the AA slowly beginning to exert a speeding up effect and the LA following some weeks later. A typical protocol is shown in Table 9.1 and 9.2. It can be seen that after 2 months (exceptionally early) the reaction with AA changed from a slowing to a speeding up. After nearly five months' treatment the LA reaction changed similarly so that by 6 months the patient reacted normally. During this period she was remarkably well. If we assume, say, 8 months, as the time for LA to have an effect, than a 2-year double-blind trial is rather a short time, especially in adults where myelin turnover is slow, for newly constituted myelin to replace the defective, susceptible, original material. Again,

Tables 9.1 and 9.2 Naudicelle begun on 27.4.76 and 24.6.76 when patient showed full multiple sclerosis result. Note persistence of this result for 2 months and gradual change in the reaction, first with arachidonic acid and then with linoleic acid in the direction of normal, so that in 5–6 months patient gives normal type of reaction, i.e. increased speed with both linoleic and arachidonic acids ($p < 0.001$). These are representative of a group of cases studied.

Table 9.1 GH (Female) (age 29)

Date	CON	SD	LA	SD	AA	SD	% change LA	% change AA
27.4.76	1·113	±·037	1·073	±0·36	1·073	±0·34	−3·64	−3·63
4.5.76	1·101	±·034	1·058	±0·35	1·068	±·032	−3·86	−3·02
18.5.76	1·108	±·036	1·074	±·040	1·075	±·035	−3·04	−2·95
8.6.76	1·172	±·035	1·117	±·037	1·166	±·030	−4·65	−0·52
28.6.76	1·144	±·030	1·091	±·029	1·162	±·029	−4·64	+1·59
26.7.76	0·902	±·024	0·879	±·030	0·970	±·041	+2·65	+7·45
6.9.76	0·980	±·031	0·994	±·034	1·024	±·032	+1·41	+4·5
4.10.76	0·970	±·041	1·036	±·043	1·043	±·037	+6·78	+7·49
8.12.76	1·002	±·024	1·042	±·035	1·047	±·035	+4·03	+4·47

Table 9.2 PP (Female) (age 24)

Date	CON	SD	LA	SD	AA	SD	% change LA	% change AA
24.6.76	1·174	±·034	1·124	±·030	1·128	±·027	−4·28	−3·88
28.7.76	0·935	±·024	0·900	±·025	0·909	±·025	−3·80	−2·77
15.9.76	0·983	±·023	0·951	±·023	1·004	±·034	−3·31	+2·15
25.10.76	0·978	±·030	0·951	±·040	0·991	±·037	−2·76	+1·31
29.11.76	1·004	±·031	1·031	±·034	1·025	±·028	+2·65	+2·12
10.1.77	1·025	±·023	1·079	±·037	1·095	±·030	+5·27	+6·83
10.2.77	1·071	±·032	1·117	±·028	1·130	±·020	+4·33	+5·49
30.2.77	0·987	±·031	1·085	±·029	1·111	±·030	+10·00	+12·64

if the defective membrane hypothesis is correct, then LA must be a lifelong therapy and should be begun as early as possible (see children scanning above). We also know that those who have been on sunflower seed oil therapy (LA) and have given it up because the dramatic improvement they expected did not occur, revert within a few months to the MS type of result (slowing by both LA and AA). Although the great majority of patients react as described there are one or two who do not respond to LA and AA fully. Two subjects have been encountered who, even after 18 months' intake of gamma linolenate, showed only partial response (AA fast but LA still slow). One has regressed somewhat and the other remained stationary. It is therefore advisable to test a patient before gamma linolenate therapy is begun and again at 6 months and one year. The biochemical basis of 'resistance' is not yet clear, nor whether additional dosage with gamma linolenate will aid them.

Finally a word may be said for the long standing case of MS where axis cylinders have probably been destroyed and where (despite current teaching) nerve cell degeneration also occurs. Clearly little is to be looked for here both because no myelin will reform around defunct axis cylinders, and because the contribution to the protein of myelin derived from the nerve cell[58] is lacking. The imposition of the neural factor probably underlies the striking manner in which long affected MS subjects may pass into a phase of steady deterioration. Rose[59] in discussing this is drawn to the conclusion that 'secondary adverse factors accumulate and cause progressive interference in the function of the neuronal systems that have been most affected by demyelination'. Clearly we must act before this stage is reached and prospects seem brighter today than ever before.

References

1. Millar, J. H. D., Zilkha, K. J., Langman, M. J. S., Payling-Wright, H., Smith, A. D., Belin, J. and Thompson, R. H. S. (1973). Double blind trial of linoleate supplementation of the diet in multiple sclerosis. *Br. Med. J.*, **1**, 765

2. Jatzkewitz, H. and Mehl, E. (1962). Zum Schicksal der C_{24}-Fettsäuren beim sudanophilen Myelinabbau im Zentralnervensystem: Teil 1 (C_{24}-Fettsäuren Defizit in den lipophilen Abbau- und Umwandlungsproduktion). *Hoppe-Seyler's Z. Physiol. Chem.*, **329**, 264

3. Baker, R. W. R., Thompson, R. H. S. and Zilkha, K. J. (1963). Fatty acid composition of brain lecithins in multiple sclerosis. *Lancet*, **i**, 26

4. Gerstl, B., Tavaststjerna, M. C., Hayman, R. B., Eng, L. F. and Smith, J. K. (1965). Alterations in myelin fatty acids and plasmalogens in multiple sclerosis. *Ann. N.Y. Acad. Sci.*, **122**, 405

5. Gerstl, B., Eng, L. F., Tavaststjerna, M. C., Smith, J. K. and Kruse, S. L. (1970). Lipids and proteins in multiple sclerosis white matter. *J. Neurochem.*, **17**, 677

6. Thompson, R. H. S. (1966). A biochemical approach to the problem of multiple sclerosis. *Proc. R. Soc. Med.*, **59**, 269

7. Thompson, R. H. S. (1973). Fatty acid metabolism in multiple sclerosis. *Biochem. Soc. Symp.*, **35**, 103

8. Clausen, J. and Hansen, I. B. (1970). Myelin constituents of human central nervous system. Studies of phospholipid, glycolipid and fatty acid pattern in normal and multiple sclerosis brains. *Acta Neurol. Scand.*, **46**, 1

9. Baker, R. W. R., Sanders, H., Thompson, R. H. S. and Zilkha, K. J. (1965). Serum cholesterol linoleate levels in multiple sclerosis. *J. Neurol. Neurosurg. Psychiatry*, **28**, 212

10. Callaghan, N., Kearney, B. and Love, W. C. (1973). Dietary intake of linoleic acid in multiple sclerosis and other diseases. *J. Neurol. Neurosurg. Psychiatry*, **36**, 668

11. Love, W. C., Cashell, M., Reynolds, M. and Callaghan, N. (1974). Linoleate and fatty acid patterns of serum lipids in multiple sclerosis and other diseases. *Br. Med. J.*, **3**, 18

12. Gul, S., Smith, A. D., Thompson, R. H. S., Payling-Wright, H. and Zilkha, K. J. (1970). The fatty acid composition of phospholipids from platelets and erythrocytes in multiple sclerosis. *J. Neurol. Neurosurg. Psychiatry*, **33**, 506

13. Mahler, R., cited by R. H. S. Thompson (1973). Fatty acid metabolism in multiple sclerosis. *Biochem. Soc. Symp.*, **35**, 103

14. Swank, R. L. (1950). Multiple sclerosis: a correlation of its incidence with dietary fat. *Am. J. Med. Sci.*, **220**, 421

15. Sinclair, H. M. (1956). Deficiency of essential fatty acids and atherosclerosis etcetera. *Lancet*, **1**, 381

16. Allison, R. S. (1963): Some neurological aspects of medical geography. *Proc. R. Soc. Med.*, **56**, 71

17. Shenton, B. K. and Field, E. J. (1975a). Lymphocyte reactivity depression by linoleic acid and related substances: an absorption study. In E. Schutter (ed.). *Immunopathologie du Système Nerveux. Colloquium*, p. 189 (Inserm)

18. David, J. R., Al-Askari, S., Lawrence, H. S. and Thomas, L. (1964). Delayed hypersensitivity *in vitro*. *J. Immunol.*, **93** (2), 264–273, 274–278

19. Bloom, B. R. and Bennett, B. (1966). Mechanism of a reaction *in vitro* associated with delayed-type hypersensitivity. *Science*, **153**, 80

20. Field, E. J. and Caspary, E. A. (1970). Lymphocyte sensitisation: an *in vitro* test for cancer. *Lancet*, **ii**, 1337

21. Caspary, E. A. and Field, E. J. (1971). Specific lymphocyte sensitisation in cancer: is there a common antigen in human malignant neoplasia? *Br. Med. J.*, **2**, 613

22. Shenton, B. K., Hughes, D. and Field, E. J. (1973). Macrophage electrophoretic migration (MEM) test for lymphocyte sensitisation: Some practical experience in macrophage selection. *Br. J. Cancer*, **28**, Suppl. 1, 215

23. Parker, J. W. and Lukes, R. J. (1971). 'Spontaneous' lymphocyte transformation following Hong Kong 'Flu'. In E. O. Ross McIntyre (ed.). *Proc. 4th Leucocyte Cult. Conf.*, p. 281 (New York: Appleton Century Croft)

24. Field, E. J. and Caspary, E. A. (1972): 'Spontaneous' lymphocyte reactivity in the presence of virus infections. *Lancet*, **1**, 963
25. Balfour, I. C., Evans, C. A., Middleton, U. L. and Pegrum, G. D. (1972). Observations on the cytotoxicity of lymphocytes to a target cell system. *Clin. Exp. Immunol.*, **10**, 67
26. Field, E. J. (1974). Effect of viruses on lymphocyte reactivity. *Br. Med. J.*, **1**, 245
27. Shenton, B. K. (1974). Diagnostic test for multiple sclerosis. *Br. Med. J.*, **2**, 574
28. Field, E. J. and Shenton, B. K. (1975a). Macrophage electrophoretic mobility (MEM) test for lymphocyte sensitisation: importance of macrophages from healthy animals. *Int. Res. Commun. Syst.*, **3**, 154
29. Field, E. J. and Shenton, B. K. (1975b). The macrophage electrophoretic mobility (MEM) test: a consideration of the practical difficulties and application of the method. *Int Res. Commun. Syst.*, 583
30. Lewkonia, R. M., Kerr, E. J. L. and Irvine, W. J. (1974). Clinical evaluation of the macrophage electrophoretic mobility test for cancer. *Br. J. Cancer*, **30**, 532
31. Shenton, B. K. and Field, E. J. (1975b). The macrophage electrophoretic mobility (MEM) test: some technical considerations. *J. Immunol. Methods*, **7**, 149
32. Caspary, E. A. and Field, E. J. (1970). Sensitisation of blood lymphocytes to possible antigens in neurological disease. *Eur. Neurol.* **4**, 256
33. Caspary, E. A. and Field, E. J. (1974). Lymphocyte sensitisation to basic protein of brain in multiple sclerosis and other neurological diseases. *J. Neurol. Neurosurg. Psychiatry*, **37**, 710
34. Turnell, R. W., Clarke, L. H. and Burton, A. F. (1973). Studies on the mechanism of corticosteroid-induced lymphocytolysis. *Cancer Res.*, **33**, 203
35. Field, E. J., Caspary, E. A., Hall, R. and Clark, F. (1970). Circulating sensitized lymphocytes in Graves' Disease. Observations on its pathogenesis. *Lancet*, **i**, 1144
36. Field, E. J., Shenton, B. K. and Joyce, G. (1974). Specific laboratory test for multiple sclerosis. *Br. Med. J.*, **1**, 412
37. Field, E. J. and Shenton, B. K. (1975c). Inhibitory effect of unsaturated fatty acids on lymphocyte-antigen interaction with special reference to multiple sclerosis. *Acta Neurol. Scand.* **52**, 121
38. Jenssen, H. L., Kohler, H., Gunther, J. and Meyer-Rienecker, H. (1974a). The specific test for multiple sclerosis. *Lancet*, **ii**, 1327
39. Jenssen, H. L., Kohler, H., Gunther, J. and Meyer-Rienecker, H. (1974b). Diagnostic test for multiple sclerosis. *Br. Med. J.*, **4**, 407
40. Mertin, J., Hughes, D., Caspary, E. A., Thomson, A. M., Foster, J. B. and Stewart-Wynne, E. G. (1974). Non specificity of laboratory test for diagnosis of multiple sclerosis. *Br. Med. J.*, **4**, 567
41. Field, E. J. and Shenton, B. K. (1975d). Diagnostic test for multiple sclerosis. *Br. Med. J.*, **i**, 92
42. Jenssen, H. L., Meyer-Rienecker, H. J., Kohler, H. and Gunther, J. K. (1976). The linoleic acid depression (LAD) test for multiple sclerosis using the macrophage electrophoretic mobility (MEM) test. *Acta Neurol. Scand.*, **53**, 51
43. Field, E. J., Caspary, E. A., Shenton, B. K. and Madgwick, H. (1973). Lymphocye

sensitisation after exposure to measles and influenza: possible relevance to patho-genesis of multiple sclerosis. *J. Neurol. Sci.*, **19,** 179

44. Field, E. J., Caspary, E. A. and Ball, E. J. (1963). Some biological properties of a highly active encephalitogenic factor isolated from human brain. *Lancet* **ii,** 11

45. Shenton, B. K., Field, E. J., Jenssen, H. L., Kohler, H., Gunther, J. and Meyer-Rienecker, H. (1974). Diagnostic test for multiple sclerosis. *Br. Med. J.*, **4,** 590–1

46. Field, E. J. and Joyce, G. (1976). A simplified laboratory test for multiple sclerosis. *Lancet* **ii,** 367

47. Field, E. J., Joyce, G. and Smith, B. M. (1976). Erythrocyte-UFA (EUFA) mobility test for multiple sclerosis: implications for pathogenesis and handling of the disease. *J. Neurol.* (in press)

48. Bretscher, M. S. (1972). Phosphatidyl-ethanolamine: differential labelling in intact cells and cell ghosts of human erythrocytes by a membrane-impermeable reagent. *J. Mol. Biol.*, **71,** 523

49. Renooij, W., van Golde, M. G., Zwaal, F. A. and van Deenen, L. L. M. (1976). Topological asymmetry of phospholipid metabolism in rat erythrocyte mem-branes: evidence for flip-flop of lecithin. *Eur. J. Biochem.*, **61,** 53

50. Plum, C. M. and Fog, T. (1959). Studies in multiple sclerosis. *Acta Neurol. Scand.* Suppl. **128,** 34

51. Prineas, J. (1968). Red blood cell size in multiple sclerosis. *Acta Neurol. Scand.*, **44,** 81

52. Laszlo, S. (1964). Fragilité osmotique des globules rouges dans la sclérose en plaques. *Acta Neurol. Belg.*, **64,** 529

53. Caspary, E. A., Sewell, F. and Field, E. J. (1967). Red blood cell fragility in multiple sclerosis. *Br. Med. J.*, **2,** 610

54. Clausen, J. and Møller, J. (1967). Allergic encephalomyelitis induced by brain antigen after deficiency in polyunsaturated fatty acids during myelination. Is multiple sclerosis a nutritive disorder? *Acta Neurol. Scand.*, **43,** 375

55. Field, E. J. (1973). A rational prophylactic therapy for multiple sclerosis? *Lancet* **ii,** 1080

56. Crombie, A. L., Shenton, N. K. and Field, E. J. (1975). Aetiology of optic neuritis. *Br. Med. J.*, **3,** 703

57. Shenton, B. K., Jenssen, H. L., Kohler, H., Meyer-Rienecker, H. and Field, E. J. (1975). Linoleic acid and multiple sclerosis: effect of prolonged administration on lymphocyte reactivity to antigen. *Int. Res. Commun. Syst.*, **3,** 503

58. Giorgi, P. P., Karlsson, J. O., Sjostrand, J. and Field, E. J. (1973). Axonal flow and myelin protein in the optic pathway. *Nature New Biology*, **244,** 121

59. Rose, A. (1972). Multiple sclerosis: a clinical interpretation. In F. Wolfgran, G. W. Ellison, J. G. Stevens and J. M. Andrews (eds.). *Multiple Sclerosis: Im-munology, Virology and Ultra-structure*. UCLA Forum in Med. Sci. No 16, p. 1 (New York: Academic Press)

60. Field, E. J. (1970) Atio-patholgische aspekte der multiplen sklerose. *Aktuelle Neurologie*, **1,** 23

ADDENDUM

Since the above was completed, a simplified laboratory test has been developed (Field and Joyce, 1977), depending upon the susceptibility of erythrocytes to prostaglandin PGE_2 with regard to their absolute electrophoretic mobility. Using this arachidonic-acid based material, it has been found that:

(1) RBC from MS patients do not change their mobility in the presence of 0·1 μg/ml PGE_2 (an enormous dose in prostaglandin work), whilst RBC from normal or OND subjects travel more rapidly ($p < 0.001$). In this work the results are always clear cut and practically all changes are significant at $p < 0.001$. The author is not prepared to accept change when $p < 0.01$.

(2) RBC from MS patients travel more rapidly in the presence of 1 μg/ml PGE_2 and diminishing concentrations of PGE_2 down to and including 0·0000625 μg/ml (62 p). Below this there is a sudden reversion and at 31 p/ml they travel more slowly. RBC from normal or OND subjects generally travel more rapidly with concentrations down to 0·0025 or 0·0005 μg/ml and below this PGE_2 makes no significant difference down to and including 61 p/ml. Below this at 31 p/ml such cells, however, begin to travel more rapidly once more.

(3) Patients who have been treated with gamma linolenate (Naudicelle) for 6–8 months change over from the MS type of effect of PGE_2 to the normal-OND. Occasionally a patient takes a little longer to make the alteration and so, if feasible, it is advisable to re-test at the end of a year, to make sure the gamma linolenate is being effective.

(4) Some patients who have been treated with gamma linolenate (2 capsules of Naudicelle, three times a day—with restriction of animal fat intake especially at the time of taking the capsules) show further interesting changes. They might be described as becoming 'more normal than normal'. With 1·0 μg/ml PGE_2 they give the speeding up shown by normals and OND, but the change occurs also at extreme dilutions of PGE_2. Whilst normal-OND subjects revert to control speeds at 61 p/ml and become faster at 31 p/ml, this speeding up only rarely persists at 15·6 p/ml. However, with patients who have been taking gamma linolenate for 2–3 years, the speeding up is persistent ($p < 0.001$) at 15·6 p/ml, 7·8 p/ml and even at 3·9 p/ml, though values return to normal in the presence of 1·85 p/l. This phenomenon which is being further explored in collaboration with Dr A. F. Rogers of the University of Bristol (to whom the author is indebted for PGE_2) might well provide the basis for an estimation method for PGE_2 very much more sensitive than those currently available.

A typical set of results is set out in Table 1.

(5) In the original MEM–LAD test (p. 247), a considerable number of MS families were studied and anomalous results were found (about 77% reduction), approximately mid-way between the 90% + reduction seen in MS and the 57% amongst normals—i.e. about 77%. A typical family tree is shown in Figure 1 and the English results (similar ones have been obtained by an independent group working in Rostock, DDR), summarised in Table 2. The same family as in Figure 1 is shown, tested 3 years later with the E–UFA test (Figure 2). Although there is similarity in the results, II, 4

C, N. (25) M

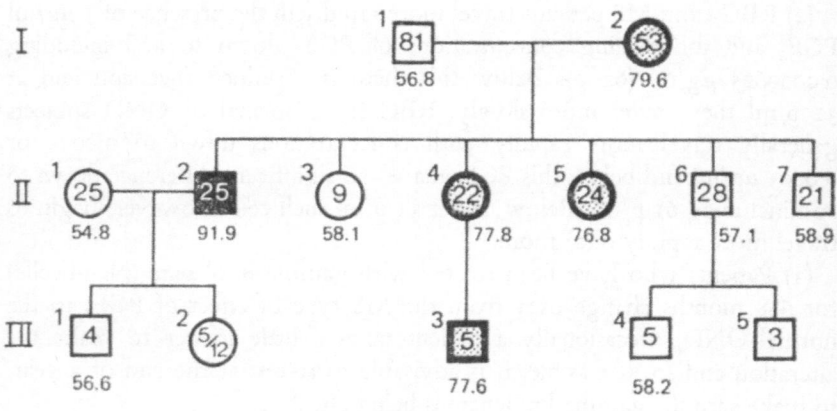

FIGURE 1

C.N. (28) M

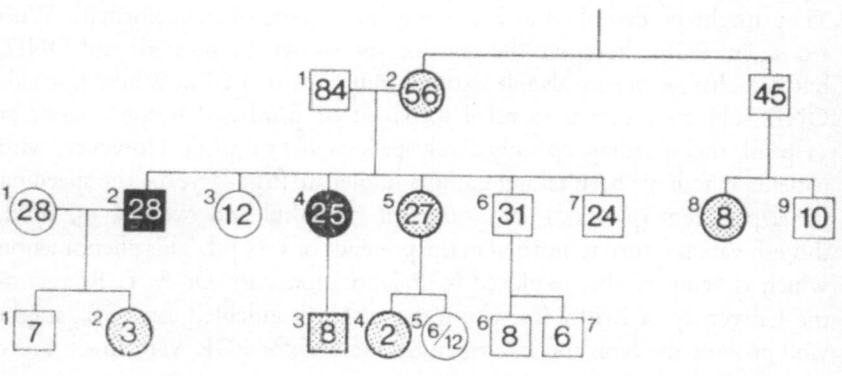

FIGURE 2

Table 1

	1·0 g/ml	62·5 p/ml	31·25 p/ml	15·625 p/ml	7·8 p/ml	3·9 p/ml	1·95 p/ml
PM F (46)	F<0·001	ns	F<0·001	F<0·001	F<0·001	F<0·001	F<0·001

Patient. F, 46. MS 10 years. Naudicelle 3 years.
Note extreme sensitivity of RBC to minute amounts of PGE_2 which cause increased speed of electrophoretic migration.
F = Significantly faster migration.

Table 2

	77% (Anomalous)	57% (Normal)	No. of subjects	Proportion of subjects with anomalous result
Fathers	0	6	6	0
Mothers	11	0	11	100%
Brothers	1	15	16	6·3%
Sisters	13	5	18	72·2%
Sons	2	11	13	15·4%
Daughters	4	1	5	80·0%
Nephews	3*	9†	12	25·0%
Nieces	7‡	8§	15	46·7%
Total	41	55	96	42·7%

* Children of a sister of a propositus.

† Four of these were children of a sister of a propositus and three belonged to a brother of a propositus.

‡ Six of these were children of a sister of a propositus and three belonged to a brother of a propositus.

§ Four of these belonged to a sister and four to a brother of a propositus.

Note uniform 'anomalous' result in the mothers of patients, and preponderance in near female relatives. None has ever developed MS (but see text[36]).

(the sister of the propositus II, 2) was found to give (on repeated examination) a full positive MS result. The girl is quite asymptomatic, but on examination shows unequal reflexes, an absent upper left abdominal reflex and on one occasion a sustained right ankle clonus. She is apparently a silent case of MS (cf. p. 4 and Chapters 6 and 7). Two other silent cases of MS (a sister and a daughter of two propositae) (so far not examined physically for psychological reasons) have also been uncovered. It seems possible that the E–UFA test is more sensitive than the original MEM–LAD. Whilst no other example of an anomalous (77% type) MEM–LAD result turning into a full-blown MS one has been found, the possibility must now be entertained. A further account of some family trees in MS of childhood is given elsewhere[60].

In conclusion it is perhaps permissible after 100 years of gloomy lack of real progress to end on a note of new optimism. The importance of UFA in MS has been realized: this in its turn has led to laboratory diagnostic procedures which are based upon the idea of an inborn mishandling of UFA reflected in abnormal cell surfaces in MS and hence in myelin produced; and this leads to the possibility that the inborn error, if recognized before myelin is properly laid down, may be biochemically corrected.

If MS develops on the basis of a 'prepared soil', it may be possible to alter this character so that the disease does not occur. Indeed its prevention may antecede an exact knowledge of its final pathogenesis. And lastly it seems possible that the additional factor needed for the development of the disease on the 'prepared soil' may be either exogenous (e.g. a virus—specially acting as a 'slow' infection) or endogenous.

Reference

Field, E. J. and Joyce, G. (1977). Prostaglandin (PGE$_2$) and human erythrocyte electrophoretic mobility: a specific test for multiple sclerosis? *IRCS Med. Sci.*, 5, 158

Acknowledgements

The editor would like to record his indebtedness to Miss Greta Joyce, AILMS for much of the recent experimental work alluded to, and to Mrs F. Hill, MA for her devoted attention to manuscript typing, scrutiny and correction.

Index